In Vitro Methods of Toxicology

Ronald R. Watson, Ph.D., Editor
University of Arizona

CRC Press
Boca Raton Ann Arbor London Tokyo

Library of Congress Cataloging-in-Publication Data

In vitro methods of toxicology / Ronald R. Watson, editor.
p. cm. — (Pharmacology/toxicology series)
Includes bibliographical references and index.
ISBN 0-8493-7298-4
1. Toxicity testing—In vitro. I. Watson, Ronald R. (Ronald Ross) II. Series: Pharmacology & toxicology (Boca Raton, Fla.)
[DNLM: 1. Cells, Cultured. 2. Tissue Culture. 3. Toxicology--methods. QV 602 I62]
RA1199.4.I5I49 1992
615.9′07—dc20
DNLM/DLC
for Library of Congress 91-48231
CIP

This book represents information obtained from authentic and highly regarded sources. Reprinted material is quoted with permission, and sources are indicated. A wide variety of references are listed. Every reasonable effort has been made to give reliable data and information, but the authors and the publisher cannot assume responsibility for the validity of all materials or for the consequences of their use.

Direct all inquiries to CRC Press, Inc., 2000 Corporate Blvd., N.W., Boca Raton, Florida, 33431.

International Standard Book Number 0-8493-7298-4
Library of Congress Card Number 91-48231

Printed in the United States of America 1 2 3 4 5 6 7 8 9 0

Printed on acid-free paper

Pharmacology and Toxicology: Basic and Clinical Aspects

Mannfred A. Hollinger, Series Editor
University of California, Davis

Published Titles

Inflammatory Cells and Mediators in Bronchial Asthma, Devendra K. Agrawal and Robert G. Townley
Pharmacology of the Skin, Hasan Mukhtar
The Basis of Toxicity Testing, Donald H. Ecobichon

Forthcoming Titles

Alcohol Consumption, Cancer, and Birth Defects, Anthony J. Garro
Beneficial and Toxic Effects of Aspirin, Susan E. Feinman
Biopharmaceutics of Ocular Drug Delivery, Peter Edman
Classical Receptor Theory, Terry P. Kenakin
Human Drug Metabolism from Molecular Biology to Man, Elizabeth Jeffreys
Neural Control of Airways, Peter J. Barnes
PAF Receptor Signal Mechanisms, Shivendra D. Shukla
Placental Pharmacology, B. B. Rama Sastry
Placental Toxicology, B. B. Rama Sastry
Preclinical and Clinical Modulation of Anticancer Drug Toxicity, Kenneth D. Tew, Peter Houghton, and Janet Houghton
Rational Drug Design, David B. Weiner and William V. Williams
Receptor Characterization and Their Modulation, Devendra K. Agrawal

CONTENTS

SERIES PREFACE

All xenobiotics can, potentially, produce toxic effects. The challenge to toxicologists is how to recognize and quantify these effects in order to assess safety. Early methods employed by toxicologists were restricted to relatively crude indices such as whole animal lethality and organ histology. As we have become more aware of the potentiality for relatively subtle toxic effects, as well as increasing our awareness of animal issues, the need to develop appropriate corresponding *in vitro* models has become recognized. The most significant methods developed over the last 20 years involve the use of isolated cells and perfused organs. These non *in vivo* techniques have been applied to a wide range of toxicologic questions and new applications are continually being sought. In the present volume, Dr. Watson has successfully organized a team of contributors whose expertise covers the most significant aspects of *in vitro* methods of toxicology. In addition to being a ''how to'' book, the volume informs readers of pitfalls and caveats involved in translating *in vitro* data to the *in vivo* situation. The descriptions contained herein will provide invaluable guidance and assistance to those health professionals ultimately responsible for assessment of toxicity.

Manfred A. Hollinger, Ph.D.
Series Editor
Professor
Department of Medical Pharmacology and Toxicology
University of California, Davis
Davis, California

THE EDITOR

Ronald R. Watson, Ph.D. initiated and directs the Specialized Alcohol Research Center at The University of Arizona College of Medicine. The main theme of this NIAAA center grant is to understand the role of ethanol-induced immunosuppression on disease and disease resistance in animals.

Dr. Watson attended the University of Idaho, but graduated from Brigham Young University in Provo, Utah with a degree in Chemistry in 1966. In 1971, he completed his Ph.D. degree in Biochemistry from Michigan State University. His postdoctoral schooling was completed at the Harvard School of Public Health in Nutrition and Microbiology, including a two-year postdoctoral research experience in Immunology. He was an Assistant Professor of Immunology and did research at the University of Mississippi Medical Center in Jackson from 1973 to 1974. He was an Assistant Professor of Microbiology and Immunology at the Indiana University Medical School from 1974 to 1978 and was an Associate Professor at Purdue University in the Department of Food and Nutrition from 1978 to 1982. In 1982, he joined the faculty at The University of Arizona in the Department of Family and Community Medicine, Nutrition Section, and is a Research Professor.

Dr. Watson has edited 24 books, including 10 on alcohol abuse and four on other drugs of abuse. He has worked for several years on research for the U.S. Navy Alcohol and Substance Abuse Program. He has published 225 research papers and review chapters.

Dr. Watson is a member of several national and international nutrition, immunology, and cancer societies, and research societies on alcoholism.

CONTRIBUTORS

Louis C. Almekinders, M.D.
Assistant Professor (Orthopaedic Surgery)
Department of Surgery
University of North Carolina
Chapel Hill, North Carolina

Harvey Babich, Ph.D.
Associate Professor
Department of Biological Sciences
Stern College, Yeshiva University
New York, New York

Michael Balls, D.Phil.
Professor
Department of Human Morphology
University of Nottingham
Nottingham, England

David J. P. Bassett, Ph.D.
Professor and Chair
Department of Occupational and Environmental Health
College of Pharmacy and Allied Health Professions
Wayne State University
Detroit, Michigan

Ellen Borenfreund, Ph.D.
Adjunct Associate Professor
Laboratory for In Vitro Toxicology Assay Development
The Rockefeller University
New York, New York

Peter Borgs, M.Sc.
Research Specialist
Department of Surgery
College of Medicine
University of Arizona
Tucson, Arizona

Matthew O. Bradley, Ph.D.
Senior Vice President
Genetic MediSyn Corporation
Rockville, Maryland

Todd C. Case, M.D.
Department of Surgery
College of Medicine
University of Arizona
Tucson, Arizona

Guan-jie Chen
Department of Family and Community Medicine
University of Arizona
Tucson, Arizona

Richard H. Clothier, Ph.D.
Senior Lecturer
Department of Human Morphology
University of Nottingham
Nottingham, England

John W. Coleman
Senior Lecturer
Department of Pharmacology and Therapeutics
University of Liverpool
Liverpool
England

Nicholas J. DelRaso
Armstrong Laboratory for Toxic Hazards
U.S. Air Force
Wright-Patterson AFB
Ohio

Sue M. Ford, Ph.D.
Department of Pharmaceutical Sciences
College of Pharmacy and Allied Health Professions
St. John's University
Jamaica, New York

R. Jerrold Fulton, Ph.D.
Director
Immunochemicals Division
Inland Laboratories, Inc.
Dallas, Texas

Gerhard Gstraunthaler, Ph.D.
Assistant Professor
Institute of Physiology
University of Innsbruck
Innsbruck
Austria

Mary J. C. Hendrix, Ph.D.
Associate Professor
Department of Anatomy
University of Arizona
Tucson, Arizona

Dennis S. Huang
Department of Family and Community Medicine
University of Arizona
Tucson, Arizona

Lawrence H. Lash, Ph.D.
Assistant Professor
Department of Pharmacology
Wayne State University School of Medicine
Detroit, Michigan

Tee-Ping Lee, Ph.D.
Director
Renal Electrolyte Laboratory
Department of Medicine
Buffalo VAMC
Buffalo, New York

Albert P. Li, Ph.D.
Fellow
Health Sciences Department
Monsanto Corporate Research
Monsanto Company
St. Louis, Missouri

Francisca Martínez, Ph.D.
Research Associate
Department of Family and Community Medicine
University of Arizona
Tucson, Arizona

Raul Martínez-Zaguilán, Ph.D.
Research Associate
Department of Biochemistry
Arizona Health Sciences Center
University of Arizona
Tucson, Arizona

Richard D. May, Ph.D.
Staff Immunologist
Chemotherapy and Toxicology Department
Southern Research Institute
Birmingham, Alabama

Walter Pfaller, M.D.
Professor
Institute of Physiology
University of Insbruck
Insbruck
Austria

Geronimo Ramirez, Jr., M.D.
Department of Surgery
College of Medicine
University of Arizona
Tucson, Arizona

Robert A. Roth, Ph.D.
Professor
Pharmacology and Toxicology Department
Michigan State University
East Lansing, Michigan

Joseph F. Sina, Ph.D.
Senior Research Fellow
Department of Safety Assessment
Merck Sharp and Dohme Research Laboratories
West Point, Pennsylvania

Toshio Sofuni, Ph.D.
Head
Division of Genetics and Mutagenesis
National Institute of Hygienic Sciences
Tokyo
Japan

Katsuyasu Tachibana
Faculty of Fisheries
Nagasaki University
Nagasaki
Japan

Annette G. Teepe
Research Biologist
Health Sciences Department
Monsanto Corporate Research
Monsanto Company
St. Louis, Missouri

Ronald R. Watson, Ph.D.
Department of Family and Community Medicine
University of Arizona
Tucson, Arizona

Bernhard Watzl
Department of Family and Community Medicine
University of Arizona
Tucson, Arizona

Dennis L. Way
Director of Lymphology Laboratories
Department of Surgery
College of Medicine
University of Arizona
Tucson, Arizona

Patricia D. Williams, Ph.D.
American Cyanamid Company
Medical Research Division
Pearl River, New York

Charles L. Witte, M.D.
Professor
Department of Surgery
College of Medicine
University of Arizona
Tucson, Arizona

Marlys H. Witte, M.D.
Professor
Department of Surgery
College of Medicine
University of Arizona
Tucson, Arizona

Steven Wood
Nutritionist
Department of Family and Community Medicine
University of Arizona
Tucson, Arizona

Chapter 1

IN VITRO MODELS FOR THE STUDY OF CANCER

Mary J. C. Hendrix

TABLE OF CONTENTS

I. INTRODUCTION

Metastasis is considered the major cause of morbidity and death for cancer patients. Hence, a critical challenge to clinical and basic scientists is the development of improved prognostic methods to better predict the metastatic aggressiveness of a patient's individual tumor and especially to control local invasion. Before effective therapeutic regimes can be planned, we must first invest more effort in understanding the pathogenesis of tumor cell dissemination.

The most critical step in metastasis has been judged to be invasion. This process involving the insidious migration of tumor cells delineates the difference between benign and malignant tumors. A three-step model describing the sequence of biochemical events during tumor cell invasion has been proposed,[1] and basically describes: (1) tumor cell attachment to a matrix *substratum;* (2) local degradation of the matrix by tumor cell-associated proteases; and (3) tumor cell locomotion into the matrix modified by proteolysis. Although simplistic in theory, these steps are quite complex to study because the mechanisms underlying metastasis occur in an intricate cascade, in which one event appears to trigger the onset of another.

Recent advances in the field of tumor cell biology have focused on the unique interactions between tumor cells and other cells, as well as extracellular barriers. In order to study various aspects of invasion dynamics *in vitro,* a plethora of invasion assays has been developed to investigate unique metastatic properties demonstrated by specific tumor cells. An account of these newly developed assays began in the late 1970s and has escalated exponentially since that time.[2] At present, it would be difficult to imagine the development of a novel invasion assay that did not incorporate or reflect some aspect of a previously documented protocol. Probably the most controversial aspect of these assays is the qualitative and quantitative analysis associated with each. If one assumes that each assay is meritorious in its own right, then rigorous interpretation of experimental data should be applied universally. Although there are numerous assays available for the study of various characteristics of tumor cell biology, this chapter will focus primarily on the invasive properties of tumor cells as they relate to metastasis.

II. SPECIFIC INVASION ASSAYS

Several *in vitro* assays focusing on the study of invasion and metastatic properties of tumor cells warrant recognition as being truly innovative as well as contributing important knowledge in a field that is exploding with discoveries. To begin with, the assay for invasion of tumor cells into blood vessels contained within the chick chorioallantoic membrane was developed to mimic the event of intravasation,[3] and led subsequently to the development of another useful model using only endothelial cells and their matrix as the tumor barrier.[4]

The next assay which has certainly left its mark in tumor cell biology is the human amnion assay using a modified Boyden chamber,[5] from which many matrix assays have been developed, including the reconstituted basement membrane matrix assay,[6-8] and collagen gels,[9] as well as other specific combinations of matrix components. Basically, these assays offer a matrix barrier, with or without associated tissue host cells, for tumor cells to penetrate. With regard to the quantitative evaluation of invasion in these assays, there is considerable debate over the most efficient method to use. Invasive cells that have successfully migrated through a specific barrier have been quantitated via cell-associated radioactivity or by direct cell counts.[10] In addition, release assays have been utilized in an attempt to derive similar information pertaining to invasive ability. In these assays, instead of radiolabeling tumor

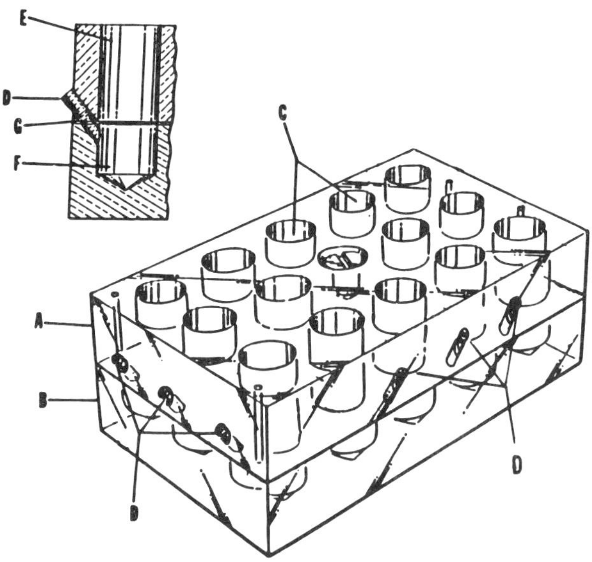

FIGURE 1. Analytical membrane invasion culture system (MICS) chamber: (A) top plate, (B) bottom plate, (C) experimental wells, (D) sampling ports, (E) upper well, (F) lower well, (G) matrigel-coated nucleopore filter is interposed between top and bottom plate. Tumor cells are then seeded into upper wells, allowed to attach to the coated filter, and subsequently assayed at 72 h in bottom wells via the side sampling ports.

cells, the matrix components are radiolabeled, and the destruction of the matrix by the confronting cells is measured from the release of radioactivity into culture medium.[4,11]

With regard to the application of the above-mentioned invasion assays, tumor cell populations essentially confronted with a matrix barrier of some known composition, and those cells which successfully migrate through the barrier, are considered more invasive than the cells which do not (within a certain time frame). Variations or discrepancies which exist in the conduct of these assays pertain to the use of chemoattractants as well as the duration of time that the assays are allowed to run. In this regard, care must be taken to ensure that complete documentation of protocols accompanies every report so that the assays may be repeated with a high degree of accuracy.

Our laboratory has developed two invasion chambers, which are essentially modifications of the Boyden chamber. These are shown in Figures 1 and 3. The assay is known as the membrane invasion culture system (MICS), and data derived from the 72-hour invasion assay have been shown to correlate with the metastatic potential of the cells tested.[8,10] The matrix barrier originally used in this assay was a human amnion.[12] More recently, a polycarbonate filter coated with matrigel,[8] which consists of laminin, type IV collagen, entactin, and heparin sulfate proteoglycan[13] has been employed. After trying numerous methods of evaluation of invasion, we have adopted the direct cell counting technique as the most accurate analysis of invading cells, shown in Figure 2. Using this method, one can precisely distinguish cellular from noncellular material. When determining the invasive rate of cell populations, we use the analytical MICS chamber, shown in Figure 1, which consists of 14 contiguous wells in the upper and lower well plates, separated by a matrigel-coated filter. Side-sampling ports communicate with the lower wells so that invasive cells can be removed from the undersurface of a filter with the addition of enzymes or chelating agents in solution. Alternatively, and more simplistically, at the termination of invasion assays, the noninvasive cells located on the upper surface of the matrigel-coated filter can be removed with a

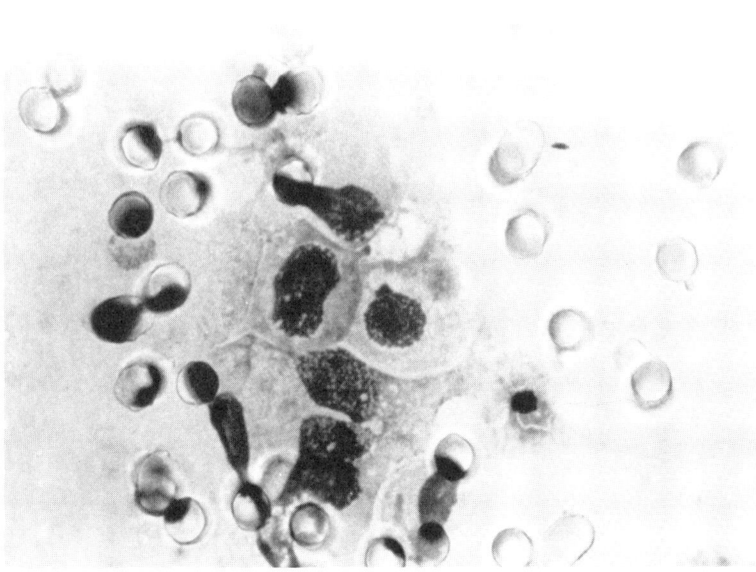

FIGURE 2. Photomicrograph of tumor cells attached to the matrigel-coated polycarbonate membrane (containing 10-μm-size pores). Several cells can be seen migrating through the pores (×1500).

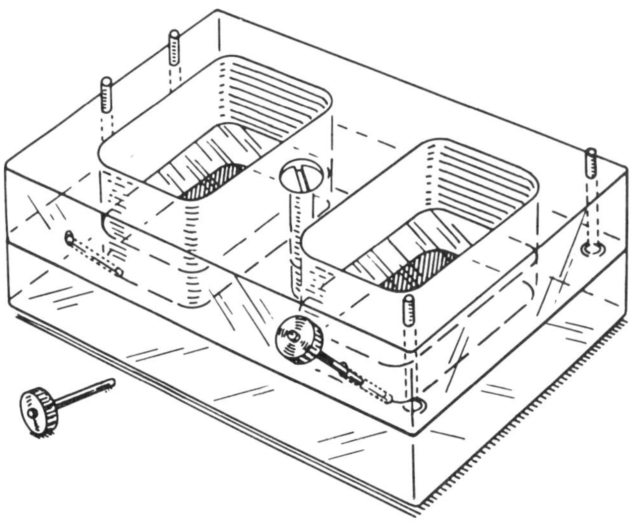

FIGURE 3. The mega membrane invasion culture system (MegaMICS) was developed for the purpose of collecting large populations of invasive tumor cells after they have invaded a membranous barrier. The chamber is composed of a top and bottom plate containing upper and lower experimental wells, respectively, with side sampling ports. Briefly, the matrigel-coated filter is interposed between the top and bottom plates. Cells are then seeded into the upper wells, and invasive cells are subsequently collected in the lower well via the side sampling ports.

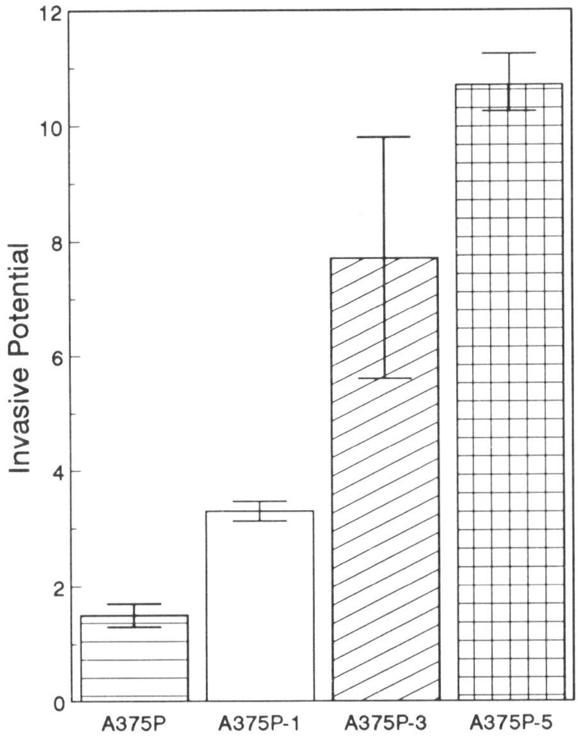

FIGURE 4. Percent invasion profiles of selected subpopulations of a poorly metastatic human melanoma cell line (A375P) that invaded a matrigel-coated filter in the analytical MICS chamber after 72 h, prior to and following selection in the MegaMICS chamber, 1, 3, and 5 times.

Kim-Wipe, and the undersurface containing the invasive cells can be stained and counted microscopically. Invasion data can subsequently be plotted using the following equation:

$$\frac{\text{Number of invasive cells counted}}{\text{Number of cells seeded onto the coated filter}} \times 100$$

These data can be corrected for proliferation during the assay using protein determinations.[12,14]

For the purpose of studying subpopulations of invasive cells, we developed the MegaMICS chamber, shown in Figure 3, which allows the selection of more invasive cells from a heterogeneous population.[14] This assay uses the same type of matrix barrier described for the analytical MICS chamber and allows the collection of preparative quantities of cells for further analyses, such as cytogenetic studies,[15] biochemical and molecular studies,[14] as well as clonogenic studies.[16] This chamber allows one to investigate unique properties inherent to invasive subpopulations that heretofore have been difficult to achieve. Furthermore, our laboratory has demonstrated that a poorly invasive tumor cell line can be selected up to five times in the MegaMICS, which results in the selection of five sublines, each one more invasive than its predecessor (Figure 4); and, most interestingly, the invasive sublines are capable of producing increased lung metastases when tested *in vivo*.[14]

The last type of invasion assay falls in the category of three-dimensional organ cultures. Noteworthy among this group is the chick heart fragment assay,[17] the previously mentioned chick chorioallantoic membrane assay[3] as well as the chick egg assay,[18] and the human brain cortex and dura mater fragment assay.[19] These assays have an advantage in that they represent a natural host cellular barrier as well as an extracellular barrier for tumor cells to penetrate. Levels of invasion can be determined histologically; however, overall quantitation is difficult.

Some of the assays described above have been adapted for the screening of anticancer drugs, which may contribute significantly to the pool of therapeutic agents selected for research, development, and clinical trials.[20-22] Furthermore, the testing of genetically manipulated cells has now been applied to these invasion assays in an attempt to elucidate specific genes and gene mutations responsible for invasion and metastasis.[14,23] Hence, it is fair to speculate that these *in vitro* tumor cell invasion assays will continue to contribute to our understanding of tumor cell dynamics and events associated with metastasis. It is important to keep in mind that these *in vitro* assays should be accompanied by corresponding *in vivo* evaluation to lend credibility to their outcome.

REFERENCES

1. **Liotta, L. A., Rao, C. N., and Wewer, U. M.,** Biochemical interactions of tumor cells with the basement membrane, *Annu. Rev. Biochem.*, 55, 1037, 1986.
2. **Post, G.,** Methods and models for studying tumor invasion, in *Tumor Invasion and Metastasis,* Liotta, L. A. and Hart, I. R., Eds., Martinus Nijhoff, The Hague, 1982.
3. **Hart, I. R. and Fidler, I. J.,** An *in vitro* quantitative assay for tumor cell invasion, *Cancer Res.*, 38, 3218, 1978.
4. **Nicolson, G. L.,** Metastatic tumor cell attachment and invasion assay utilizing vascular endothelial cell monolayers, *J. Histochem. Cytochem.*, 30, 214, 1982.
5. **Liotta, L. A., Lee, C. W., and Morakis, D. J.,** New method for preparing large surfaces of intact human basement membrane for tumor invasion studies, *Cancer Lett.*, 11, 141, 1980.
6. **Albini, A., Iwamoto, Y., Kleinman, H. K., Martin, G. R., Aaronson, S. A., Kozlowski, J. M., and McEwan, R. N.,** A rapid *in vitro* assay for quantitating the invasive potential of tumor cells, *Cancer Res.*, 47, 3239, 1987.
7. **Kramer, R. H., Bensch, K. G., and Wong, J.,** Invasion of reconstituted basement membrane matrix by metastatic human tumor cells, *Cancer Res.*, 46, 1980, 1986.
8. **Hendrix, M. J. C., Seftor, E. A., Seftor, R. E. B., and Fidler, I. J.,** A simple quantitative assay for studying the invasive potential of high and low human metastatic variants, *Cancer Lett.*, 38, 137, 1987.
9. **Schor, S. L., Schor, A. M., Winn, B., and Rushton, G.,** The use of three-dimensional collagen gels for the study of tumor cell invasion *in vitro:* experimental parameters influencing cell migration into the gel matrix, *Int. J. Cancer,* 29, 57, 1982.
10. **Hendrix, M. J. C., Seftor, E. A., Seftor, R. E. B., Misiorowski, R. L., Saba, P. Z., Sundareshan, P., and Welch, D. R.,** Comparison of tumor cell invasion assays: human amnion versus reconstituted basement membrane barriers, *Invasion Metastasis,* 9, 278, 1989.
11. **Bogenmann, E., Mark, C., Isaacs, H., Neustein, H. B., DeClerck, Y. A., Laug, W. E., and Jones, P. A.,** Invasive properties of primary pediatric neoplasms *in vitro, Cancer Res.*, 43, 1176, 1983.
12. **Hendrix, M. J. C., Gehlsen, K. R., Wagner, H. N., Rodney, S. R., Misiorowski, R. L., and Meyskens, F. L.,** *In vitro* quantification of melanoma tumor cell invasion, *Clin. Expl. Metastasis,* 3, 221, 1985.
13. **Kleinman, H. K., McGarvey, M. L., Liotta, L. A., Robey, P. G., Tryggvason, K., and Martin, G. R.,** Isolation and characterization of type IV procollagen, laminin, and heparan sulfate proteoglycan from the EHS sarcoma, *Biochemistry,* 21, 6188, 1982.
14. **Seftor, E. A., Seftor, R. E. B., and Hendrix, M. J. C.,** Selection of invasive and metastatic subpopulations from a heterogeneous human melanoma cell line, *Biotechnology,* 9, 324, 1990.
15. **Bevacqua, S. J., Greeff, C. W., and Hendrix, M. J. C.,** Cytogenetic evidence of gene amplification as a mechanism for tumor cell invasion, *Somatic Cell Mol. Genet.*, 14, 83, 1988.
16. **Yohem, K. H., Seftor, E. A., Meyskens, F. L., Jr., and Hendrix, M. J. C.,** Cloning efficiency of human melanoma cells modulated after invasion through a reconstituted basement membrane, *Cancer Lett.*, 45, 135, 1989.
17. **Mareel, M. M., DeBruyne, G. K., Vandesande, F., and Dragonetti, C.,** Immunohistochemical study of embryonic chick heart invaded by malignant cells in three-dimensional culture, *Invasion Metastasis,* 1, 195, 1981.

18. **Chambers, A. F., Denhardt, G. H., and Wilson, S. M.,** Ras-transformed NIH 3T3 cell lines, selected for metastatic ability in chick embryos, have increased proportions of p21-expressing cells and are metastatic in nude mice, *Invasion Metastasis,* 10, 225, 1990.
19. **Ibayashi, N., Herman, M. M., Boyd, J. C., and Rubinstein, L. J.,** Relationship of invasiveness to proliferating activity and to cytoskeletal protein production in human neuroepithelial tumors maintained in an organ culture system: use of human cortex and dura as supporting matrices, *Neurosurgery,* 26, 629, 1990.
20. **Welch, D. R., Lobl, T. J., Seftor, E. A., Wack, P. J., Aeed, P. A., Yohem, K. H., Seftor, R. E. B., and Hendrix, M. J. C.,** Use of the Membrane Invasion Culture System (MICS) as a screen for anti-invasive agents, *Int. J. Cancer,* 43, 449, 1989.
21. **Mareel, M. M. and DeMets, M.,** Anti-invasive activities of experimental chemotherapeutic agents, *Crit. Rev. Oncol. Hematol.,* 9, 263, 1989.
22. **Seftor, R. E. B., Seftor, E. A., Grimes, W. J., Liotta, L. A., Stetler-Stevenson, W. G., Welch, D. R., and Hendrix, M. J. C.,** Human melanoma cell invasion is inhibited *in vitro* by swainsonine and deoxymannojirimycin with a concomitant decrease in collagenase IV expression, *Melanoma Res.,* 1, 43, 1991.
23. **Chu, Y.-W., Duffy, J. J., Seftor, R. E. B., Nagle, R. B., and Hendrix, M. J. C.,** Transfection of a deleted CK18 cDNA into a highly metastatic melanoma cell line decreases the invasive potential, *Clin. Biotech.,* 3, 27, 1991.

Chapter 2

IN VITRO TUMOR TOXICITY WITH ANTIBODY-TOXIN CONJUGATES

Richard D. May and R. Jerrold Fulton

TABLE OF CONTENTS

I. INTRODUCTION

Over the past two decades, a number of laboratories have approached the treatment of neoplastic disease by means of immunotherapy in order to minimize the nonspecific cytotoxic side effects of radiotherapy and chemotherapy (reviewed in Reference 1). Such modalities include the use of cytokines,[2,3] cellular therapy,[3,4] and antibody-directed therapy.[5-9] As early as 1906, Paul Ehrlich envisioned the use of this latter approach, which he referred to as "magic bullets", to specifically treat disease.[10] However, the first antibody-toxin conjugates, or immunotoxins (ITs), were not developed until the late 1970s to early 1980s.[11-19] With the advent of monoclonal antibody (mAb) technology[20] and many important advances and refinements in the IT and toxin fields, highly specific mAbs and potent toxins, or their subunits, can be used to create what today may be considered "patriot missiles" to treat neoplastic disease, autoimmune disease and immune dysfunction, graft-versus-host disease (GVHD), and even AIDS.

The purpose of this chapter is not to review the IT field. A number of excellent reviews have been published in recent years, which provide ample background information.[21-28] Rather, this chapter is designed to provide specific information and methodology to enable the reader to construct, analyze, and test ITs for their selective toxicity to tumor or normal cells using appropriate *in vitro* techniques.

II. PREPARATION OF IMMUNOTOXINS

The general approach is to select a mAb with specificity for the target cell, couple it to the desired toxin, purify the IT, and then verify its specificity and determine its potency by a number of *in vitro* assays. In theory, this is straightforward. However, not all mAbs function as potent ITs, despite their antibody (Ab) specificity.[29,30] In addition, a number of considerations should be made during the selection of Ab and toxin for the development of a useful IT.

A. CHOICE OF ANTIBODY

Generally, purified mAbs of mouse or rat origin are selected, although heterologous Abs can also be useful, depending on the application. For example, in the indirect IT assay (see below), purified Fab′ fragments of goat anti-mouse immunoglobulin are the reagent of choice.[31] While the immunoglobulin (Ig) isotype is not usually critical, IgG mAbs are preferable over IgM mAbs, due mainly to size (molecular weight) considerations. Cell-reactive mAbs are usually chosen, based on their known specificity, or following some simple selection criterion, e.g., flow cytometry, to demonstrate specific binding to the appropriate target cell.

Despite their specific binding, not all mAbs will function as effective ITs.[29,30] A variety of factors are involved in determining whether a given mAb will make a potent IT. These include Ab affinity,[32-34] the nature and density of the surface Ag bound by the mAb,[30,32,35,36] the determinant (epitope) on the target Ag bound by the mAb,[37-40] the characteristics of the tumor target cell,[29,33,41] and the rate and route of internalization of the bound IT.[30,37,39,42-44] For example, IT cytotoxicity requires that the cell internalizes the bound IT so that the toxin reaches the cytoplasm.[45] Therefore, the target cell Ag should be one that is endocytosed following incubation with the Ab being tested. Thus, these factors, when known, should be kept in mind during the selection and screening of mAbs for use as ITs.

A useful assay which predicts the ability of mAbs to function as potent ITs, known as the "indirect IT assay", has been described[31,46] and provides a simple, rapid, and reliable screening method for choosing a good mAb for toxin conjugation. In addition, the indirect

IT assay does not require that the prospective mAb be purified to determine if it is worth pursuing as an IT. However, once the mAb has been selected, it must be used in purified form. A quantity of at least 10 mg is recommended to begin the conjugation procedure.

For development of ITs for eventual clinical use, a panel of normal human tissues should be screened for binding with the mAb of interest at the outset of the study to avoid use of a mAb with undesirable cross-reactivity.

It is essential to obtain a negative control Ab, which should also be conjugated to the toxin. This Ab can be a mAb with irrelevant specificity for the target cell(s) (e.g., an antibacterial or antiviral mAb), or a myeloma protein with no known specificity can be used (e.g., MOPC-21 as a mouse IgG1k, RPC-5 as a mouse IgG2ak, etc. Purified myeloma proteins may be purchased from East Acres Biologicals, Southbridge, MA or Organon Teknika, West Chester, PA. Many hybridoma and myeloma cell lines are available from American Type Culture Collection, Rockville, MD if you are inclined to ''grow your own''.) In either case, the Ig isotype of the negative control mAb or myeloma protein should match that of the mAb used to construct the IT with tumor cell specificity.

B. CHOICE OF TOXIN

The choice of a toxin for IT construction requires consideration of (1) the theoretical attributes which are desirable for the resulting conjugate, and (2) the practical limitations resulting from the innate properties of the individual toxins and target antigens (Ags). The major choices available are either one of the bacterial toxins, primarily diphtheria toxin (DT) or pseudomonas exotoxin A (PE), or one of the plant toxins or their enzymatic subunits, such as ricin or ricin A chain. Table 1 lists many of the toxins which have been used in the construction of ITs.

Although the mechanisms of action and internalization differ between the bacterial and the plant toxins, all are proteins or glycoproteins which inhibit cellular protein synthesis after translocation to the cytoplasm.[45] The major functions expressed by these toxins are (1) cell surface binding, (2) membrane translocation, and (3) enzymatic inhibition of protein synthesis. The ideal toxin for IT construction should lack appreciable ''nonspecific'' cellular binding and toxicity and rapidly inhibit protein synthesis, indicating efficient membrane translocation.

Several mutants of DT and PE, such as CRM-45, CRM-107, and PE40, lack appreciable cell surface binding, but retain most of the translocation activity of the native toxin.[47-49] Thus, these mutant toxins are well suited for IT production, and potent and specific ITs have been prepared with them (see Table 1). Unfortunately, similar mutants are not available for the plant toxins. ITs prepared with whole ricin (IT-Rs) express extremely rapid kinetics for inhibition of cellular protein synthesis, implying efficient membrane translocation. However, IT-Rs also express a high degree of nonspecific toxicity due to the galactose binding activity of the B chain subunit and, hence, their ability to bind to cell surfaces. For *in vitro* purposes, the ricin binding site can be effectively blocked by the addition of excess lactose or galactose.[57] A chemical method for covalently blocking the galactose binding sites of ricin has recently been developed,[58] and IT-Rs prepared with blocked ricin express specificity in the absence of galactose.[58,59]

Preparation of ITs with the purified A chain subunit (IT-As) results in an IT with extremely low nonspecific toxicity, but slower kinetics of killing, presumably due to the lack of efficient membrane translocation. In this regard, the other plant toxin A chains and the single chain ribosome inactivating proteins (RIPs) express the same advantages and disadvantages as ricin A chain.

One other source of potential nonspecificity results from the high mannose carbohydrates present on both the A and B chains of some of the plant toxins, such as ricin. These carbohydrate structures are recognized specifically by surface receptors on reticuloendothelial

TABLE 1
Bacterial and Plant Toxins Commonly Used to Construct Immunotoxins

Toxin	Mol wt (kDa)	Structure[a]	Toxicity[b]	Ref.
	A. Bacterial Toxins			
Diphtheria toxin	62	P	High	11,14
CRM 45	45	P′	Low	47
CRM 107	62	P′	Low	48
Pseudomonas exotoxin A	66	P	High	49
PE40	40	P′	Low	49
	B. Plant Toxins			
Ricin	62	A-B	High	15
Abrin	65	A-B	High	19
Viscumin	64	A-B	High	50
Ricin A chain	30–32	A	Low	13,51
Abrin A chain	30	A	Low	51,52
Gelonin	30	A′	Low	44,53
Saporin	30	A′	Low	52,54
Pokeweed antiviral protein	27	A′	Low	33
Trichosanthin	30	A′	Low	55
Momordin	31	A′	Low	52,56
Bryodin	30	A′	Low	56

[a] Structure designations are P — single chain protein containing functionally distinct domains for enzymatic activity, translocation, and binding activities; P′ — single chain mutant protein in which receptor binding activity is largely deleted; A-B — two-subunit protein containing an enzymatically active A chain and a receptor-binding B chain; A — purified A subunit of A-B dimer; A′ — single chain protein containing enzymatic activity, but no receptor binding activity.

[b] High toxicity indicates ability of unconjugated toxin to bind cell surface receptors. Low toxicity indicates the toxin, or toxin subunit, is unable to bind and penetrate the cell on its own.

cells, which reside primarily in the liver and spleen.[60] This results in rapid clearance of the IT from the circulation following intravenous administration. Chemical "deglycosylation" greatly reduces the liver clearance of ricin A chain without altering its enzymatic activity.[61] While this problem is largely restricted to *in vivo* use of IT-As, it should be considered at the outset if the long-term research goal is directed toward *in vivo* use.

Because of its ready availability, ease of use, low nonspecific toxicity *in vitro* and *in vivo,* and high potency for inhibition of protein synthesis, ricin A chain is a useful toxin for IT construction. The major problem encountered with ricin A chain is that not all mAbs will function as potent A chain ITs. In many cases, it is necessary to screen several mAbs to the same Ag in order to find one which makes a potent IT-A. In some cases, the use of a different toxin may result in a potent IT, whereas the same mAb did not make a potent ricin A chain IT;[52] however, in this instance, it is unlikely that another plant toxin A chain or RIP will give different results, and it may be necessary to use intact ricin or one of the bacterial toxins. Nevertheless, because of its eventual usefulness for *in vivo* purposes, as well as its availability and relative safety for laboratory personnel, we will describe the preparation of IT-As made with either native or deglycosylated ricin A chain.

C. ANTIBODY-TOXIN CONJUGATION

The development of heterobifunctional cross-linkers was a crucial step in the early development of ITs. This allowed the efficient and reproducible production of protein heteroconjugates, without the formation of undesirable homopolymers, and large molecular weight aggregates which are generated with homobifunctional cross-linkers. Two basic types of intermolecular bonds have been widely used in the construction of ITs, namely, reducible disulfide bonds and nonreducible thioether bonds. It is necessary to employ a reducible disulfide bond in the preparation of ITs with the plant toxin A chains and single chain RIPs, whereas ITs containing intact toxins can be prepared with a thioether bond since a reducible disulfide is present between the enzymatic fragment and the rest of the toxin.

The general approach is to react a free thiol group on one protein with a thiol-reactive group on the second. In the case of the plant toxin A chains, such as ricin A or abrin A, a single free cysteine is available and thiolation is not necessary. With intact toxins and single chain RIPs, where a thiol is not present, thiolation is most easily accomplished with 2-iminothiolane, which substitutes free amino groups, preserving the positive charge and introducing the desired thiol directly.[62]

There are a large number of heterobifunctional cross-linkers available for the introduction of thiol reactive groups (Sigma, St. Louis, MO or Pierce, Rockford, IL); however, the most widely used are SPDP [*N*-succinimidyl 3-(2-pyridyldithio)propionate] for disulfide linkages[63] and MBS (*m*-maleimidobenzoyl-*N*-hydroxy-succinimide ester) for thioether linkages[15] or derivatives of these with increased stability, water solubility, or extended chain length. Of particular note is SMPT [4-succinimidyl-oxycarbonyl-α-methyl-α-(2-pyridyldithio)-toluene], which yields disulfide conjugates with increased stability *in vivo*.[64]

The preparation of a ricin IT-A involves substitution of the Ab with SPDP or SMPT, removal of excess cross-linkers, reaction of the substituted Ab with reduced ricin A chain, and subsequent purification of the conjugate to remove unconjugated Ab and A chain. The Ab is prepared in a phosphate buffer (e.g., PBS or 50 m*M* sodium phosphate, pH 7 to 8) at 1 to 10 mg/ml. SPDP is dissolved in dimethylformamide at 10 mg/ml, and added to the Ab solution in a 4- to 5-fold molar excess. The mixture is then incubated for 30 min at room temperature. Next, the reaction mixture is desalted on a column of Sephadex G-25M that is equilibrated in the same buffer. An equal milligram amount of ricin A chain, representing a 5-fold molar excess, is reduced with 5 m*M* dithiothreitol for 30 min at room temperature, desalted as above, mixed with the SPDP-substituted Ab, and then allowed to react overnight at 4°C. Excess ricin A is removed by size exclusion chromatography on a column of Sephacryl S-200 HR, or similar resin, that is equilibrated in 50 m*M* phosphate buffer, pH 7. The first eluted peak, containing IT-A and unconjugated Ab, is then applied to a column of Blue Sepharose CL-6B that is equilibrated in the same buffer. Unconjugated Ab will not bind Blue Sepharose and passes through with the starting buffer.[64] The IT-A is then eluted in the same buffer containing 1.0 *M* NaCl. Finally, the purified IT-A is dialyzed or desalted into PBS, or another physiological buffer, concentrated to at least 1 mg/ml for stability, and stored in frozen aliquots. An exact determination of the concentration of the IT-A is somewhat difficult, although a close approximation can be obtained spectrophotometrically by simply averaging the extinction coefficients for IgG (OD_{280} of 1.4 = 1.0 mg/ml) and ricin A chain (OD_{280} of 0.77 = 1.0 mg/ml) in proportion to the molar ratio present in the conjugate. An extinction coefficient of OD_{280} of 1.0 = 1.0 mg/ml represents a close approximation for conjugates containing 1 to 2 moles A chain per mole of Ab. Determination of the molar ratio of A chain to Ab is discussed below.

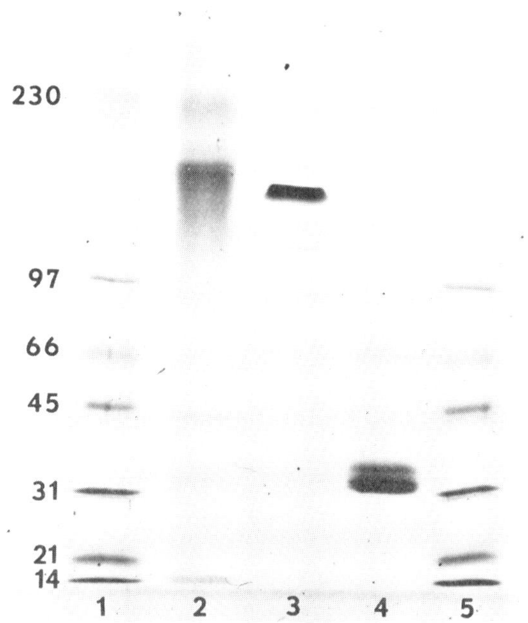

FIGURE 1. SDS-PAGE analysis of immunotoxin samples. Samples, approximately 1 μg each, were electrophoresed on a 4–15% gradient gel run under nonreduced conditions using a PhastSystem (Pharmacia) and stained with Coomassie Blue R-350. Contents of lanes: 1, Mol wt standards of 230, 97, 66, 45, 31, 21, and 14 kDa; 2, purified IT-A; 3, unconjugated IgG; 4, unconjugated ricin A chain; 5, mol wt standards of 97, 66, 45, 31, 21, and 14 kDa.

III. *IN VITRO* TESTING

A. BIOCHEMICAL CHARACTERIZATION

The purity of the IT-A is determined by SDS-PAGE or by analytical HPLC size exclusion analysis. This permits one to (1) confirm conjugation of Ab and toxin, (2) determine if any unconjugated Ab or free A chain is present in the preparation, and (3) quantitate conjugate species containing one, two, or more A chains per Ab molecule. Figure 1 shows an SDS-PAGE gel in which an IgG Ab was conjugated to ricin A chain using SPDP as a cross-linker. This gel demonstrates that the IT-A primarily contains conjugates with 1 A chain per IgG, lesser amounts of higher molecular weight conjugates, and virtually undetectable amounts of free IgG and A chain. The relative proportions of conjugate containing one, two, or more A chains per IgG can be quantitated by densitometric scanning of the gel. This information can then be used to calculate the average A chain content.

B. ANTIBODY ACTIVITY

Following IT-A preparation and purification, it is important to demonstrate that the Ab activity of the IT-A has not been significantly impaired during the conjugation process. The same binding assay used for selection and/or testing of the starting mAb can be used to show Ab activity in the IT-A. For instance, this may involve determination of the relative binding avidity by flow cytometry to determine the concentration of mAb or IT-A needed to achieve 50% of the maximal mean fluorescence intensity (MFI_{50})[38] or a competitive inhibition assay in which various concentrations of native mAb and IT-A are used to inhibit binding of radiolabeled mAb.[38] Decreases in Ab activity following conjugation to A chain are routinely 0- to 10-fold. Large decreases in Ab activity would dictate lowering the cross-linker substitution of the Ab.

C. RICIN A CHAIN ENZYMATIC ACTIVITY

The activity of the A chain in the IT-A conjugate is determined by reducing the conjugate and comparing the enzymatic activity of the released A chain with that of the unconjugated A chain used to construct the IT-A. This involves using a cell-free rabbit reticulocyte assay as described by Press et al.[66] The A chain activity should not be significantly altered by the conjugation procedure.

D. CYTOTOXIC ACTIVITY OF THE IT-A: THE DIRECT IT-A ASSAY

Like most RIPs or toxin subunits, ricin A chain is an inhibitor of protein synthesis.[45] Therefore, the target cell should actively make protein so that the toxin can cause inhibition. This is usually not a problem if the target cell is a tumor cell line. However, normal cells may require some stimulus for the bound IT-A to manifest its cytotoxicity. For example, resting T or B lymphocytes may be stimulated with mitogens to activate them following incubation with IT-A. Technically, a protein synthesis assay, e.g., ^{3}H-leucine incorporation, should be used. However, a cell proliferation assay can also be used, e.g., ^{3}H-thymidine incorporation, a tetrazolium assay, such as MTT,[67] or neutral red dye uptake.[68] ^{3}H-leucine and ^{3}H-thymidine incorporation data following IT-A treatment of Daudi cells are equivalent.[68a] Alternatively, a clonogenic assay may be used to assess IT cytotoxicity with tumor cells.[69] A target cell line lacking the target Ag is frequently used to demonstrate further specificity of the IT-A.

The most reproducible cytotoxicity results are obtained when tumor target cells are in log growth phase. Thus, cell passage should occur 1 to 2 days prior to the IT-A killing assay. To perform the assay, tumor cells are washed with medium 2 to 3 times, and a constant number of cells are added to wells of a 96-well microtiter plate (usually 1 to 2×10^5 cells per well). The IT-A preparations should be centrifuged at high speed (e.g., $20{,}000 \times g$ for 20 min) prior to use to remove any Ab aggregates that may have formed. Such aggregates could nonspecifically bind to cells to give misleading results. Serial dilutions of control and specific IT-As are made in medium and added to the cells. Replicates of at least three should be performed.

Recommended IT-A concentrations range from 10^{-7} *M* (18 μg/ml for an IgG IT-A containing 1 A chain per IgG molecule) to 10^{-13} *M*. In addition to equivalent dilutions of the irrelevant negative control IT-A, dilutions of free A chain and free Ab should also be included to demonstrate that these reagents alone have no toxic effects on the cells. Dilutions of whole ricin toxin can be used as a positive cytotoxic control. Cells treated with medium alone are used to establish 100% of control values in the direct IT assay.

The time of incubation of cells at 37°C with IT-As may vary and usually depends on the target cells used. Most experiments incubate for 1 to 2 days before harvest. If the nature of the experiment calls for a pulse of the cells with IT-A, cells may be incubated for 60 min at 4°C with IT-A to allow binding, and then washed to remove unbound IT-A prior to incubation at 37°C.

When plotted, results are routinely expressed as "percent of control", using the cpm incorporated in cells treated with medium alone as 100% of control. It is helpful to the reader to indicate the number of cpm in medium-treated cells in the figure legend. A representative cytotoxicity experiment is shown in Figure 2. The concentration of IT which inhibits protein synthesis or cellular proliferation by 50% is termed the "IC_{50}". IC_{50} values are routinely used to compare the potency of IT-As and are expressed in tabular form. IT-As with IC_{50} values less than 10^{-10} *M* are generally considered good. Although values

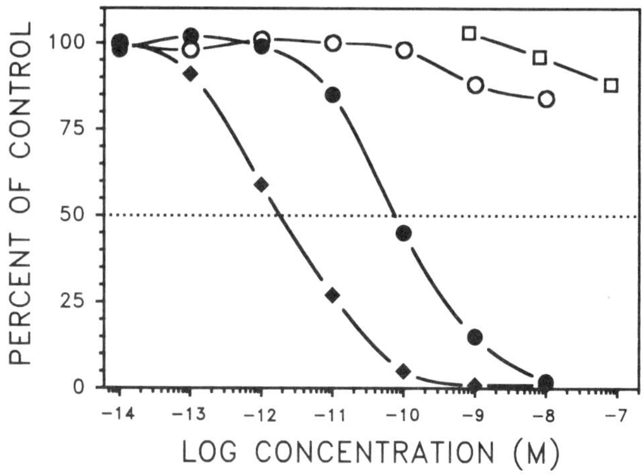

FIGURE 2. *In vitro* direct IT-A proliferation/cytotoxicity assay. Mouse Ig^+ WEHI-279 cells, 1×10^5 cells per well in triplicate, were placed into wells of a 96-well plate in 100 μl RPMI 1640 medium containing 5% fetal bovine serum and incubated for 18 h at 37°C in 5% CO_2 with the indicated concentrations of whole native ricin (♦), goat anti-mouse Ig IT-A (●), normal goat IgG IT-A (negative control) (○), or free ricin A chain (□). Cultures were pulsed for 4 h with 50 μg MTT per well, followed by addition of 150 μl acidic isopropanol per well to dissolve the insoluble formazan product. The plates were then read on a Molecular Devices 96-well plate reader at a wavelength of 570 nm, using 650 nm as reference. The mean absorbance of untreated cultures (100% of control) was 1.6 ± 0.09.

depend on the tumor cell used, whole ricin usually has an IC_{50} of 10^{-11} *M* or less. In the experiment in Figure 2, the specific IT-A has an IC_{50} of approximately 8×10^{-11} *M*, while ricin has an IC_{50} of approximately 2×10^{-12} *M*. The controls (irrelevant IT-A and free A chain) were not toxic ($IC_{50} > 10^{-7}$ *M*).

IV. DISCUSSION AND CONCLUSION

In this chapter, we have described how to prepare and test ITs for killing tumor cells *in vitro*. The selection of toxin and Ab are crucial for constructing a successful IT. We have provided detailed methodology for constructing an IT-A using ricin A chain, which is widely used in this field. The purity, Ab binding activity, and cytotoxic efficacy of the IT-As are tested by appropriate *in vitro* methods. Specificity of killing is demonstrated by a direct IT-A assay, which includes using an isotype-matched negative control IT-A, as well as an Ag-negative cell line.

ITs have shown promise for a variety of *in vivo* and *in vitro* settings, including malignancy,[21-28,70-72] autoimmunity and immune regulation,[73,74] bone marrow transplantation and GVHD,[57,69,75,76] and AIDS.[77-79] Careful *in vitro* testing of ITs can predict some of the problems associated with their *in vivo* applications, such as liver toxicity, and nonspecific binding to nontarget tissues. However, *in vitro* efficacy may not always be translated into *in vivo* usefulness.[40] Thus, preclinical *in vivo* animal models must eventually be developed and tested prior to using ITs clinically.

ABBREVIATIONS USED

Ab, antibody; Ag, antigen; DT, diphtheria toxin, GVHD, graft-vs.-host disease; HPLC, high performance liquid chromatography; IC_{50}, concentration that inhibits protein synthesis by 50% compared to untreated cells; Ig, immunoglobulin; IT, immunotoxin; IT-A, ricin A chain-containing IT; IT-R, whole ricin-containing IT; mAb, monoclonal antibody; MBS, *M*-maleimidobenzoyl-*N*-hydroxy-succinimide ester; PBS, phosphate buffered saline; PE, pseudomonas exotoxin A; RIP, ribosome inactivating protein; SDS-PAGE, sodium dodecyl sulfate polyacrylamide gel electrophoresis; SMPT, 4-succinimidyloxycarbonyl-α-methyl-α-(2-pyridyldithio)-toluene; SPDP, *N*-succinimidyl 3-(2-pyridyldithio)propionate.

REFERENCES

1. **Foon, K. A.,** Biological response modifiers: the new immunotherapy, *Cancer Res.*, 49, 1621, 1989.
2. **Ratain, M. J., Golumb, H. M., Bardawil, R. G., et al.,** Durability of responses to interferon alfa-2b in advanced hairy cell leukemia, *Blood,* 69, 872, 1987.
3. **Rosenberg, S. A., Lotze, M. T., Muul, L. M., et al.,** A progressive report on the treatment of 157 patients with advanced cancer using lymphokine-activated killer cells and interleukin-2 or high-dose interleukin-2 alone, *N. Engl. J. Med.*, 316, 889, 1987.
4. **Topalian, S. L., Solomon, D., Avis, F. P., et al.,** Immunotherapy of patients with advanced cancer using tumor-infiltrating lymphocytes and recombinant interleukin-2: a pilot study, *J. Clin. Oncol.*, 6, 839, 1988.
5. **Miller, R. A., Maloney, D. G., Warnke, R., and Levy, R.,** Treatment of B-cell lymphoma with monoclonal anti-idiotype antibody, *N. Engl. J. Med.*, 306, 517, 1982.
6. **Kramer, E. L. and Larson, S. M.,** Tumor targeting with radiolabeled antibody for diagnosis and therapy, *Immunol. Allergy Clin. N. Amer.*, 11, 301, 1991.
7. **Reisfeld, R. A., Mueller, B. M., Schrappe, M., Wargalla, U., Yang, H. M., and Wrasidlo, W.,** Antibody-drug conjugates for cancer therapy. Promises and problems, *Immunol. Allergy Clin. N. Amer.*, 11, 341, 1991.
8. **Pietersz, G. A., Smyth, M. J., Kanellos, J., Cunningham, Z., Sacks, N. P. M., and McKensie, I. F. C.,** Preclinical and clinical studies with a variety of immunoconjugates, *Antibody, Immunoconjugates, and Radiopharm.*, 1, 79, 1988.
9. **Möller, G., Ed.,** Antibody carriers of drugs and toxins in tumor therapy, *Immunological Reviews,* Vol. 62, Munksgaard, Copenhagen, 1982, 1.
10. **Ehrlich, P.,** Address delivered at the dedication of the Georg Speyer House, in *The Collected Papers of Paul Ehrlich,* Himmelweit, F., Ed., Vol. 3., Pergamon Press, New York, 1960, 53.
11. **Moolten, F. L., Capparell, N. J., Zajdel, S. H., and Cooperband, S. R.,** Anti-tumor effects of antibody-diphtheria toxin conjugates. II. Immunotherapy with conjugates directed against tumor antigens induced by Simian virus 40, *J. Natl. Cancer Inst.*, 55, 473, 1975.
12. **Masuho, Y., Hara, T., and Noguchi, T.,** Preparation of a hybrid of fragment Fab′ of antibody and fragment A of diphtheria toxin and its cytotoxicity, *Biochem. Biophys. Res. Commun.*, 90, 320, 1979.
13. **Krolick, K. A., Villemez, C., Isakson, P., Uhr, J. W., and Vitetta, E. S.,** Selective killing of normal or neoplastic B cells by antibodies coupled to the A chain of ricin, *Proc. Natl. Acad. Sci. U.S.A.*, 77, 5419, 1980.
14. **Ross, W. C. J., Thorpe, P. E., Cumber, A. J., Edwards, D. C., Hinson, C. A., and Davies, A. J. S.,** Increased toxicity of diphtheria toxin for human lymphoblastoid cells following covalent linkage to anti-(human lymphocyte) globulin or its $F(ab')_2$ fragment, *Eur. J. Biochem.* 104, 381, 1980.
15. **Youle, R. J. and Neville, D. M., Jr.,** Anti-Thy 1.2 monoclonal antibody linked to ricin is a potent cell-type-specific toxin, *Proc. Natl. Acad. Sci. U.S.A.*, 77, 5483, 1980.
16. **Raso, V. and Griffin, T.,** Specific cytotoxicity of a human immunoglobulin-directed Fab′-ricin A chain conjugate, *J. Immunol.*, 125, 2610, 1980.
17. **Gilliland, D. G., Steplewski, Z., Collier, R. J., Mitchell, K. F., Chang, T. H., and Koprowski, H.,** Antibody-directed cytotoxic agents: use of monoclonal antibody to direct the action of toxin A chain to colorectal carcinoma cells, *Proc. Natl. Acad. Sci. U.S.A.*, 77, 4539, 1980.
18. **Blythman, H. E., Casellas, P., Gros, O., et al.,** Immunotoxins: hybrid molecules of monoclonal antibodies and a toxin subunit specifically kill tumor cells, *Nature,* 290, 145, 1981.
19. **Thorpe, P. E., Cumber, A. J., Williams, N., Edwards, D. C., Ross, W. C. J., and Davies, A. J. S.,** Abrogation of the non-specific toxicity of abrin conjugated to anti-lymphocyte globulin, *Clin. Exp. Immunol.*, 43, 195, 1981.

20. **Köhler, G. and Milstein, C.,** Continuous cultures of fused cells secreting antibody of predefined specificity, *Nature,* 256, 495, 1975.
21. **Vitetta, E. S., Fulton, R. J., May, R. D., Till, M., and Uhr, J. W.,** Redesigning nature's poisons to create anti-tumor reagents, *Science,* 238, 1098, 1987.
22. **Frankel, A. E., Ed.,** *Immunotoxins,* Kluwer Academic Publishers, Boston, 1988.
23. **Byers, V. S. and Baldwin, R. W.,** Therapeutic strategies with monoclonal antibodies and immunoconjugates, *Immunology,* 65, 329, 1988.
24. **Blakey, D. C., Wawrzynczak, E. J., Wallace, P. M., and Thorpe, P. E.,** Antibody toxin conjugates: a perspective, *Prog. Allergy,* 45, 50, 1988.
25. **Hertler, A. A. and Frankel, A. E.,** Immunotoxins: a critical review of their use in the treatment of malignancies, *J. Clin. Oncol.,* 7, 1932, 1989.
26. **FitzGerald, D. and Pastan, I.,** Targeted toxin therapy for the treatment of cancer, *J. Natl. Cancer Inst.,* 81, 1455, 1989.
27. **Lord, J. M., Spooner, R. A., and Roberts, L. M.,** Immunotoxins: monoclonal antibody-toxin conjugates — a new approach to cancer therapy, *Adv. Biotechnol.,* 11, 193, 1989.
28. **Press, O. W.,** Immunotoxins, *Biotherapy,* 3, 65, 1991.
29. **Bjorn, M. J., Ring, D., and Frankel, A.,** Evaluation of monoclonal antibodies for the development of breast cancer immunotoxins, *Cancer Res.,* 45, 1214, 1985.
30. **Press, O. W., Vitetta, E. S., Farr, A. G., Hansen, J. A., and Martin, P. J.,** Evaluation of ricin A-chain immunotoxins directed against human T cells, *Cell Immunol.,* 102, 10, 1986.
31. **Till, M., May, R. D., Uhr, J. W., Thorpe, P. E., and Vitetta, E. S.,** An assay that predicts the ability of monoclonal antibodies to form potent ricin A chain-containing immunotoxins, *Cancer Res.,* 48, 1119, 1988.
32. **Youle, R. J. and Neville, D. M., Jr.,** Kinetics of protein synthesis inactivation by ricin-anti-Thy 1.1 monoclonal antibody hybrids. Role of the ricin B subunit demonstrated by reconstitution, *J. Biol. Chem.,* 257, 1598, 1982.
33. **Ramakrishnan, S. and Houston, L. L.,** Comparison of the selective cytotoxic effects of immunotoxins containing ricin A chain or pokeweed antiviral protein and anti-Thy 1.1 monoclonal antibodies, *Cancer Res.,* 44, 201, 1984.
34. **Shen, G.-L., Li, J.-L., Ghetie, M.-A., et al.,** Evaluation of four CD22 antibodies as ricin A chain-containing immunotoxins for the *in vivo* therapy of human B-cell leukemias and lymphomas, *Int. J. Cancer.,* 42, 792, 1988.
35. **Griffin, T. W., Haynes, L. R., and Levin, L. V.,** Selective cytotoxicity of ricin A chain-anti carcinoembryonic antibody conjugates to human adenocarcinoma cells, in *Receptor-mediated Targeting of Drugs,* Gregoriadis, G., Poste, G., Senior, J., and Trouer, A., Eds., Plenum Press, New York, 1984, 187.
36. **Embleton, M. J., Byers, V. S., Lee, H. M., Scannon, P., Blackhall, N. W., and Baldwin, R. W.,** Sensitivity and selectivity of ricin toxin A chain-monoclonal antibody 791T/36 conjugates against human tumor cell lines, *Cancer Res.,* 46, 5524, 1986.
37. **Press, O. W., Martin, P., Thorpe, P. E., and Vitetta, E. S.,** Ricin A-chain containing immunotoxins directed against different epitopes on the CD2 molecule differ in their ability to kill normal and malignant T cells, *J. Immunol.,* 141, 4410, 1988.
38. **May, R. D., Finkelman, F. D., Wheeler, H. T., Uhr, J. W., and Vitetta, E. S.,** Evaluation of ricin A chain-containing immunotoxins directed against different epitopes on the δ-chain of cell surface-associated IgD on murine B cells, *J. Immunol.,* 144, 3637, 1990.
39. **May, R. D., Wheeler, H. T., Finkelman, F. D., Uhr, J. W., and Vitetta, E. S.,** Intracellular routing rather than cross-linking or rate of internalization determines the potency of immunotoxins directed against different epitopes of sIgD on murine B cells, *Cell Immunol.,* 135, 490, 1991.
40. **Luo, Y. and Seon, B. K.,** Marked difference in the *in vivo* antitumor efficacy between two immunotoxins targeted to different epitopes of common acute lymphoblastic leukemia antigen (CD10), *J. Immunol.,* 145, 1974, 1990.
41. **Raso, V., Ritz, J., Basala, M., and Schlossman, S. F.,** Monoclonal antibody-ricin A chain conjugate selectively cytotoxic for cells bearing the common acute lymphoblastic leukemia antigen, *Cancer Res.,* 42, 457, 1982.
42. **Casellas, P., Brown, J. P., Gros, O., et al.,** Human melanoma cells can be killed *in vitro* by an immunotoxin specific for melanoma-associated antigen p97, *Int. J. Cancer.,* 30, 437, 1982.
43. **Preijers, F. W. M. B., Tax, W. J. M., De Witte, T., et al.,** Relationship between internalization and cytotoxicity of ricin A-chain immunotoxins, *Br. J. Haematol.,* 70, 289, 1988.
44. **Goldmacher, V. S., Scott, C. F., Lambert, J. M., et al.,** Cytotoxicity of gelonin and its conjugates with antibodies is determined by the extent of their endocytosis, *J. Cell. Physiol.,* 141, 222, 1989.

45. **Olsnes, S. and Sandvig, K.,** How protein toxins enter and kill cells, in *Immunotoxins,* Frankel, A. E., Ed., Kluwer Academic Publishers, Boston, 1988, 39.
46. **Weltman, J. K., Pedroso, P., Johnson, S.-A., Davignon, D., Fast, L. D., and Leone, L. A.,** Rapid screening with indirect immunotoxin for monoclonal antibodies against human small cell lung cancer, *Cancer Res.,* 47, 5552, 1987.
47. **Colombatti, M., Greenfield, L., and Youle, R. J.,** Cloned fragment of diphtheria toxin linked to T-cell specific antibody identifies regions of B chain active in cell entry, *J. Biol. Chem.,* 261, 3030, 1986.
48. **Greenfield, L., Johnson, V. G., and Youle, R. J.,** Mutations in diphtheria toxin separate binding from entry and amplify immunotoxin selectivity, *Science,* 238, 536, 1987.
49. **Pai, L. H., Batra, J. K., FitzGerald, D. J., Willingham, M. C., and Pastan, I.,** Anti-tumor activities of immunotoxins made of monoclonal antibody B3 and various forms of *Pseudomonas* exotoxin, *Proc. Natl. Acad. Sci. U.S.A.,* 88, 3358, 1991.
50. **Wiedlocha, A., Sandvig, K., Walzel, H., Radzikwosky, C., and Olsnes, S.,** Internalization and action of an immunotoxin containing mistletoe lectin A-chain, *Cancer Res.,* 51, 916, 1991.
51. **Thorpe, P. E. and Ross, W. C. J.,** The preparation and cytotoxic properties of antibody-toxin conjugates, *Immunol. Rev.,* 62, 119, 1982.
52. **Blakey, D. C., Wawrzynczak, E. J., Stirpe, F., and Thorpe, P. E.,** Anti-tumour activity of a panel of anti-Thy 1.1 immunotoxins made with different ribosome-inactivating proteins, in *Membrane-Mediated Cytotoxicity,* Bonavida, B., Collier, R. J., Eds., Alan R. Liss, New York, 1987, 195.
53. **Scott, C. F., Jr., Goldmacher, V. S., Lambert, J. M., et al.,** The antileukemic efficacy of an immunotoxin composed of a monoclonal anti-Thy-1 antibody disulfide linked to the ribosome-inactivating protein gelonin, *Cancer Immunol. Immunother.,* 25, 31, 1987.
54. **Bregni, M., Siena, S., Formosa, A., et al.,** B-cell restricted saporin immunotoxins: activity against B-cell lines and chronic lymphocytic leukemia cells, *Blood,* 73, 753, 1989.
55. **Wang, O. C., Ying, W. B., Xie, H., Zhang, Z. C., Yang, Z. H., and Ling, L. O.,** Trichosanthin-monoclonal antibody conjugate specifically cytotoxic to human hepatoma cells *in vitro, Cancer Res.,* 51, 3353, 1991.
56. **Stirpe, F., Wawrzynczak, E. J., Brown, A. N., et al.,** Selective cytotoxic activity of immunotoxins composed of a monoclonal anti-Thy 1.1 antibody and the ribosome inactivating proteins bryodin and momordin, *Br. J. Cancer.,* 58, 558, 1988.
57. **Vallera, D. A., Ash, R. C., Zanjani, E. D., et al.,** Anti-T-cell reagents for human bone marrow transplantation: ricin linked to three monoclonal antibodies, *Science,* 222, 512, 1983.
58. **Lambert, J. M., McIntyre, G., Gauthier, M. N., et al.,** The galactose-binding sites of the cytotoxic lectin ricin can be chemically blocked in high yield with reactive ligands prepared by chemical modification of glycopeptides containing triantennary N-linked oligosaccharides, *Biochemistry,* 30, 3234, 1991.
59. **Roy, D. C., Griffin, J. D., Belvin, M., Blättler, W. A., Lambert, J. M., and Ritz, J.,** Anti-MY9-blocked-ricin: an immunotoxin for selective targeting of acute myeloid leukemia cells, *Blood,* 77, 2404, 1991.
60. **Fodstad, Ø., Olsnes, S., and Pihl, A.,** Toxicity, distribution and elimination of the cancerostatic lectins abrin and ricin after parenteral injection into mice, *Br. J. Cancer,* 34, 418, 1976.
61. **Blakey, D. C., Watson, G. J., Knowles, P. P., and Thorpe, P. E.,** Effect of chemical deglycosylation of ricin A chain on the *in vivo* fate and cytotoxic activity of an immunotoxin composed of ricin A chain and anti-Thy-1.1 antibody, *Cancer Res.,* 47, 947, 1987.
62. **Marsh, J. W., Srinivasachar, K., and Neville, D. M., Jr.,** Antibody-toxin conjugation, in *Immunotoxins,* Frankel, A. E., Ed., Kluwer Academic Publishers, Boston, 1988, 213.
63. **Carlsson, J., Drevin, H., and Axén, R.,** Protein thiolation and reversible protein-protein conjugation. *N*-succinimidyl 3-(2-pyridyldithio)propionate, a new heterobifunctional reagent, *Biochem. J.,* 173, 723, 1978.
64. **Thorpe, P. E., Wallace, P. M., Knowles, P. P., et al.,** New coupling agents for the synthesis of immunotoxins containing a hindered disulfide bond with improved stability *in vivo, Cancer Res.,* 47, 5924, 1987.
65. **Knowles, P. P. and Thorpe, P. E.,** Purification of immunotoxins containing ricin A-chain and abrin A-chain using Blue Sepharose CL-6B, *Anal. Biochem.,* 160, 440, 1987.
66. **Press, O. W., Vitetta, E. S., and Martin, P. J.,** A simplified microassay for inhibition of protein synthesis in reticulocyte lysates by immunotoxins, *Immunol. Lett.,* 14, 37, 1986.
67. **Mosmann, T.,** Rapid colorimetric assay for cellular growth and survival: application to proliferation and cytotoxicity assays, *J. Immunol. Meth.,* 65, 55, 1983.
68. **Kull, F. C., Jr. and Cuatrecasas, P.,** Estimation of cell number by neutral red content. Applications for proliferative and survival assays, *Appl. Biochem. Biotech.,* 8, 97, 1983.

68a. **May, R.,** unpublished observations.

69. **Uckun, F. M., Gajl-Peczalska, K., Meyers, D. E., et al.,** Marrow purging in autologous bone marrow transplantation for T-lineage acute lymphoblastic leukemia: efficacy of *ex vivo* treatment with immunotoxins and 4-hydroperoxycyclophosphamide against fresh leukemic marrow progenitor cells, *Blood,* 69, 361, 1987.
70. **Weiner, L. M., O'Dwyer, J., Kitson, J., et al.,** Phase I evaluation of an anti-breast carcinoma monoclonal antibody 260F9-recombinant ricin A chain immunoconjugate, *Cancer Res.,* 49, 4062, 1989.
71. **Oratz, R., Speyer, J. L., Wernz, J. C., et al.,** Antimelanoma monoclonal antibody-ricin A chain immunoconjugate (XMMME-001-RTA) plus cyclophosphamide in the treatment of metastatic malignant melanoma: results of a phase II trial, *J. Biol. Response Mod.,* 9, 345, 1990.
72. **Vitetta, E. S., Stone, M., Amlot, P., et al.,** Phase I immunotoxin trial in patients with B-cell lymphoma, *Cancer Res.,* 51, 4052, 1991.
73. **Street, N. E., Fulton, R. J., Sanders, V. M., and Vitetta, E. S.,** Inhibition of the helper function of murine T cells with Fab′-anti-L3T4 ricin A chain immunotoxin, *J. Immunol.,* 139, 1734, 1987.
74. **Krolick, K. A.,** Selective elimination of autoreactive lymphocytes with immunotoxins, *Clin. Immunol. Immunopathol.,* 50, 273, 1989.
75. **Vallera, D. A., Carroll, S. F., Snover, D. C., Carlson, G. J., and Blazar, B. R.,** Toxicity and efficacy of anti-T-cell ricin toxin A chain immunotoxins in a murine model of established graft-versus-host disease induced across the major histocompatibility barrier, *Blood,* 77, 182, 1991.
76. **Kernan, N. A., Byers, V., Scannon, P. J., et al.,** Treatment of steroid-resistant acute graft-vs-host disease by *in vivo* administration of an anti-T-cell ricin A chain immunotoxin, *JAMA,* 259, 3154, 1988.
77. **Chaudhary, V. K., Mizukami, T., Fuerst, T. R., et al.,** Selective killing of HIV-infected cells by recombinant human CD4-*Pseudomonas* exotoxin hybrid protein, *Nature,* 335, 369, 1988.
78. **Till, M. A., Ghetie, V., May, R. D., et al.,** Immunoconjugates containing ricin A chain and either human anti-gp41 or CD4 kill H9 cells infected with different isolates of HIV, but do not inhibit normal T or B cell function, *J. AIDS,* 3, 609, 1990.
79. **Matsushita, S., Koito, A., Maeda, Y., Hattori, T., and Takatsuki, K.,** Selective killing of HIV-infected cells by anti-gp120 immunotoxins, *AIDS Res. Hum. Retrovir.,* 6, 193, 1990.

Chapter 3

IMMUNOGLOBULIN PRODUCTION BY B CELLS: *IN VITRO* TOXICOLOGY

Francisca Martínez and John W. Coleman

TABLE OF CONTENTS

I. INTRODUCTION

A. FOREWORD

As a process evolved primarily for the elimination of harmful foreign organisms, the mammalian immune system comprises a complexity of cellular interactions which requires constant regulation to ensure that cellular activity is maintained at a level appropriate to the circumstances. The mechanism of regulation in a healthy individual may encompass modulation of the activity of cytotoxic T lymphocytes, which are specialized for the destruction of virus-infected host cells, or the cooperative activity of T and B lymphocytes, cells jointly responsible for the production of antibodies. Regulation of the immune system, and of antibody production in particular, is dependent upon a carefully balanced network of cells and soluble modulatory factors (cytokines) which operate mainly in the microenvironment of lymphoid organs and peripheral circulation.

The B lymphocyte lineage of immunocompetent cells is characterized by the production of immunoglobulin (Ig) molecules which are secreted upon activation of these cells by specific antigen. Secreted Igs recognize and bind to the same circulating foreign proteins that induced their synthesis and, thus, by acting on antibodies, provide the means by which antigens are eliminated from the host system, a process that involves recognition of the Fc portion of antibody molecules by phagocytic cells. Ig production by B cells represents the final step in a process which begins with internalization of foreign antigen by accessory cells, recognition of processed antigen by MHC II-restricted T lymphocytes, cytokine release, and clonal expansion of antigen-specific T and B cells. Impairment of accessory cell or T cell functions may affect B cell function in such a way as to inhibit Ig synthesis, resulting in an attenuation of antibody-mediated immunity. On the other hand, deregulation of T cells involved in maintenance of tolerance to self (suppression) may result in a disproportionate increase in the levels of antibodies that recognize self-antigens and, consequently, the onset of autoimmunity.

B. POLYCLONAL ACTIVATION

Much of the understanding of mechanisms of growth and differentiation of lymphocytes (and hence insight into immune cell dysfunction) has been gained through the *in vitro* use of polyclonal activators (mitogens), proteins or polysaccharides that trigger cell division and effector functions of resting cells. Particularly useful in this respect have been the plant-derived lectins concanavalin A (Con A), phytohemagglutinin (PHA), and pokeweed mitogen (PWM). Mitogenic lectins appear to have no specific endogenous cellular receptor but bind to a wide range of mono- and oligosaccharides linked via asparagine residues to the protein moiety of cell surface molecules.[1,2] However, there is a distinction of cellular targets for different mitogens; thus PHA and Con A preferentially stimulate T lymphocytes whereas PWM activates B cells via a prior stimulation of T cell responses.[3,4] Generally, mitogens activate most cellular processes upon prolonged cell contact. Binding is virtually complete within 30 min and results in a ''trigger'' type signal which commits the lymphocyte to G_1 of the cell cycle; events following this activation signal are similar to those observed in the first step of antigen-stimulated lymphocyte responses and involve the *de novo* generation of intracellular second messenger molecules (chiefly 1,4,5-inositol trisphosphate and diacylglycerol) and an increased influx of calcium ions.[5]

The cellular interactions that govern Ig synthesis in response to PWM closely resemble those operating in antigen-driven systems for the generation of a specific antibody. Both processes require the presence of monocytes[6,7] and T cells.[8-10] Similarly, there is widespread evidence to suggest that soluble, lymphocyte-derived growth factors involved in antigen-specific antibody secretion have a comparable role in antigen- and PWM-driven responses.

Thus, antigen-T cell receptor (TCR) interactions result in the appearance of early activation markers on the T lymphocyte surface in the presence of the macrophage-derived factor interleukin (IL) 1.[11] PWM-induced differentiation of human B lymphocytes into Ig-secreting cells is greatly enhanced by the addition of recombinant IL-1.[10] IL-1 augments transcription and release of another soluble mediator, IL-2,[12] and induces expression of membrane receptors for this factor on T cells.[11,13,14] Expression of the IL-2 receptor is upregulated further by interaction with IL-2, which leads to clonal expansion of effector T cells with helper, suppressor, and cytotoxic characteristics.[15,16] The promotion of T helper cell functions early on in culture results in the development of Ig synthesis in response to both specific[15] and polyclonal stimuli;[17] IL-2 has also been reported to directly augment Ig production by highly purified, polyclonally activated human B cells *in vitro*.[18]

The first class of Ig to be expressed by any B cell is IgM; membrane expression of IgM normally precedes Ig class-switching.[19] Class-switching and the subsequent production of particular Ig isotypes by surface IgM$^+$ murine B cells has been shown to be influenced by soluble T cell- or macrophage-derived cytokines such as IL-4 (IgE, IgG1),[20] IFN τ (IgG2a),[21] and transforming growth factor β (IgA).[22] IL-4 also directs switching to IgE synthesis in human B cells.[23] IL-5 is reported to promote growth and differentiation of IgA-precommitted B cells, rather than to induce a class-switch to IgA production.[24] IL-6 increases secretion of all three isotypes (IgM, IgG, IgA) in PWM-stimulated human B cells[25] but has also been suggested to induce preferential class-switching of IgM$^+$ B cells to IgG1-secreting cells in human IL-6 transgenic mice.[26] On the other hand, there is a requirement for polyclonal activation of B cells before signals for Ig class-switching may be translated.[27] It has been suggested that polyclonal activation is a primative defense mechanism against infection: the rapid induction of large quantities of low affinity cross-reactive antibodies is sufficient to "contain" the infection until high avidity antibodies appear in the specific immune response mounted against the infecting agent.[28]

Responses to antigenic and polyclonal stimuli are distinguished primarily on the basis of internalization and presentation of the protein eliciting the response. In the first stages of antigen-induced antibody production, antigen is internalized either nonspecifically, by macrophages,[29] or specifically, via the Ig surface receptors of B cells.[30] Subsequent to intracellular proteolytic degradation, antigen peptides become associated with products of the major histocompatibility complex (MHC) class II genes and are presented, in the context of these MHC proteins, to T lymphocytes bearing receptors for the antigen-MHC complex. Antigen recognition by T cells is therefore restricted to antigenic peptides presented in conjunction with self class II molecules. Clonal expansion of these antigen-specific T helper lymphocytes and production of soluble factors for B cell growth and differentiation leads to the synthesis of antibody which exhibits an antigen-binding site (idiotype) identical to that of the surface Ig on the original antigen-presenting B cell. Theoretically, the number of T and B cells that take part in the response is restricted to those bearing receptors specific for any determinant of that particular antigen, so that the number of different idiotypes of the resulting antibodies produced is limited. In contrast, polyclonal activation by lectins may occur in the absence of internalization and proteolytic processing of the molecule: provided cell-to-cell interaction is allowed, lymphocyte targets can be activated by lectins immobilized on sepharose beads.[31] Second, the effect of PWM on T and B cell responses is neither antigen-specific nor MHC-restricted. Lectins interact with certain sugar residues that are more or less equally represented on all lymphocyte membranes[32] and therefore bind irrespective of the antigen specificity of that cell. In addition, allogeneic (histoincompatible) normal T cells (and their soluble products) provide as much help to PWM-stimulated B cells as do autologous (histocompatible) T cells,[33,34] which suggests that Ig synthesis in PWM-stimulated systems is independent not only of antigen specificity but also of MHC class II haplotype.

C. CLINICAL CORRELATIONS

Measurement of Ig production *in vitro* is useful for the identification of defects in B lymphocytes that may arise either as a result of trauma or which may be the basis of immunodeficiency or autoimmune diseases, and can often be correlated with manifestations of clinical symptoms. Being MHC-unrestricted and with an inherent T helper cell requirement, the PWM system is especially useful for the elucidation of disease states arising from a defect in cellular components: since allogeneic normal T cells can provide help to the same extent as autologous T cells, one may identify defects in B cell activity if, on addition of normal T cells to allogeneic B cells from a patient with immune-based disease, synthesis of Ig is modified. Yu and Ziff[35] combined T and B cells from individuals with procainamide-induced lupus erythematosus (LE) patients with their counterparts from normal subjects and observed that not only did all patients have diminished B cell responses, but also that 50% exhibited a reduction in T cell activity. In earlier reports, Jasin and Ziff[36] and Budman et al.[37] demonstrated that the increased amounts of circulating Ig in patients with systemic (nondrug-induced) lupus erythematosus (SLE) was reflected in an enhanced Ig production by PWM-stimulated peripheral blood mononuclear cells (PBMC) of these patients, which in turn correlated with disease activity assessed both clinically and from a serological standpoint. From their results the authors proposed an excessive B cell activity in these patients which reflects onset of autoimmunity *in vivo* but which is not restricted to autoantibody production.

Defective responses to PWM have been observed in patients whose cells show normal responses to other mitogens. Eck et al.[38] reported that a return to normal levels of plasma glutamate in tumor-resected colorectal carcinoma patients correlated with a recovery of reactivity to the T cell mitogen Con A but not to PWM, suggesting that this differential responsiveness might reflect a differential recovery of lymphocyte subsets *in vivo*. Another study[39] found that the release of IgG by PWM-stimulated PBMC from patients with juvenile rheumatoid arthritis (JRA) was significantly lower than that from normal subjects, but that IgG released in response to stimulation by the T cell-independent B cell mitogen *Staphylococcus aureus* (SA) did not differ greatly between patient and control groups. Again, clinical estimations indicated both a greater number of affected joints and higher severity scores for those with low responses to PWM. Since the target B lymphocyte of PWM activity is preferentially a mature, low density IgD^-IgM^- cell[40,41] while that of SA is less mature, denser, and $sIgD^-IgM^+$ or $sIgD^+IgM^+$,[41] the data of Oen and Krzekotowska[39] suggest that the defect in some autoimmune states may be due to alterations in the relative proportions and/or function of B cell subsets.

Responses to PWM *in vitro* can be influenced not only as a result of spontaneous disease activity but also by perturbation of the immune system by drugs and external influences. In a recent study, PBMC of SLE patients treated with prostaglandin E1[42] exhibited a decreased ability to release IgG in response to PWM stimulation *in vitro*. These findings were associated with a concurrent decrease in serum levels of circulating immune complexes and anti-DNA antibodies (a marker of SLE) and reduced glomerular IgG deposits. Similarly, the alleviation of both clinical symptoms and a return to normal responses to PWM in the JRA patients investigated by Oen and Krzekotowska[39] could be accomplished by the administration of slow-acting, antirheumatic drugs. On the other hand, many drugs have been implicated in the progression to autoimmune disease in predisposed individuals, the most notable of these being the antiarrhythmic drug procainamide, reported to cause LE-like symptoms in 20 to 30% of treated individuals,[43-45] and the antihypertensive hydralazine, treatment with which has been reported to induce LE symptoms in as many as 44% patients.[46] Tissue-damaging, antinuclear antibodies (ANA) have likewise been detected in some individuals treated with the antirheumatic drug D-penicillamine[47] and D-penicillamine-L-cysteine disulfide is the metabolite of this drug implicated in pathogenesis.[48] Earlier studies showed that B lymphocytes releasing antibodies that react with host tissues (autoreactive clones) are not eliminated in healthy individuals.[49] It is now believed that self-constituent-reactive IgM and IgG antibodies secreted by B cells of normal unimmunized animals do in fact have a variety of biological roles.[50] The differentiation of autoreactive precursors into effector cells in disease states (whether arising spontaneously or induced by external factors) may result from a defect of the regulatory mechanism that operates in normal individuals. Other authors[51,52] suggest that autoimmune disease may combine hyperstimulation of a normal B cell pool with the positive selection of autoreactive B cell clones. Significantly, abnormal polyclonal B cell activation may be responsible for the excessive production of autoantibodies in mice with spontaneous LE-like disease.[53,54] With regard to adverse drug effects, it is possible that an interaction of drug or drug metabolites with membrane determinants of potential stimulatory cells (such as dendritic or B cells) may form the basis of an abnormal polyclonal B cell activation ultimately responsible for the elicitation of an autoreactive antibody. Gleichman and colleagues[55] suggest that recognition by helper T cells of drug-modified membrane determinants associated with MHC molecules may elicit a chronic graft-vs.-host-like response, in which all host B cells expressing the altered antigen undergo clonal expansion with help provided directly from the drug-specific T cells. This postulate was used to explain the significant increase in B cell proliferation and polyclonal IgG secretion in mice injected with syngeneic spleen cells previously treated with phenytoin,[55] an anticonvulsant that has been associated with the induction of ANA in humans.[56] A breakdown of T cell tolerance to self-antigen presented in association with products of the MHC is likely to be the trigger for the autoimmune response; this loss of tolerance may result from a more direct pharmacological action of drugs on the immune cells themselves.

II. *IN VITRO* IgG SYNTHESIS BY B LYMPHOCYTES

A. MEASUREMENT OF TOTAL IgG

The content of antibody in a biological sample may be quantified by one of a range of immunochemical techniques which exhibit different degrees of sensitivity. By virtue of its convenience and versatility, the enzyme-linked immunosorbent assay (ELISA or EIA) has become the assay of choice for studies which require the measurement of low concentrations of antigen in biological fluids or cell culture supernatants. This technique, which uses antibodies coupled to an easily measured enzyme, combines the sensitivity of simple spectrophotometric enzyme assays with the specificity of antibody/antigen interactions and in addition is rapid, safe, and reasonably economical.

To measure the release of IgG by B cells in culture, we developed an amplified ELISA which incorporates a biotin-streptavidin peroxidase detection system.[57] Streptavidin (a product of *Streptomyces avidinii*) exhibits a particularly high binding affinity for biotin (a low molecular weight vitamin). Antibodies labeled with biotin may be subsequently detected by enzyme-labeled streptavidin, the low dissociation constant of the interaction allowing high sensitivity of detection. Streptavidin exhibits both a lower degree of glycosylation and a lower pI than a related protein, avidin,[58] and we have found that the levels of nonspecific interactions, or background noise (often a problem in ELISA techniques), are reduced if streptavidin is used in preference to avidin. In the experiments described here, 96-well ELISA microtiter plates are coated overnight with affinity-purified goat anti-human IgG in carbonate buffer (0.05 *M*, pH 9.6) at 4°C. Plates are then washed 3 times in phosphate-buffered saline (PBS) + 0.05% Tween 20 (PBS-Tween) and shaken to remove the residual wash buffer. Culture supernatant samples and a human serum standard are added to the first row of wells in the plate and diluted downwards in complete medium (see below). After

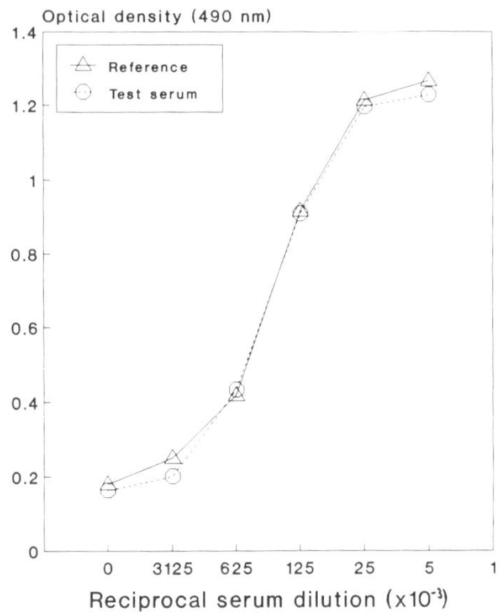

FIGURE 1. Determination of IgG content of normal human serum using a commercial reference standard. Reference and test sera were assayed for total IgG by sandwich ELISA. Values are means of duplicate columns, with differences between duplicates consistently less than 5% of the mean.

incubation (1 h, room temperature) and washing (PBS-Tween), we add biotin-labeled anti-human IgG antibody for 1 h. The plates are washed again and then streptavidin-horseradish peroxidase is added (1 h), before color development with substrate solution (400 μg/ml *O*-phenylenediamine dihydrochloride in citrate buffer + 0.1% hydrogen peroxide). The reaction is stopped with 25% sulfuric acid and optical density determined at 490 nm. A typical standard curve generated by this method, both for original reference (commercially available serum) and test serum, is shown in Figure 1. The detection range for IgG in this ELISA is generally 3.5 to 440 ng/ml.

B. CELL CULTURE

To enable a valid investigation of the effect of drugs or other exogenous factors on lymphocyte function to be related to activation of the cell, rather than to a nonspecific action on the release of preformed material associated with cell cytoplasm or membrane, it is necessary to examine the kinetics of the response in the presence and absence of a protein synthesis inhibitor (e.g., cyclohexamide or puromycin) added to cells at the beginning of culture. The PBMC used in these studies are obtained from whole human blood by a now well-established procedure. Sodium heparin-treated, diluted whole blood is layered over density gradient medium, centrifuged, and PBMC separated into a buffy layer (between gradient medium and plasma) removed by gentle aspiration. The buffy layer, which also contains platelets, is washed with PBS and the pellet resuspended, washed once more with PBS, and finally with incomplete medium (RPMI-1640 containing 2.0 m*M* L-glutamine and 40 μg/ml gentamicin). PBMC are resuspended finally in complete medium (incomplete medium plus 5 to 10% fetal calf serum) and viability determined by dye exclusion following incubation of cells with 0.04% trypan blue dye for 1 to 2 min. Cell viability should be 97% or higher.

In our experiments, PBMC (1×10^6 cell per ml) were incubated (37°C, 5% CO_2) in the presence of PWM (5.0 μg/ml) and in the presence and absence of puromycin (10 μg/ml) in 24-well sterile culture plates (1.0 ml per well). Supernatant fractions were harvested

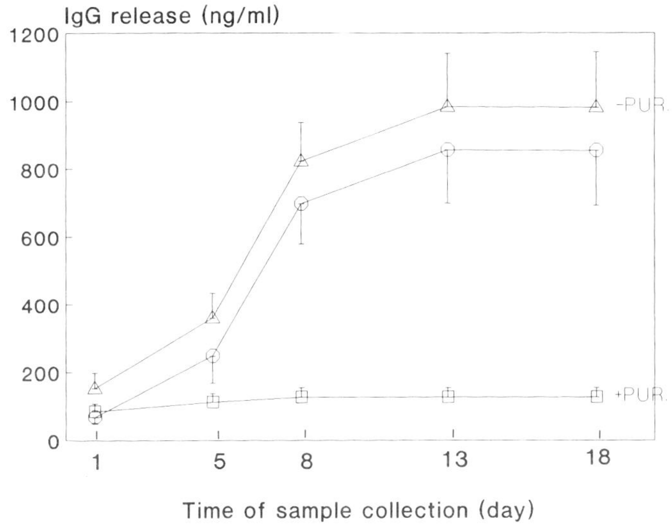

FIGURE 2. The kinetics of IgG synthesis in the presence and absence of puromycin. Values are means ± SD of 12 replicate cultures and represent cumulative total (△) and cumulative passive (☐) release over the incubation period shown. Active synthesis (○) is derived as the difference of the means of total and passive release.

at different time periods from cells incubated for 18 to 20 days and stored at −20°C for later assay for total IgG by the amplified ELISA described above. IgG content of test samples was obtained by measuring the parallel shift between standard and test dilution curves.

The cumulative release of IgG over this period is shown for one experiment in Figure 2. Cells incubated in the presence of puromycin do not synthesize antibody *de novo;* any activity measured represents preformed Ig released from cytoplasm or membrane of B cells into culture fluid. Active synthesis was determined as the difference between total Ig produced and passively released (preformed) material. The proportion of the latter (in total IgG released) declines to negligible levels by day 5, while active antibody synthesis continues up until day 8 or 9 before reaching a plateau. In these experiments significant IgG synthesis was not observed after day 10 of culture. Thus, for best results (maximum IgG synthesis, minimum contamination with preformed IgG), supernatant fluid from each well should be replaced with fresh complete medium at day 4 or 5 of culture, and supernatant samples for assay of active IgG production harvested not less than 3 days following this exchange.

C. EFFECT OF DRUGS ON TOTAL IgG SYNTHESIS *IN VITRO*

1. Drugs Implicated in ANA Formation

With the development and optimization of cell culture system and assay, one may rapidly screen a wide selection of drugs for their effects on one of the important functions of B cells, Ig synthesis, whether or not they have been previously implicated in immune-mediated disorders. In our own experiments, we were interested primarily in the effects on this parameter of drugs reported to induce nonorgan specific autoimmune disorders (e.g., SLE, rheumatoid arthritis [RA]), or at least the production of autoantibodies found most often in these disorders (i.e., ANA), with the proposal that induction of such autoreactive proteins *in vivo* might correlate with an effect on total IgG synthesis *in vitro*. The list of drugs screened in the experiments described here is shown in Table 1.

For experiments to investigate the effects of drugs on IgG synthesis, compounds were dissolved initially to high concentrations in RPMI or in organic solvent before extensive further dilution in complete medium. Each drug was serially diluted tenfold in sterile

TABLE 1
Drugs Implicated in Autoimmune Disorders and Tested for Effect on IgG Synthesis *In Vitro*

Drug	Abnormality *in vivo*	Ref.
Chlorpromazine	↑ serum ANA ↑ serum IgM SLE, agranulocytosis	59–61
D-Penicillamine	↑ serum ANA ↓ T helper cell function	47, 63
Phenytoin	↑ serum ANA ↓ B cell number Hypogammaglobulinemia	56, 64
Procainamide	↑ serum ANA SLE, thrombocytopenia, agranulocytosis	43–45
Thiouracils (methimazole, propylthiouracil)	↑ serum ANA ↑ antigranulocyte and antimonocyte antibodies Agranulocytosis	64, 65

96-well culture plates in complete medium (100 μl). PBMC were obtained as described above, treated with 0.5 μg/ml PWM, and then added to each well of the prepared culture plates (2×10^6 cell per ml in 100 μl complete medium). After 7 to 8 days at 37°C/5% CO_2, culture plates were centrifuged and harvested supernatant samples stored at −20°C before measurement of total IgG by ELISA. Experiments were repeated at least four times for each drug, using PBMC obtained from different donors.

The control regulator drug used in these studies was the immunosuppressant agent cyclosporin A (CsA). This drug has been well characterized as an inhibitor of PWM-induced IgG synthesis *in vitro*.[66] Consistent with this report, CsA was shown to suppress IgG synthesis in our own studies in a concentration-dependent manner (Figure 3), thus validating the culture system and ELISA for "test" drugs. Of the drugs reported to induce ANA *in vivo* and tested in our system, the antipsychotic agent chlorpromazine (CPZ), in the concentration range 0.19 to 1.67 μ*M*, significantly ($p < 0.05$) augmented IgG synthesis with maximum effect at 1.67 μ*M* (Table 2).[57] The observed inhibition of synthesis at 5 μ*M* CPZ was attributed to a decline in cell viability, since we found CPZ was cytotoxic at 10 μ*M* as assessed by trypan blue exclusion. Further experiments showed the enhancing effect of CPZ (at 2.0 μ*M*) to be maximal when the drug was added at the start of culture and less marked or absent if the drug was added 24 h later (Figure 4). Further, augmentation of synthesis was retained if CPZ was washed from cells after the first 24 h (Table 3). Since the onset of antibody production depends on early cellular events such as lymphokine release,[67] it is possible that the effects of CPZ derives from an action on secretion of these proteins (although we showed subsequently that IL-1 release is not affected by the presence of CPZ in culture; thus other early-production cytokines involved in B cell regulation — for example, IL-6 — might be involved in the drug-mediated response). The competitive inhibition of the binding of endogenous mediators to cellular receptors must also be considered a possibility for the action of some drugs on the immune system and this can be verified by investigation of the effects both of more specific agonists and antagonists. Since CPZ blocks receptors for histamine and 5-hydroxytryptamine (5-HT) *in vivo,* and because these receptors are present on lymphocyte surfaces,[68-70] we investigated the effects of these agonists, along with a number of more specific antagonists, on IgG synthesis *in vitro,* but showed that the effect of CPZ could not, in fact, be attributed to an interaction of this drug with lymphocyte receptors for histamine and 5-HT.[71]

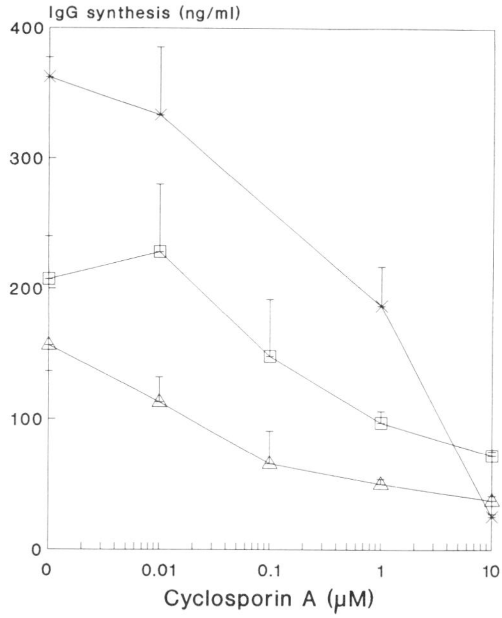

FIGURE 3. The effect of cyclosporin A (CsA) on PWM-stimulated IgG synthesis by human PBMC in three separate experiments. Values shown are means ± SD of quintuplicate cultures of cells incubated in CsA.

TABLE 2
The Effect of CPZ on PWM-Stimulated IgG Synthesis *In Vitro*

Conc of CPZ (μM)	IgG synthesis (% control)[a]
0	100
0.19	136 ± 28.7
0.55	163 ± 39.5
1.67	200 ± 35.3
5.00	143 ± 38.5

[a] Means ± SD of quadruplicate experiments; $p < 0.05$ by one-way ANOVA.

Other compounds implicated in ANA induction and investigated here did not (in the absence of cytotoxicity) have significant, consistent effects on IgG synthesis *in vitro* (data not shown). Thus the reported actions of these drugs and others[72] on physiological immune responses do not always extend to a modulation of all immune parameters *in vitro*. This suggests that certain cofactors present only in the physiological environment are necessary for drugs to affect lymphocyte function: Lipsky and Ziff[62] found, for example, that therapeutic concentrations of D-penicillamine could inhibit the PWM-induced generation of antibody-forming cells only if copper sulfate was also present in culture. Alternatively, it is possible that certain drugs require prior transformation to metabolites for adverse effects on the immune system to be manifested.[73,74] Monocytes and lymphocytes contain a limited number of enzyme systems for the metabolism of some compounds,[75] but the majority of biotransformation reactions that occur *in vivo* will be represented to a more limited extent (or not

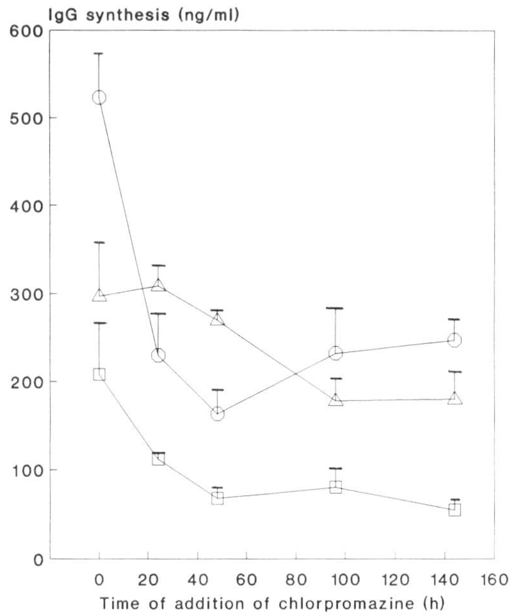

FIGURE 4. Chlorpromazine-mediated enhancement of IgG synthesis is influenced by the time of addition of the drug. PBMC were incubated in 2.0 μM CPZ for different time periods and IgG synthesis determined by ELISA. Values shown are means ± SD of quintuplicate cultures in three experiments. Modified from Reference 57.

TABLE 3
The Effect of CPZ on IgG Synthesis *In Vitro* Is Exerted in the First 24 h of Culture

Conc of CPZ (μM)	IgG Synthesis (ng/ml) Continuous culture[a]	Interrupted culture[b]
0	203 ± 11.9	166 ± 22.7
0.55	288 ± 42.7	222 ± 41.7
1.67	444 ± 163	308 ± 104

Note: PWM-stimulated cells were incubated with CPZ for 7 days[a] or 24 h[b] (cells then washed free of drug) before IgG content of supernatant samples was assayed for all cells at day 7 of culture by ELISA. Values are means ± SD of triplicate cultures ($p < 0.05$ by one-way ANOVA).

at all) in isolated lymphoid cells. This detail might be regarded as a drawback of *in vitro* systems since a drug with suggested physiological immune modulatory activity may be unable to exert similar effects *in vitro;* on the contrary, any metabolite generated by isolated preparations of immunocompetent cells will be formed at a site relevant in terms of immune system modulation, whereas metabolites generated by liver microsomal preparations — which have been used by some authors to examine the immunotoxicological properties of certain drugs[74] — may not necessarily enter the circulation or lymphoid tissues. The *in vitro* cell preparation has an added advantage in its autonomy from the various *in vivo* regulatory processes which may be susceptible to intraindividual variation and/or drug interactions.

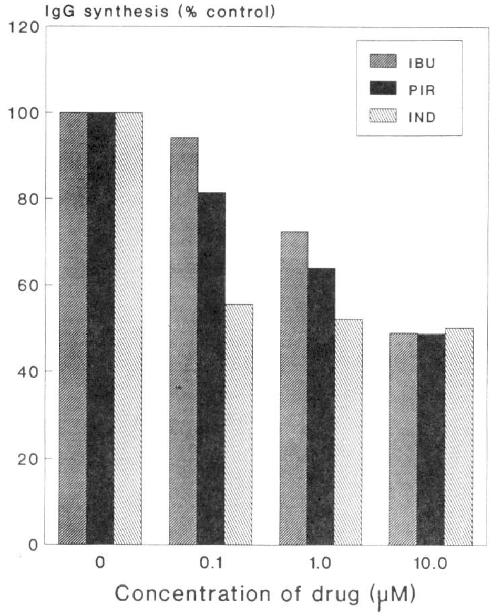

FIGURE 5. Comparison of the potency of inhibition of IgG synthesis by nonsteroidal anti-inflammatory drugs. Values shown are means of three separate experiments (quintuplicate cultures per drug concentration per experiment). Modified from Reference 57.

2. Nonsteroidal Anti-Inflammatory Drugs

The Ig synthesis/assay system described here was also used to investigate the effects of nonsteroidal anti-inflammatory drugs (NSAIDs) on the human immune system. NSAIDs inhibit the synthesis of prostaglandin (PG) E_2 by a selective inhibition of arachidonate cyclooxygenase, the enzyme involved in the transformation of arachidonic acid to PGs and thromboxane A_2. PGs are important mediators of the inflammatory response, and there is now clear evidence that they are also important in the regulation of immune responses *in vivo* and *in vitro*. Knudsen et al.[76] reported that PGE_2 exerted a negative feedback effect on the release of IL-1 by monocytes *in vitro* and showed that suppression was due to a PGE_2-mediated elevation of cAMP in the responding cells; cAMP is in fact associated with decreased immune responsiveness.[77] An earlier study[78] indicated a role for PGE in the enhancement of cell-mediated immunity *in vivo* by the observation that antibodies to PGE prevent the generation of host-vs.-graft and graft-vs.-host reactions in mice. More recently it has been shown that PGE_2 may downregulate expression of IL-2 and transferrin receptors.[79] Thus a study of PG-synthesis inhibitors might facilitate elucidation of the role of PGs on immune function. Since NSAIDs depress serum rheumatoid factor (RF) levels of patients with RA,[80] we considered that a similar effect might be observed on IgG production *in vitro*, with potential relevance to the effects of PGE_2 on this parameter.

Indomethacin, piroxicam, and ibuprofen induced a significant ($p < 0.01$ to $p < 0.05$) concentration-dependent inhibition of IgG synthesis *in vitro*, within the range of concentrations attained *in vivo* during normal dosage (10^{-4} to 10^{-8} *M*), and furthermore, with relative order of potency for inhibition of synthesis (indomethacin > piroxicam > ibuprofen), concordant with the inhibition of arachidonate cyclooxygenase by NSAIDs *in vivo*[81-83] (Figure 5).[57] Since IgG synthesis could not be completely abrogated by the action of indomethacin (an observation made also by Ceuppens and Goodwin),[84] the likelihood is that PGE_2, which is produced by monocytes in PWM-stimulated cell culture, does not provide an obligatory signal for antibody synthesis but acts instead as a potentiator. According to Ceuppens and

Goodwin,[84] PGE_2 mediates its effects on antibody synthesis via an inhibition of the function of $CD8^+$ (suppressor) T cells. Since T cells with suppressor characteristics have been reported to express a high density of PGE_2 receptors,[85] it is possible that inactivation of these cells may occur subsequent to a PGE_2-mediated downregulation of activation-related receptors, a hypothesis that would concur with the observations of Chouaib et al.[79] on the effects of PGE_2 on IL-2 and/or transferrin receptors, as described above.

III. CONCLUSION

In vitro studies have, over the years, become increasingly useful in the elucidation of mechanisms by which drugs exert immune modulatory effects. The model of lymphocyte activation by pokeweed mitogen is a good representation of the series of immune events that culminate *in vivo* in antibody production: PWM provides one of the signals for maturation of resting B lymphocytes into IgG-secreting plasma cells via an obligatory prior activation of T cells. However, it is clear that, while some drugs with demonstrable activity on the immune system *in vivo* also exert modulation *in vitro,* this is not an obligate finding. We have suggested that metabolism or the presence of other cofactors may be required for immune perturbation to be manifested *in vitro*. On the other hand, cell culture systems allow a precise investigation of drug action on isolated cells of the immune system, thus removing the problem of extraneous activity caused by unknown variables (e.g., presence of other drugs, variable levels of endogenous immunomodulatory factors such as neurotransmitters and hormones) and thus provide some indication as to how these agents may perturb the immune system *in vivo* and precipitate the disorders and debilitating syndromes occasionally associated with their use.

REFERENCES

1. **Barondes, S. H.,** Lectins: their multiple endogenous cellular functions, *Annu. Rev. Biochem.*, 50, 207, 1981.
2. **Osawa, T. and Tsuji, T.,** Fractionation and structural assessment of oligosaccharides and glycopeptides by use of immobilized lectins, *Annu. Rev. Biochem.*, 56, 21, 1987.
3. **Douglas, S. D.,** Electron microscope and functional aspects of human lymphocyte responses to mitogens, *Transplant. Rev.*, 11, 39, 1972.
4. **Greaves, M. and Janossy, G.,** Elicitation of selective T and B lymphocyte responses by cell surface binding ligands, *Transplant. Rev.*, 11, 87, 1972.
5. **Hadden, J. W.,** Transmembrane signals in the activation of T lymphocytes by mitogenic antigens, *Immunol. Today,* 9, 235, 1988.
6. **Rosenberg, S. A. and Lipsky, P. E.,** Monocyte dependence of pokeweed mitogen-induced differentiation of immunoglobulin-secreting cells from human peripheral blood mononuclear cells, *J. Immunol.*, 122, 926, 1979.
7. **Lane, H. C., Volkman, D. J., Whalen, G., and Fauci, A. S.,** *In vitro* antigen-induced, antigen-specific antibody production in man, *J. Exp. Med.*, 154, 1043, 1981.
8. **Mitchison, N. A.,** The carrier effect in the secondary response to hapten-protein conjugates. II. Cellular cooperation, *Eur. J. Immunol.*, 1, 18, 1971.
9. **Janossy, G., de la Concha, E. G., Luguetti, A., Snajdr, M. J., Waxdal, M. J., and Platts-Mills, T. A. E.,** T cell regulation of immunoglobulin synthesis and proliferation in pokeweed (PA-1)-stimulated human lymphocyte cultures, *Scand. J. Immunol.*, 6, 109, 1977.
10. **Jelinek, D. F. and Lipsky, P. E.,** Enhancement of human B cell proliferation and differentiation by tumor necrosis factor-α and interleukin 1, *J. Immunol.*, 139, 2970, 1987.
11. **Williams, J. M., Deloria, D., Hansen, J. A., Dinarello, C. A., Loertscher, R., Shapiro, H. M., and Strom, T. P.,** The events of primary T cell activation can be staged by use of sepharose-bound anti-T3 (64.1) monoclonal antibody and purified interleukin 1, *J. Immunol.*, 135, 2249, 1985.

12. **Gillis, S. and Mizel, S. B.,** T-cell lymphoma model for the analysis of interleukin 1-mediated T cell activation, *Proc. Nat. Acad. Sci. U.S.A.*, 78, 1133, 1981.
13. **Hoffman, M. K.,** Macrophages and T cells control distinct phases in B cell differentiation in the humoral immune response *in vitro*, *J. Immunol.*, 125, 2076, 1980.
14. **Kaye, J., Gillis, S., Mizel, S. B., Sherach, E. M., Dinarello, C. A., Lachman, L. B., and Janeway, C. A.,** Growth of a cloned helper T cell line induced by a monoclonal antibody specific for the antigen receptor: interleukin-1 is required for the expression of receptors for interleukin-2, *J. Immunol.*, 133, 1339, 1984.
15. **Watson, J. and Mochizuki, D.,** Interleukin 2: a class of T cell growth factors, *Immunol. Rev.*, 51, 257, 1980.
16. **Robb, R. J., Munck, A., and Smith, K. A.,** T cell growth factor receptors, *J. Exp. Med.*, 154, 1455, 1981.
17. **Nakagawa, N., Nakagawa, T., Volkman, D. J., Ambrus, J. T., and Fauci, A. S.,** The role of interleukin 2 in inducing Ig production in a pokeweed mitogen-stimulated mononuclear cell system, *J. Immunol.*, 138, 795, 1987.
18. **Splawski, J. B., Jelinek, D. F., and Lipsky, P. E.,** Immunomodulatory role of IL-4 on the secretion of Ig by human B cells, *J. Immunol.*, 142, 1569, 1989.
19. **Abney, E. R., Cooper, M. D., Kearney, J. F., Lawton, A. R., and Parkhouse, R. M. E.,** Sequential expression of immunoglobulin in developing mouse lymphocytes: a systemic survey that suggests a model for the generation of immunoglobulin isotype diversity, *J. Immunol.*, 120, 2041, 1978.
20. **Snapper, C. M., Finkelman, F. D., and Paul, W. E.,** Regulation of IgG1 and IgE production by interleukin 4, *Immunol. Rev.*, 102, 51, 1988.
21. **Snapper, C. M., Peschel, C., and Paul, W. E.,** IFN-τ stimulates IgG2a secretion by murine B cells stimulated with bacterial lipopolysaccharide, *J. Immunol.*, 140, 2121, 1988.
22. **Coffman, R. L., Lebman, D. A., and Shrader, B.,** Transforming growth factor β specifically enhances IgA production by lipopolysaccharide-stimulated murine B lymphocytes, *J. Exp. Med.*, 170, 1039, 1989.
23. **Sarfati, M. and Delapese, G.,** Possible role of human lymphocyte receptor for IgE (CD23) or its soluble fragments in the *in vitro* synthesis of human IgE, *J. Immunol.*, 141, 2195, 1988.
24. **Harriman, G. R., Kunimoto, D. Y., Elliott, J. F., Paetkau, V., and Strober, W.,** The role of IL-5 in IgA B cell differentiation, *J. Immunol.*, 140, 3033, 1988.
25. **Muraguchi, A., Hirano, T., Tang, B., Matsuda, T., Horii, Y., Nakajima, K., and Kishimoto, T.,** The essential role of B cell stimulatory factor 2 (BSF-2/IL-6) for the terminal differentiation of B cells, *J. Exp. Med.*, 167, 332, 1988.
26. **Suematsu, S., Matsuda, T., Aozasa, K., Akira, S., Nakano, N., Ohno, S., Miyazaki, J., Yamamura, K.-I., Hirano, T., and Kishimoto, T.,** IgG1 plasmacytosis in interleukin 6 transgenic mice, *Proc. Natl. Acad. Sci. U.S.A.*, 86, 7547, 1989.
27. **O'Garra, A., Umland, S., de France, T., and Christiansen, J.,** 'B-cell factors' are pleiotropic, *Immunol. Today*, 9, 45, 1988.
28. **Clagett, J. A. and Engel, D.,** Polyclonal activation: a form of primitive immunity and its possible role in pathogenesis of inflammatory diseases, *Dev. Comp. Immunol.*, 2, 235, 1978.
29. **Unanue, E. R.,** Antigen-presenting function of the macrophage, *Annu. Rev. Immunol.*, 2, 395, 1984.
30. **Lanzavecchia, A.,** Antigen-specific interaction between T and B cells, *Nature*, 314, 537, 1985.
31. **Greaves, M. and Janossy, G.,** Elicitation of selective T and B lymphocyte responses by cell surface binding ligands, *Transplant Rev.*, 11, 87, 1972.
32. **Severinson, E. and Larsson, E. L.,** Lymphocyte responses to polyclonal T and B cell activators, in *Handbook of Experimental Immunology*, Vol. 2, Weir, D. M., Ed., Blackwell Scientific, Oxford, 1986, 63.1.
33. **Saxon, A., Stevens, R. H., and Ashman, R. F.,** Regulation of immunoglobulin production in human peripheral blood leukocytes: cellular interactions, *J. Immunol.*, 118, 1872, 1977.
34. **Stevens, R. H., Thiele, C. J., and Saxon, A.,** The production of a soluble T-lymphocyte-derived factor which substitutes for helper T lymphocytes in the *in vitro* production of immunoglobulin, *Immunology*, 36, 407, 1979.
35. **Yu, C. and Ziff, M.,** Effects of long-term procainamide therapy on immunoglobulin synthesis, *Arthritis Rheum.*, 28, 276, 1985.
36. **Jasin, H. E. and Ziff, M.,** Immunoglobulin synthesis by peripheral blood cells in systemic lupus erythematosus, *Arthritis Rheum.*, 18, 219, 1975.
37. **Budman, D. R., Merchant, E. B., Steinberg, A. D., Doft, B., Gershwin, M. E., Lizzio, E., and Reeves, J. P.,** Increased spontaneous activity of antibody-forming cells in the peripheral blood of patients with active SLE, *Arthritis Rheum.*, 20, 289, 1977.

38. **Eck, H.-P., Betzler, M., Schlag, P., and Dröge, W.,** Partial recovery of lymphocyte activity in patients with colorectal carcinoma after curative surgical treatment and return of plasma glutamate concentrations to normal levels, *J. Cancer Res. Clin. Oncol.*, 116, 648, 1990.
39. **Oen, K. and Krzekotowska, D.,** *In vitro* immunoglobulin production by lymphocytes of patients with juvenile rheumatoid arthritis: effects of *Staphylococcus aureus* Cowan I stimulation and monocyte depletion, *J. Rheumatol.*, 15, 1539, 1988.
40. **Kuritani, T. and Cooper, M. D.,** Human B cell differentiation, *J. Exp. Med.*, 155, 1561, 1982.
41. **Mudde, G. C., Verberne, C. J. M., Groeneveld, K., and DeGast, G. C.,** Human tonsil B lymphocyte function. I. The proliferative response to *Staphylococcus aureus* and pokeweed mitogen in relation to surface heavy chains μ and δ, *Clin. Exp. Immunol.*, 56, 709, 1984.
42. **Lin, C. Y.,** Improvement in steroid and immunosuppressive drug resistant lupus nephritis by intravenous prostaglandin E1 therapy, *Nephron,* 55, 258, 1990.
43. **Blomgren, S. E., Condemi, J. J., Bignall, M. C., and Vaughan, J. H.,** Antinuclear antibodies induced by procainamide, *New Engl. J. Med.*, 281, 64, 1969.
44. **Woosley, R. L., Drayer, D. E., Reidenberg, M. M., Nies, A. S., Carr, K., and Oats, J. A.,** Effect of acetylator phenotype on the rate at which procainamide induces ANA and the lupus syndrome, *New Engl. J. Med.*, 298, 1157, 1978.
45. **Rubin, R. L., Reimer, G., McNally, E. M., Nusinow, S. R., Searles, R. P., and Tan, E. M.,** Procainamide elicits a selective autoantibody immune response, *Clin. Exp. Immunol.*, 63, 58, 1986.
46. **Condemi, J. J., Moore-Jones, D., Vaughan, J. H., and Perry, H. M.,** Antinuclear antibodies following hydralazine toxicity, *New Engl. J. Med.*, 276, 486, 1967.
47. **Harkcom, T. M., Conn, D. L., and Holley, K. E.,** Penicillamine and lupus erythematosus-like syndrome, *Ann. Intern. Med.*, 89, 1012, 1978.
48. **Naikaike, S., Tanaka, C., Tomita, N., Umemoto, M., Otomo, S., and Aihara, H.,** Immunopharmacologic studies of D-penicillamine-L-cysteine disulphide, *Jpn. J. Pharmacol.*, 33, 983, 1983.
49. **Sawada, S. and Talal, N.,** Characteristics of *in vitro* production of antibodies to DNA in normal and autoimmune mice, *J. Immunol.*, 122, 2309, 1979.
50. **Avrameas, S.,** Natural autoantibodies: from 'horror autotoxicus' to 'gnothi seauton', *Immunol. Today,* 12, 154, 1991.
51. **Schlomchik, M. J., Marshall-Rothstein, A., Wolfowicz, C. B., Rothstein, T. L., and Weigart, M. G.,** The role of clonal selection and somatic mutation in autoimmunity, *Nature,* 328, 805, 1987.
52. **Klinman, D. M. and Steinberg, A. D.,** Acquisition and maturation of expressed B cell repertoires in normal and autoimmune mice, *J. Immunol.*, 141, 801, 1988.
53. **Dziarski, R.,** Preferential induction of autoantibody secretion in polyclonal activation by peptidoglycan and lipopolysaccharide, *J. Immunol.*, 128, 1017, 1982.
54. **Hang, L. M., Slack, J. H., Amundson, C., Izui, S., Theofilopoulos, A. N., and Dixon, F. J.,** Induction of murine autoimmune disease by chronic polyclonal B cell activation, *J. Exp. Med.*, 157, 874, 1983.
55. **Gleichmann, E., Pals, S. T., Rolink, A. G., Radaszkiewicz, T., and Gleichmann, H.,** Graft-versus-host reactions: clues to the etiopathology of a spectrum of immunological diseases, *Immunol. Today,* 5, 324, 1984.
56. **Singsen, B. H., Fishbein, L., and Hanson, V.,** Antinuclear antibodies and lupus-like syndromes in children receiving anticonvulsants, *Paediatrics,* 57, 529, 1976.
57. **Martinez, F. and Coleman, J. W.,** The effect of selected drugs, including chlorpromazine and non-steroidal, anti-inflammatory agents, on polyclonal IgG synthesis and interleukin-1 production by human peripheral blood mononuclear cells *in vitro, Clin. Exp. Immunol.*, 76, 252, 1989.
58. **Green, N. M.,** Avidin. I. The use of [^{14}C] biotin for kinetic studies and for assay, *Biochem. J.*, 89, 585, 1963.
59. **Alarcon-Segovia, D., Fishbein, E., Cetina, J. A., Raya, R. J., and Barrera, E.,** Antigenic specificity of chlorpromazine-induced ANA, *Clin. Exp. Immunol.*, 12, 39, 1973.
60. **Canoso, R. T. and Sise, H. S.,** Chlorpromazine-induced lupus anticoagulant and associated immunological abnormalities, *Am. J. Hematol.*, 13, 121, 1982.
61. **Zarrabi, M. H., Zucker, S., Miller, F., Derman, R. M., Romano, G. S., Hartnett, J. A., and Varma, A. O.,** Immunologic and coagulation disorders in chlorpromazine-treated patients, *Ann. Intern. Med.*, 91, 194, 1979.
62. **Lipsky, P. E. and Ziff, M.,** Inhibition of human helper T cell function *in vitro* by D-penicillamine and $CuSO_4$, *J. Clin. Invest.*, 65, 1069, 1980.
63. **Guerra, I. C., Fawcett, W. A., Redmon, A. H., Lawrence, E. C., Rosenblatt, R. M., and Shearer, W. T.,** Permanent intrinsic B cell immunodeficiency caused by phenytoin hypersensitivity, *J. Allergy Clin. Immunol.*, 77, 603, 1986.

64. **Faber, V. and Preben, E.,** Leukocyte-specific anti-nuclear factors in patients with Felty's syndrome, rheumatoid arthritis, systemic lupus erythematosus and other diseases, *Acta Med. Scand.*, 179, 257, 1966.
65. **Fibbe, W. E., Claas, F. H., van der Star-Dijkstra, W., Meyboom, R. H. B., and Falkenburg, J. H. F.,** Agranulocytosis induced by propylthiouracil: evidence of a drug-dependent antibody reacting with granulocytes, monocytes and haematopoeitic progenitor cells, *Br. J. Haematol.*, 64, 363, 1986.
66. **Tosato, G., Pike, S. E., Koski, L. R., and Blaese, R. M.,** Selective inhibition of immunoregulatory cell functions by cyclosporin A, *J. Immunol.*, 128, 1986, 1982.
67. **Jelinek, D. F. and Lipsky, P. E.,** Regulation of human B lymphocyte activation, proliferation and differentiation, *Adv. Immunol.*, 40, 1, 1987.
68. **Osband, M. E., Cohen, E. B., Miller, B. R., Shen, Y. J., Cohen, L., Flescher, L., Brown, A. E., and McCaffrey, R. P.,** Biochemical analysis of specific histamine H_1 and H_2 receptors on lymphocytes, *Blood*, 58, 87, 1981.
69. **Bonnet, M., Lespinats, G., and Burtin, C.,** Evidence for serotonin (5-HT) binding sites on murine lymphocytes, *Int. J. Immunopharmacol.*, 9, 551, 1987.
70. **Khan, M. M., Wilson, A. L., and Melmon, K. L.,** Characterization of histamine type 1 receptors on natural suppressor lymphoid cells, *Biochem. Pharmacol.*, 36, 3867, 1987.
71. **Martinez, F. and Coleman, J. W.,** A comparison of the effects of chlorpromazine and more selective histamine and 5-hydroxytryptamine antagonists on human IgG synthesis *in vitro, Int. J. Immunopharmacol.*, 12, 185, 1990.
72. **Martinez, F. and Watson, R. R.,** Effects of cocaine and morphine on IgG production by human peripheral blood lymphocytes *in vitro, Life Sciences,* 47 PL59, 1990.
73. **Fritzler, M. J. and Tan, E. M.,** Antibodies to histones in drug-induced and idiopathic lupus erythematosus, *J. Clin. Invest.*, 62, 560, 1978.
74. **Spielberg, S. P., Gordon, G. B., Blake, D. A., Goldstein, D. A., and Herlong, H. F.,** Predisposition to phenytoin hepatotoxicity assessed *in vitro, New Engl. J. Med.*, 305, 722, 1981.
75. **Karki, N. T., Pokela, R., Nuutinen, L., and Pelkonen, O.,** Aryl hydrocarbon hydroxylase in lymphocytes and lung tissue from lung cancer patients and controls, *Int. J. Cancer,* 39, 565, 1987.
76. **Knudsen, P. J., Dinarello, C. A., and Strom, T. B.,** Prostaglandins posttranscriptionally inhibit monocyte expression of interleukin 1 activity by increasing intracellular cyclic adenosine monophosphate, *J. Immunol.*, 137, 3189, 1986.
77. **Bourne, H. R., Lichtenstein, L. M., Melmon, K. L., Henney, C. S., Weinstein, Y., and Shearer, G. M.,** Modulation of inflammation and immunity by cAMP, *Science,* 184, 19, 1974.
78. **Mertin, J. and Stackpoole, A.,** Anti-PGE antibodies inhibit *in vivo* development of cell-mediated immunity, *Nature,* 294, 456, 1981.
79. **Chouaib, S., Robb, R. J., Welte, K., and Dupont, B.,** Analysis of prostaglandin E_2 effect on T lymphocyte activation, *J. Clin. Invest.*, 80, 333, 1987.
80. **Goodwin, J. S., Ceuppens, J. L., and Rodriguez, M. A.,** Administration of nonsteroidal anti-inflammatory agents in patients with rheumatoid arthritis, *J. Am. Med. Assoc.*, 250, 2485, 1983.
81. **Flower, R. J.,** Drugs which inhibit prostaglandin biosynthesis, *Pharmacol. Rev.*, 26, 33, 1974.
82. **Brune, K., Rainsford, K. D., Wagner, K., and Peskar, B. A.,** Inhibition by anti-inflammatory drugs of prostaglandin production in cultured macrophages, *Naunyn-Schmiedebergs Arch. Pharmacol.*, 315, 269, 1981.
83. **Neuman, R. G., Wilson, B. D., Barkley, M., Kimball, E. S., Weichman, B. M., and Wood, D. D.,** Inhibition of prostaglandin biosynthesis by etodolac. I. Selective activities in arthritis, *Agents Actions,* 21, 160, 1987.
84. **Ceuppens, J. L. and Goodwin, J. S.,** Endogenous prostaglandin E_2 enhances polyclonal immunoglobulin production by tonically inhibiting T suppressor cell activity, *Cell. Immunol.*, 70, 41, 1982.
85. **Goodwin, J. S., Kaszubowski, P. A., and Williams, R. C.,** cAMP response to PGE_2 in subpopulations of human lymphocytes, *J. Exp. Med.*, 150, 1260, 1979.

Chapter 4

CYTOTOXICITY ASSAYS FOR INTRINSIC TOXICITY AND IRRITANCY

Michael Balls and Richard H. Clothier

TABLE OF CONTENTS

I. INTRODUCTION

Cytotoxicology is the study of toxic effects of chemicals and other materials at the cellular level, and cytotoxicity is the expression of adverse effects on the structural and/or functional properties of one or more cell components. General cytotoxicity (or basic cytotoxicity) is the result of toxic effects on structures and functions common to all the cells of the body, such as DNA, chromosomes, mitochondria, the cytoskeleton, and various membranes. Tissue-specific cytotoxicity involves adverse effects on particular types of differentiated cells, in terms of either their tissue-type specific properties (e.g., hormone production, conductivity, contractility) or their modulation of general cytotoxic effects (e.g., via the metabolic activation or detoxification of xenobiotics).

The last 20 years or so have witnessed increasing interest in *in vitro* cytotoxicology, and much attention is currently focused on 3 levels of cytotoxicity testing. First, tens, if not hundreds, of general cytotoxicity tests have been developed for a wide range of purposes; they usually involve relatively undifferentiated, permanent cell lines.[1] Second, target cell or target organ toxicity tests are becoming available for the major body organs, including the liver,[2] kidneys,[3] lungs,[4] and endocrine organs;[5] they usually involve primary cell cultures or cultures of finite-lived cell strains, which must retain an acceptable proportion of the specific properties of the tissue of origin, if they are to be of value. Third, target system tests are also in the course of development, with particular emphasis on the nervous,[6,7] immune,[8] and reproductive systems;[9] they usually involve tiered testing schemes, comprising cell cultures, organotypic cultures, and/or cell cocultures. Nevertheless, despite the progress that is being made, significant new developments in tissue culture methodology are necessary before the full potential of *in vitro* toxicology and *in vitro* toxicity testing can be realized.[10]

General cytotoxicity tests have three main uses. First, they can be used to compare directly the toxic potencies of certain types of chemicals and materials in relation to particular kinds of toxicity, e.g., intrinsic toxicity (or acute lethal potency) and irritancy. Second, they can provide baseline data essential to the meaningful interpretation of the results of target cell, organ, or system studies. For example, the effects of a chemical on cultured hepatocytes cannot be identified as hepato-specific, unless its effects on cells in general are known. Third, they can be used to screen large numbers of candidate compounds in order to determine priorities for further, more sophisticated testing, and to assist in the selection of appropriate doses to be applied in subsequent studies.

This chapter will be concerned with the development of cytotoxicity tests and their modification for special purposes and for testing certain types of materials. Three particular examples of general cytotoxicity tests (the FRAME kenacid blue test, the FRAME neutral red release test, and the FRAME fluorescein leakage test) will be described. Finally, the current status and the future potential of the general cytotoxicity approach in *in vitro* toxicology will be discussed.

II. FUNDAMENTAL QUESTIONS IN THE DEVELOPMENT OF CYTOTOXICITY TESTS

Before a cytotoxicity test can be developed, attention must be given to a wide range of biological and practical considerations and to the question of validation.

The biological considerations include choice of cell type (Table 1) and choice of endpoint and endpoint measurement (Table 2).[11] For example, human cells are preferable when human safety is the ultimate concern, but fish cells would clearly be more suitable if the goal were to replace the use of live fish in ecotoxicity testing. Again, if cell proliferation is the chosen endpoint, there are at least five different types of measurement for this endpoint (Table 2).

TABLE 1
Criteria for Choice of Cells

Human or animal origin
Adult or fetal origin
Normal or neoplastic tissue origin
Primary culture, cell strain, or continuous cell lines
Euploid or aneuploid karyotype
Recognizable morphology
Fibroblast-like or epithelial-like
Short-term or long-term stability
Growth rate
Suitability for endpoint measurements
Presence or absence of capacity to metabolize xenobiotics
Compatability with other metabolism and/or response systems

TABLE 2
Biological Endpoints for Detecting Cytotoxicity

Endpoint	Endpoint measurement
Cell morphology	Cell size and shape
	Cell-cell contacts
	Nuclear size, shape, and inclusions
	Nuclear number, size, shape, and inclusions
	Cytoplasmic vacuolation
Cell viability	Vital dye uptake
	Trypan blue exclusion
	Cell number
	Replating efficiency
Cell adhesion	Attachment to culture surface
	Detachment from culture surface
	Cell-cell adhesion
Cell proliferation	Increase in cell number
	Increase in total DNA
	Increase in total RNA
	Increase in total protein
	Colony formation
Membrane damage	Loss of enzymes (e.g., LDH)
	Loss of ions or cofactors (e.g., Ca^{2+}, K^+, NADPH)
	Leakage from preloaded cells (e.g., vital dye, ^{51}Cr)
Uptake or incorporation of radioactive precursors	Thymidine and DNA synthesis
	Uridine and RNA synthesis
	Amino acids and protein synthesis
Metabolic effects	Inhibition of metabolic cooperation
	Cofactor depletion (e.g., ATP)
	Mitochondrial function

Further, if determination of total cellular protein is the chosen endpoint measurement, there are at least two ways of performing this measurement — the Lowry method and a dye-binding method.[11]

One of the most important questions concerns the length of exposure of the cells to the test material. Many general cytotoxicity tests, designed to detect the acute cytotoxicities of test materials, have involved exposure periods as short as 4 h or 24 h. However, when Riddell et al.[12] conducted a study on 50 chemicals, they found that the values obtained for 25 of them were very similar after 24 h or 72 h, but that the shorter exposure period appeared to be an insufficient time for 24 of the other 25 chemicals to exert their full cytotoxic effects (Table 3). Only one chemical, acrylonitrile, which is highly volatile, appeared to be more toxic after 24 h than after 72 h.

TABLE 3
Comparison of 24- and 72-h Exposure Periods

Chemicals with different cytotoxicities after 24 and 72 h

Chemical	Exposure period[a] 72 hour	24 hour
Acrolein	<0.01	36 ± 4
6-Mercaptopurine	<0.01	>1000
Cycloheximide	<0.1	19 ± 4
Colchicine	8 ± 1	>1000
Bendiocarb	30 ± 5	179 ± 6
Butylated hydroxyanisole	45 ± 1	544 ± 115
Phenylbutazone	45 ± 1	768 ± 25
2,4-Dinitrophenol	72 ± 9	213 ± 18
Acetaminophen	90 ± 10	>1000
Phenacetin	95 ± 1	>1000
Methylparaben	105 ± 16	301 ± 34
Acrylamide	123 ± 8	583 ± 59
2,4-Dichlorophenoxyacetic acid	162 ± 19	557 ± 9
6-Methylcoumarin	169 ± 16	452 ± 85
Phenytoin	265 ± 44	>1000
Chloramphenicol	226 ± 41	>1000
Thioacetamide	274 ± 8	>1000
Warfarin	285 ± 26	>1000
Acetyl salicyclic acid	465 ± 86	>1000
Phenobarbital	543 ± 15	>1000
Lithium chloride	544 ± 45	>1000
Bromobenzene	641 ± 128	>1000
Isoxepac	644 ± 38	925 ± 15
Frusemide	756 ± 52	>1000
Acrylonitrile	>1000	530 ± 83

Chemicals with similar cytotoxicities after 24 and 72 h

Chemical	Exposure period[a] 72 hour	24 hour
p-Chloromercuribenzoic acid	3 ± 0.5	16 ± 0.8
Chlorpromazine	5 ± 0.6	11 ± 2
Chloroquine sulfate	7 ± 0.4	58 ± 2
Benzalkonium chloride	7 ± 0.3	8 ± 0.5
p-Aminophenol	10 ± 1	23 ± 6
Propranolol	12 ± 1	35 ± 3
Diethylstilboestrol	14 ± 3	27 ± 9
Versalide (AETT)	45 ± 1	71 ± 1
Ioxynil	47 ± 1	85 ± 11
Retinoic acid	49 ± 10	55 ± 5
Sodium dodecyl sulfate	94 ± 12	70 ± 2
L-Ascorbic acid	323 ± 58	272 ± 34
Sodium chloride	888 ± 41	>1000
Acetonyl acetone	937 ± 23	>1000

TABLE 3 (continued)
Comparison of 24- and 72-h Exposure Periods

Note: ID_{50} values for the following chemicals were >1000 μg/ml for assays performed at both 24 and 72 h after addition of test chemicals:

Acetonitrile	Ethanol	Isoniazid
Aniline	D-Fructose	Methanol
Cyclophosphamide	Glucose	Potassium iodide
Dimethyl sulfoxide	Iproniazid	

[a] Results are given as mean ID_{50} values (μg/ml) ± standard error of the mean, listed in order of KB 72-h values. Data from Riddell et al.[12]

The practical considerations include the commercial availability on a long-term basis of all that is required for conducting the test, including cells, media, cell culture apparatus, and materials required for endpoint measurements. In less than 10 years, we have had problems with all of these requirements! Ease of culture and storage of the cells must also be considered, as must the rate of test material throughput, the cost of testing each material, and the safety of all the materials used in the test.

Validation is the process whereby the reliability and relevance of a procedure are established for a particular purpose.[13] It follows test development and precedes acceptance and consists of three main stages, namely, intralaboratory assessment, interlaboratory assessment, and test data base development. Intralaboratory assessment involves the establishment of the reproducibility of the test performance within the laboratory of origin and the solving of any technical problems associated with the endpoint measurement and the spectrum of materials to which it is to be applied. Interlaboratory assessment is concerned with establishing the interlaboratory transferability of the method and the interlaboratory reproducibility of the results obtained. This stage should involve a blind trial, normally with at least 30 to 50 coded test materials, and independent assessment of the outcome of the study. The development of the test data base should involve larger numbers of materials — as many as 250 for a test designed for widespread applicability — and will provide the information upon which the performance of the test and its acceptability for use in toxicology and/or toxicity testing can be decided.

Modifications of the basic test protocol may also be necessary, for all kinds of reasons. These will include the types of materials to be tested and their physicochemical properties. For example, insolubility in aqueous media, high volatility, instability, binding to medium components or to the plastic of the culture dish surface will affect the results obtained. In addition, special considerations apply where medical devices are concerned, e.g., when dental materials, prosthetic implants, and surgical dressings are to be tested. This often involves placing pieces of the material in the culture medium, to see whether any components leach out and affect the cultured cells.

III. EXAMPLES OF GENERAL CYTOTOXICITY TESTS

Three tests developed as part of the FRAME Research Program will be discussed in detail. The detailed protocols for all of them are available from INVITTOX, the ERGATT/FRAME data base on *in vitro* toxicology (34 Stoney Street, Nottingham NG1 1NB, U.K.), as are protocols for many other tests.[14]

A. THE FRAME KENACID BLUE (KB) TEST[11,15]

The basis of this method is that, regardless of their precise cellular targets or mechanisms of action, cytotoxic chemicals will interfere with cell proliferation in cultures of continuous cell lines. The degree of interference observed will be an indication of the degree of cytotoxicity and can be quantified by counting cells or measuring their total DNA, vital dye uptake, or total protein content. The KB method is based on direct relationships between cell number, total protein, and the binding of certain dyes, such as kenacid blue R (no longer available) or Coomassie brilliant blue (which we now use instead). Originally developed for application to human fibroblast-like BCL-D1 cells grown in 24-well plates, the method has now been adapted for 3T3-L1 or V79 cells grown in 96-well plates.[15]

1. Cell Culture

3T3-L1 cells (ATCC CCL 92.1) are maintained in Dulbecco's minimum essential medium, supplemented with 10% newborn calf serum, 100 μg/ml streptomycin sulfate, 100 IU/ml benzylpenicillin, and 2 μg/ml Fungizone (Amphotericin B). A cell suspension is made from stock cell cultures to give a final concentration of 1.5×10^4 cells per ml for the standard 72-h KB test. The cells are then dispensed in 150 μl volumes into 95 of the wells of a 96-well tissue culture plate (the 96th well is the medium-only control well). The cells are then incubated for 24 h, when the test material is added at appropriate concentrations in culture medium.

2. Range-Finding Experiment

So that appropriate concentrations can be added in the definitive tests, a range-finding study is first conducted with seven concentrations of test material, namely, 0.01, 0.1, 1.0, 10, 100, 1000, and 10,000 μg/ml. The cells are examined by phase-contrast microscopy with an inverted microscope after 24, 48, and 72 h. It is usually possible to obtain an indication of the approximate toxicity of the chemical from the appearance of the cell cultures. After 72 h, the KB assay is performed. If no toxicity is found at the highest concentration, a second range-finding experiment is conducted, with concentrations between 1000 and 100,000 μg/ml (or the maximum solubility of the material, if it is less than 100,000 μg/ml).

3. Definitive Test

In the definitive test, seven concentrations of test material, selected according to the result of the range-finding study, are applied to three wells per concentration on three separate occasions (i.e., nine wells per concentration in all), with appropriate controls, including a time zero control, which involves removing the medium and allowing the cells to dry in air. After 72 h, total cellular protein is measured by the KB assay method.

4. The KB Assay

The culture medium is removed from the cells, which are then washed twice with warm phosphate-buffered saline (PBS, pH 7.4). Approximately 150 μl of fixative (1% glacial acetic acid, 50% ethanol, 40% distilled water) is then added to each well. The KB stain is prepared immediately before use by adding 12 ml glacial acetic acid to 88 ml KB stock solution (0.4 g Coomassie brilliant blue R, 250 ml ethanol, 630 ml distilled water). 150 μl KB stain is added to each well; then the tissue culture plate is rocked on a shaker for 3 h, after which the stain is removed and the cells are rinsed with washing solution (50% glacial acetic acid, 10% ethanol, 85% distilled water), then rocked in fresh washing solution for a further 20 min. The washing solution is then replaced with precisely 150 μl of desorbing solution (98.15 g potassium acetate, 300 ml distilled water, 700 ml ethanol). The absorbance of each well is then read at 570 nm in an Anthos 2001 plate-reader with a 404-nm reference blank, against the reference well containing no cells, which is set at zero. The absorbance correlates linearly with cell number.[11] Readings should be in the range 0.4 to 1.2. In addition, the air-dried control should be 30% or less of the final total protein in the untreated control cultures, i.e., the cells should have gone through two cell cycles during the 72-h period. If either of these conditions is not satisfied, then the results should be discarded and the test repeated.

5. Calculation of Results

The mean values for each set of triplicate wells are plotted on a graph as concentration *vs.* total cellular protein. The ID_{20}, ID_{50}, and ID_{80} values (i.e., the concentrations of test material which reduced the final cellular protein contents of test wells by 20%, 50%, or 80%, respectively, in comparison with untreated control wells) can then be read from the curve or calculated directly.

6. Status of the KB Method

The KB method has now been applied to about 300 pure chemicals and 250 formulations in the FRAME Alternatives Laboratory, where it is used as a standard *in vitro* test to provide data for comparison with the results of other *in vitro* tests. The KB method has been employed in a number of international validation studies, including evaluations of alternatives to the Draize eye irritancy test by the CTFA[16] and the EEC,[17] and the MEIC (multi-center evaluation of *in vitro* cytotoxicity)[18] approach of the Scandinavian Society for Cell Toxicology. Good *in vivo/in vitro* correlations have been found for metal salts and chlorides and for cosmetic formulations in the form of shampoos and oil/water emulsions.

7. Special Modifications of the KB Method

Many compounds and formulations are not readily soluble in or miscible with aqueous cell culture media. Organic solvents, such as ethanol, methanol, or dimethyl sulfoxide, can often be used to overcome this problem. Dilutions are made in such a way that the final concentration of organic solvent is always 1%, which is not toxic to cells. A solvent control (i.e., wells containing cells and solvent, but no test material) must be included when organic solvents are used, and the results are disregarded if the solvent alone reduces the final total protein by more than 15%.

In an attempt to overcome the problem for cell culture cytotoxicity tests represented by highly volatile test materials, the wells of 96-well tissue culture plates were sealed individually by the addition of a small amount of paraffin oil to each well. Of 27 liquids tested in a preliminary study,[19] 9 (namely, acetaldehyde, acetone, acetonitrile, allyl alcohol, ethanol, ethyl acetate, methanol, pyrrole, and propan-1-ol) were significantly *more* toxic in oil-sealed than in unsealed wells. The cytotoxicities of acetic acid, aniline, butanol, 1,2-dibromomethane, dimethyl formamide, dimethyl sulfoxide, glycerol, hydrochloric acid, 2-methoxyethanol, octanol, pentanol, sulfuric acid, tributyltin chloride, trichlorobenzene, trifluoracetic acid, and Tween 20 were not affected by the layer of paraffin oil. Heptanol and hexanol were significantly *less* toxic in oil-sealed than in unsealed wells, possibly because of absorption of these alcohols into the oil. Only 1 of 11 solid materials tested, sodium hydroxide, was more toxic in oil-sealed wells, probably because of an effect on the buffering system of the culture medium.

Rat oral LD_{50} values were available for eight of the nine liquids that were more toxic in sealed than in unsealed wells. The r value for the *in vivo/in vitro* comparison was 0.70 when data from unsealed wells were used and 0.85 when data from oil-sealed wells were used.[19]

B. THE FRAME NEUTRAL RED RELEASE (NRR) TEST[20]

This test was designed to mimic accidental exposure of cells in the eye to very high concentrations of materials for relatively brief periods. Thus, while the KB method involves exposure of proliferating cell cultures to μg/ml quantities of test materials for 72 h, the NRR method involves the exposure of confluent cells to mg/ml quantities for only 1 min. The 3T3-L1 cells are preloaded with a vital dye, neutral red (NR), and loss of the vital dye as a result of direct exposure to the test material is an indication of its short-term cytotoxicity.

1. Cell Culture and Vital Dye Loading

3T3-L1 cells are maintained as stock cultures in Dulbecco's minimum essential medium supplemented with 10% newborn calf serum and antibiotics, then subcultured into 96-well tissue culture plates (150 μl per well, 1.5×10^4 cells per ml, and allowed to grow to confluency [3 to 4 days]). The culture medium is then removed and replaced with NR medium (50 μg/ml NR in culture medium, made from an NR stock solution produced by adding 5 mg/ml NR to distilled water and filtering through filter paper).

2. The NRR Assay

At the end of the dye-loading period, the NR medium is replaced with fresh medium and the cells are used in the NRR assay within 2 h. Each test involves three control wells and three test wells for each concentration of the test material and is repeated on three separate occasions, as follows. First, the culture medium is removed and the cells are washed with 200 μl PBS. The PBS is then removed and 50 μl of the test material solution is added for precisely 1 min, after which the material is removed and the cells are briefly washed with 200 μl PBS. The PBS is removed and precisely 100 μl of NR destain solution (1% glacial acetic acid, 50% ethanol, 49% distilled water) is added. This both fixes the cells and removes any remaining NR. The plate is then rocked on a shaker for 20 min, to ensure that the vital dye is evenly dispersed in the NR destain solution. The optical density of each well is then read at 546 nm against a 404-nm reference filter in the plate-reader, which is zeroed on the reference well (i.e., the well containing no cells).

The mean optical density for each set of triplicate wells is determined, and the amount of NR released from each set of test wells is compared with that released from the PBS-treated control wells. The results are expressed as NRR_{20}, NRR_{50}, and NRR_{80} values (i.e., the concentrations of test material causing release of 20%, 50%, and 80% of the preloaded dye, respectively).

3. Status of the NRR Method

The NRR method has now been applied to about 200 pure chemicals and about 100 formulations in the FRAME Alternatives Laboratory. It is also being used in a number of validation studies on alternatives to the Draize eye irritancy test, including the CTFA[16] and EEC[15] studies. In Phase I of the CTFA program,[16] the NRR method was selected as a promising method for testing alcohol-based cosmetic formulations, because of the good correlation of the results obtained with Draize eye test scores.

C. THE FRAME FLUORESCEIN LEAKAGE (FL) TEST[21]

This method is based on the approaches of Tchao[22] and Reader et al.[20] and involves evaluating the effects of test materials on the permeability of a barrier of confluent epithelial cells to a nontoxic dye, fluorescein.

1. Cell Culture

Madin-Darby canine kidney cells (MDCK cells, ECACC 841903) are maintained in Dulbecco's modification of Eagle:Ham F12 medium, supplemented with 10% fetal calf serum, 100 μg/ml streptomycin sulfate, 100 IU/ml benzylpenicillin, and 2 μg/ml Fungizone (Amphotericin B). About 10^5 cells in 400 μl culture medium are then placed in Nunc 10 (Nunclon) or Millicell HA-12 (Millipore) tissue culture inserts, which are placed inside the wells of 24-well plates, which contain 500 μl of culture medium only.

2. The FL Assay

When they have grown to confluency, i.e., after about 4 days, the MDCK cell layers within the inserts are washed; then 100 μl volumes of the test materials are added (4 concentrations per test material, 2 inserts per concentration, 2 test materials per 24-well plate), either neat or dissolved in distilled water. Control inserts with and without cells receive distilled water only.

After precisely 1 min, the test materials are removed, and the cells are washed with distilled water. The water is then removed and the inserts are removed to clean 24-well plates with 500 μl warm PBS in each well. 500 μl of fluorescein in PBS (0.02%, w/v) is then added to each insert. After incubation of the plate at room temperature for 1 h, the leakage of dye from the inserts is measured by placing samples of the solutions in each well of a 96-well plate and measuring their optical densities in a plate-reader at 492 nm (reference filter 620 nm). The plate reader is zeroed on the mean optical densities of the control wells containing untreated cells. From the optical density values obtained, the concentrations of test samples are calculated which would cause 20% (FL_{20}) and 50% (FL_{50}) leakage of fluorescein across the cellular layer on the filter, in comparison with that across the inserts containing no cells (i.e., maximum leakage).

3. Status of the FL Method

This is a relatively new method, as it has as yet only been used with about 60 pure chemicals and about 20 formulations.

The FL and NRR assays measure the injurious effects of the test materials on different parts of the cell, namely the cell membrane and tight junctions or intracellular lysosomes, respectively. Despite this, both assays produced remarkably complementary results for a set of 22 test chemicals, and the ranked results correlated well with the available *in vivo* ocular irritancy data.[21]

One of our principal aims in developing the FL method was to see whether it could be used as a basis for studies on recovery from cytotoxic damage. Fluorescein is a nontoxic dye; so, after the assay, cells can be washed and placed in fresh culture medium and retested again after 24, 48, 72 or more hours. Any significant decrease in fluorescein leakage, such as increase in FL_{20}/FL_{50} concentrations, would indicate recovery from damage, i.e., the restoration of cell monolayer and cell-cell junctions.[21]

A further use for the cell monolayers on filter inserts may be in repeat-dose studies, since the cell monolayers remain stable and physiologically impermeable for several weeks. This could contribute usefully to a move away from the more or less exclusive use of general cytotoxicity tests in acute studies to their application to questions related to subchronic or chronic toxicity.

As performed at present, the FL method is relatively expensive, because of the cost of the filter inserts and the 24-well plates. Attempts are therefore being made to adapt the method for use with 96-well plates.

IV. THE CURRENT STATUS AND FUTURE POTENTIAL OF GENERAL CYTOTOXICITY TESTS

The value of cytotoxicity tests in general, and of cytotoxicity tests involving the use of permanent cell lines in particular, is a controversial issue. Flint[1,24] has argued that toxicity is a complex event; so simple tests involving the kinds of general endpoints illustrated in Table 2 are unlikely to be useful, because the cells used are usually functionally remote from cells and tissues as they exist in the whole animal. He considers that, by contrast, an *in vitro* test that gives an indication of impaired cellular function which is specific to one class of cell (e.g., the hepatocyte or the cardiac myocyte) can make a clear contribution to risk evaluation. The contrary view has been expressed by Ekwall and Ekwall,[25] who argued in favor of the combined use of general cytotoxicity tests and tests involving specific target cells, particularly as a means of identifying specific target cell/organ toxicity.

In our opinion, the *in vitro* cytotoxicity data base available to us is not yet sufficient for this controversy to be resolved. However, as evidence accumulates, it appears to support the contention of Ekwall and Ekwall, among others, that both acute systemic toxicity and local toxicity (expressed *in vivo* as irritancy or corrosivity) can be predicted by tests on relatively simple cell culture systems.

A. CYTOTOXICITY TESTS AND ACUTE LETHAL POTENCY

In some of our own studies,[26] we found that comparisons between the KB ID_{50} values and rat oral LD_{50} values and mouse i.p. LD_{50} values for 59 chemicals of various types gave r values of 0.76 and 0.80, respectively. In a second study[27] involving 28 metallic compounds, again tested *in vitro* by the KB method, r values of 0.73 and 0.86, respectively, were obtained in comparisons with rat oral and mouse i.p. LD_{50} values. When 18 metal chlorides were considered, *in vivo/in vitro* r values of 0.75 and 0.90, respectively, were obtained in comparisons with the rat and mouse LD_{50} values.

Fry et al.[28] reported similar results from *in vivo/in vitro* comparisons involving rat and mouse LD_{50} data. They obtained r values of 0.49 and 0.68, respectively, when they compared the data from a 72-h cytotoxicity test with rat oral and mouse i.p. LD_{50} values. The correlation coefficient improved to 0.82 for 18 of the 21 compounds involved, when the 3 for which metabolism is known to be a major determinant of toxicity *in vivo* were omitted from the comparison with i.p. values. When the *in vitro* cytotoxicities of six antimetabolites and six alkylating agents were compared with i.p. LD_{50} values, the correlation coefficients were 0.94 and 0.96, respectively. Fry et al. concluded that the precise relationship between LD_{50} values and *in vitro* cytotoxicities is determined by the modes of toxicity involved. They had earlier proposed[29] that i.p. LD_{50} values were the most appropriate measure of *in vivo* acute toxicity for use in *in vivo/in vitro* comparisons of acute intrinsic toxic potency.

Another line of evidence in support of the significance of general cytotoxicity tests is emerging from the MEIC project. The 50 compounds selected for study were chosen because data on them are available concerning human acute lethal dosage, human acute lethal blood concentrations, as well as rat and/or mouse LD_{50} values. The results for the first 10 compounds from 38 cytotoxicity tests are now available[30] and indicate that various combinations of the tests were able to predict the toxicity to humans of 9 of them (acetaminophen, aspirin, ferrous sulfate, diazepam, amitriptyline, ethylene glycol, methanol, ethanol, and isopropanol). This was taken to indicate that basal toxicity is the main factor in the acute *in vivo* toxicity of these compounds. The exception was digoxin, and this was taken to be an example of compounds that have more specific biological targets (i.e., related to the expression of specific receptors in the case of digoxin).

A number of authors have suggested that structure-activity relationship (SAR) data could usefully be combined with cytotoxicity data in predicting the toxicities of chemicals (e.g., References 30 and 31) and that *in vitro* methods could be useful in evaluating SAR predictions.[27,32]

B. THE CASE FOR USING TEST BATTERIES

Many authors refer to the need for test batteries to be developed and evaluated, since no one test is likely to replace the use of animal test procedures for any particular purpose. This is the basis of the MEIC approach,[30] and Halle and Spielmann[33] have also shown how the prediction of acute *in vivo* toxicity can be improved if the results of two or more cytotoxicity tests are combined.

The principles of test battery selection have recently been discussed[13,34] and can be summarized as follows:

1. Tests should have reached a satisfactory stage of development and validation before they are considered for inclusion in a battery (ideally, at least one interlaboratory validation study should have been conducted).
2. The component tests in a battery should be complementary and independent of each other and should not be duplicative (e.g., they should be concerned with different mechanisms, or should respond to different classes of test materials, or the high sensitivity of one test should be combined with the high specificity of another).
3. Three or four component tests should be sufficient in any one battery, but selection from a larger number of tests (say, six or eight) may be necessary, according to the type of material under test, likely degree of toxicity, etc.
4. The predictive performance of a battery must be subjected to evaluation with respect to an appropriate number of reference chemicals, according to the same criteria as are applied to the evaluation of individual tests.

C. *IN VITRO* TESTS FOR IRRITANCY POTENCY

The status of alternatives to acute ocular and dermal toxicity tests in animals has recently been reviewed by Frazier,[35] who found that a variety of general cytotoxicity tests show promise as screening tests for irritancy potency evaluation (i.e., for determining the relative irritancies of chemicals).

Our own three cytotoxicity tests are involved in a number of validation projects. As has already been mentioned, the NRR method was selected as one of the most promising tests in phase I of the CTFA program, which involved 10 ethanol-based cosmetic formulations, whereas the KB method was one of the tests which performed well in phase II of the CTFA program, when *in vitro* results and Draize eye scores were compared for 18 oil-water emulsions.

A particularly interesting set of results was obtained when the FL, NRR, and KB tests were used in an evaluation of 18 chemicals, selected for use in a pilot study funded by the EEC, for which *in vivo* eye irritancy evaluations based on historical data were independently provided by the technical information service of a chemical company. As can be seen from Table 4, the NRR method failed to identify silver nitrate and mercuric chloride as irritants, probably because the high concentrations of these salts applied "fixed" the vital dye within the cells. The KB method failed to identify sodium hydroxide and acetic acid as irritants, presumably because the buffering system in the medium was able to neutralize much of the alkali and acid, before the cells began to be affected. The FL method successfully identified all these four chemicals as severe irritants. None of the three methods were able to identify acetaldehyde, a highly volatile chemical, as an irritant. However, when the new modification of the KB method for volatile materials was used (i.e., with added paraffin oil as a well sealant),[19] the ID_{50} value fell to 36 μg/ml, which brought it well below the arbitrary irritant/nonirritant threshold (100 μg/ml) applied to the other chemicals.

TABLE 4
Results for Three Cytotoxicity Tests in Relation to Ocular Irritancy

Test material and class	FL_{20} (mg/ml)	I/N[b]	NRR_{50} (mg/ml)	I/N[c]	$KB\text{-}ID_{50}$ (μg/ml)	I/N[d]
R41[a]						
Tributyltin chloride	0.029	I	150	I	0.21	I
Silver nitrate	0.053	I	>2,000	N	3	I
Mercuric chloride	0.063	I	>100	N	7	I
Benzalkonium chloride	0.089	I	0.44	I	1.38	I
Sodium dodecyl sulfate	0.19	I	1	I	72	I
Sodium hydroxide	0.48	I	0.53	I	1,544	N
Acetic acid	12	I	148	I	1,259	N
Acetaldehyde	94	N	263	N	266[e]	N
R36[a]						
Chloroform	<25	I	108	I	>2,500	N
Butanol	28	I	31.6	I	7,355	N
Nonirritant[a]						
Brij 35	60	N	116	I	52	I
Toluene	65	N	857	N	857	N
2-Methoxyethanol	88	N	327	N	>9,000	N
Fluorescein	245	N	>200	N	510	N
Triacetin	494	N	>1,155	N	5,205	N
Dimethyl sulfoxide	584	N	503	N	18,349	N
Triethanolamine	680	N	234	N	2,502	N
n-Hexane	710	N	659	N	68	I

[a] The test materials were classified independently by the Central Toxicology Laboratory, Imperial Chemical Industries plc, following the eye hazard classification scheme specified by EEC Directive 83/467, Appendix 6, Part II (B): R36 = irritating to eyes; R41 = risk of serious damage to eyes. *In vitro* results were classified as indicators of irritancy (I) or nonirritancy (N) according to the following criteria: [b]I = $FL_{20} < 50$ mg/ml, N = $FL_{20} > 50$ mg/ml in the FL test; [c]I = $NRR_{50} < 150$ mg/ml, N = $NRR_{50} > 150$ mg/ml in the NRR test; [d]I = $ID_{50} < 100$ μg/ml, N = $ID_{50} > 100$ μg/ml in the 72-h KB test. [e] = 36 μg/ml (I) in the modified KB test.[19]

On the basis of our experience with these methods and with a physicochemical method, namely, EYTEX,[36] and our participation in a number of validation studies, we suggest that the following would be likely to comprise a useful battery of tests for use in predicting eye irritancy:

1. The EYTEX test
2. A short-term, high concentration cytotoxicity test (e.g., exposure for 1 min or 10 min to mg quantities), as in the NRR method or the FL method
3. A long-term, low concentration cytotoxicity test (e.g., exposure for 24 h or 72 h to μg quantities), as in the KB method or the NR uptake method[37]
4. An organotypic test, based on a chick chorioallantoic membrane[38] method or the isolated, enucleated eye method[39]
5. A test designed to provide information on recovery from damage (such methods are awaiting development and validation)

Of equal importance to its composition is how the battery of tests should be used. The key words here are flexibility combined with experience and scientific justification. The precise tests to be used should not be rigidly laid down as regulatory requirements. The particular combination of methods which will be appropriate will depend on the type of material under test, the purpose of the test, and the experience of the testing laboratory, where, ultimately, the responsibility will, and should, lie.

D. CYTOTOXICITY TESTS AND METABOLISM-MEDIATED TOXICITY

The toxicity of many xenobiotics is mediated through the production of reactive metabolites, and much effort has been put into detecting such metabolism-mediated toxicity in *in vitro* systems.[40] However, such systems must reflect the balance between activation and inactivation pathways, which determines the outcome of the interaction between the xenobiotic and the metabolism-competent cell.[40]

Quantitatively, hepatic microsomal P450-mediated monooxygenase (P450-MMO) activity and conjugation with glutathione (GSH) are the major routes of activation and inactivation, respectively. Because of this, much attention has been paid to the development of short-term or long-term hepatocyte culture systems.[2]

Another approach, which has been successfully employed in the *in vitro* detection of genotoxicity, has been to try to use a liver 9000-g supernatant fraction with added cofactors (the S9 mix), together with fibroblast-like cells as a response system, in the *in vitro* assessment of metabolism-mediated toxicity. Pretreatment of the animals providing tissue for the S9 fraction can be used to increase P450-MMO activity and/or to decrease GSH.

Various reports have suggested that this approach, which has advantages in terms of speed, species comparisons, and the use of human tissue as a source of the S9 fraction, could be used to study a wide range of compounds. However, our experience has been that the complexity of activation/inactivation will frustrate the general applicability of the S9 approach until more is known about mechanisms of metabolism-mediated toxicity. There is also the technical problem that S9 fractions and microsome fractions are themselves toxic to the cells used as the response system.

In studies on three compounds, we identified three completely different situations.[40] Cytotoxicity caused by the reactive metabolites of cyclophosphamide could be readily detected in an S9/V79 cell test, without modification of the S9. However, cytotoxicity due to reactive metabolites of bromobenzene could only be detected if the S9 fraction used was taken from rats pretreated with diethyl maleate to deplete hepatic GSH content. Finally, we could not detect the metabolism-mediated toxicity of acetaminophen, because of insufficient generation of free reactive metabolites and/or their instability.

There are three main ways forward. First, the problems associated with the use of S9 fractions could be overcome, e.g., by the manipulation of GSH levels *in vitro;* second, culture methods for hepatocytes, with retention of an appropriate complement of enzyme activities, could be improved; or, third, cell lines could be produced by using gene cloning or cell immortalization techniques, so that they expressed selected activation and/or inactivation pathways and could be used as complementary components in a test battery.

E. GENERAL CYTOTOXICITY TESTS AND OTHER TYPES OF TOXICITY

The importance of general cytotoxicity tests in providing baseline data essential to the identification of target cell/organ-specific or target system-specific toxicity has already been discussed. But could such tests be useful for predicting forms of toxicity other than acute effects? In a recent paper, Shrivastava et al.[41] considered retrospectively whether *in vitro* cytotoxicity data could predict the maximum tolerated dose to rats and dogs, as obtained in conventional 4-week *in vivo* procedures. The analysis involved 25 compounds, randomly selected and possessing a wide range of pharmacological activities. A better than 80% correlation was found; so this may represent both a technical and a conceptual breakthrough in the application of *in vitro* cytotoxicity tests.

V. THE VALIDATION AND ACCEPTANCE OF CYTOTOXICITY TESTS

Before cytotoxicity tests can be accepted, both for basic toxicology research purposes and for regulatory testing, they must become established in terms of their relevance according to certain criteria,[13] such as level of toxicity assessment (toxic potential, toxic potency, toxic hazard, and risk), type of testing (screening, adjunct, or replacement), type of toxicity (e.g., irritancy, nephrotoxicity, neurotoxicity), and chemical spectrum of applicability (i.e., general or specific to particular classes). It is easier to envisage a screening test for the irritant potency of surfactants in the eye than a replacement test for predicting the neurotoxic hazards represented by the full spectrum of chemicals.

The promotion of acceptance should be preceded by validation, which is essentially a scientific process whereby relevance and reliability are established. Many cytotoxicity tests exist, but few of them have been validated, even to a minimal degree. This is partly because of a failure to recognize the importance of validation and partly because of a tendency to make unjustified claims for particular procedures, before interlaboratory blind trials have been conducted and before an adequate data base has been established.[13,42]

One of the major impediments to progress in validation is the need for access to compounds for which adequate *in vivo* toxicological data are available. For this reason, the establishment of an international reference chemical data bank has been proposed.[13,43]

Once a test has been adequately validated as useful for particular purposes, its acceptance should be formally proposed and considered by the appropriate authorities. Proposals on how this process of acceptance should take place were recently published.[44] Independent assessment of the outcome of validation studies, and of the value of the validated test or battery of tests in competition with others, was seen as an essential part of the process. Finally, if the quality of information used in risk assessment and safety assessment is to be improved, while at the same time the dependence of toxicity testing on conventional animal procedures is to be reduced, intelligent strategies must be developed for the integrated use of batteries of complementary general and target cell/organ/system-specific *in vitro* tests. In addition, *in vitro* tests must be used in combination with other nonanimal approaches, such as the computer modeling of SAR and of physiological systems and processes.[10]

REFERENCES

1. **Flint, O. P.,** *In vitro* toxicology: a commercial proposition?, *Xenobiotica,* 18, 707, 1988.
2. **Guillouzo, A., Morel, F., Ratanasavanh, D., Chesne, C., and Guguen-Guillouzo, C.,** Long-term culture of functional hepatocytes, *Toxicol. in Vitro,* 4, 415, 1990.
3. **Gandolfi, A. J. and Brendel, K.,** *In vitro* systems for nephrotoxicity studies, *Toxicol. in Vitro,* 4, 337, 1990.
4. **Ryrfeldt, A., Cotgreave, I. A., and Moldéus, P.,** *In vitro* models to study mechanisms of lung toxicity, *ATLA,* 18, 267, 1990.
5. **Atterwill, C. K. and Fowler, K. F.,** A comparison of cultured rat FRTL-5 and porcine thyroid cells for predicting the thyroid toxicity of xenobiotics, *Toxicol. in Vitro,* 4, 369, 1990.
6. **Walum, E., Hansson, E., and Harvey, A. L.,** *In vitro* testing of neurotoxicity, *ATLA,* 18, 153, 1990.
7. **Atterwill, C. K., Simpson, M. G., Evans, R. J., Allen, S. L., and Ray, D.,** Alternative methods and their application in neurotoxicity testing, *Animals and Alternatives in Toxicology: Present Status and Future Prospects,* Balls, M., Southee, J. A., and Bridges, J. W., Eds., Macmillan, London, 1991, 121.
8. **Botham, P. and Kimber, I.,** Immunotoxicology and allergy: options for *ex vivo* and *in vitro* experimentation, *Animals and Alternatives in Toxicology: Present Status and Future Prospects,* Balls, M., Southee, J. A., and Bridges, J. W., Eds., Macmillan, London, 1991, 153.

9. **Duffy, P., Freeman, S., and Newall, D.,** The future of alternative approaches in reproductive toxicity testing, *Animals and Alternatives in Toxicology: Present Status and Future Prospects,* Balls, M., Southee, J. A., and Bridges, J. W., Eds., Macmillan, London, 1991, 177.
10. **Balls, M., Garle, M., and Clothier, R.,** Future developments in *in vitro* methodology, *Animals and Alternatives in Toxicology: Present Status and Future Prospects,* Balls, M., Southee, J. A., and Bridges, J. W., Macmillan, London, 1991, 313.
11. **Knox, P., Uphill, P. F., Fry, J. R., Benford, J., and Balls, M.,** The FRAME multicentre project on *in vitro* cytotoxicology, *Food Chem. Toxicol.,* 24, 457, 1986.
12. **Riddell, R. J., Panacer, D. S., Wilde, S. M., Clothier, R. H., and Balls, M.,** The importance of exposure period and cell type in *in vitro* cytotoxicity tests, *ATLA,* 14, 86, 1986.
13. **Balls, M., Blaauboer, B., Brusick, D., Frazier, D., Lamb, D., Pemberton, M., Reinhardt, C., Roberfroid, M., Rosenkranz, H., Schmid, B., Spielmann, H., Stammati, A.-L., and Walum, E.,** Report and recommendations of the CAAT/ERGATT workshop on the validation of toxicity test procedures, *ATLA,* 18, 313, 1990.
14. **Warren, M., Atkinson, K., and Steer, S.,** INVITTOX: The ERGATT/FRAME data bank of *in vitro* techniques in toxicology, *Toxicol. in Vitro,* 4, 707, 1990.
15. **Clothier, R. H., Hulme, L., Ahmed, A. B., Reeves, H. L., Smith, M., and Balls, M.,** *In vitro* cytotoxicity of 150 chemicals to 3T3-L1 cells, assessed by the FRAME kenacid blue method, *ATLA,* 16, 84, 1988.
16. **Gettings, S. D., DiPasquale, L. C., Bagley, D. M., Chudkowski, M., Demetrulias, J. L., Feder, P. I., Hintze, K. L., Marenus, K. D., Pape, W., Roddy, M. T., Schnetzinger, R., Silber, P. M., Teal, J. J., and Weise, S. L.,** The CTFA evaluation of alternatives program: an evaluation of potential *in vitro* alternatives to the Draize primary eye irritation test. (Phase I) Hydroalcoholic formulations: a preliminary communication, *In Vitro Toxicol.,* 3, 293, 1990.
17. Anon, Collaborative study on the evaluation of alternative methods to the eye irritation test, part I (54 pp) and part II (296 pp), document XI/632/91/V/E/1/131/91, CEC, Brussels, 1991.
18. **Ekwall, B., Bondesson, I., Castell, J. V., Gómez-Lechón, M. J., Hellberg, S., Högberg, J., Jover, R., Ponsoda, X., Romert, L., Stenberg, K., and Walum, E.,** Cytotoxicity evaluation of the first ten MEIC chemicals: acute lethal toxicity in man predicted by cytotoxicity in five cellular assays and by oral LD_{50} tests in rodents, *ATLA,* 17, 83, 1989.
19. **Smith, L. M., Clothier, R. H., Hillidge, S., and Balls, M.,** Modification of the FRAME kenacid blue method for cytotoxicity tests on volatile materials, *ATLA,* 20, in press.
20. **Reader, S. J., Blackwell, V., O'Hara, R., Clothier, R. H., Griffin, G., and Balls, M.,** A vital dye release method for assessing the short-term cytotoxic effects of chemicals and formulations, *ATLA,* 17, 28, 1989.
21. **Shaw, A. J., Clothier, R. H., and Balls, M.,** Loss of trans-epithelial impermeability of a confluent monolayer of Madin-Darby canine kidney (MDCK) cells as a determinant of ocular irritancy potential, *ATLA,* 18, 145, 1990.
22. **Tchao, R.,** Trans-epithelial permeability in fluorescein *in vitro* as an assay to determine eye irritants, *Alternative Methods in Toxicology, Progress in In Vitro Toxicology,* Vol. 6, Goldberg, A. M., Ed., Mary Ann Liebert Inc., New York, 1988, 271.
23. **Shaw, A. J., Balls, M., Clothier, R. H., and Bateman, N. D.,** Predicting ocular irritancy and recovery from injury using Madin-Darby canine kidney (MDCK) cells, *Toxicol. in Vitro,* 5, 569, 1991.
24. **Flint, O. P.,** *In vitro* toxicity testing: purpose, validation and strategy, *ATLA,* 18, 11, 1990.
25. **Ekwall, B. and Ekwall, K.,** Comments on the use of diverse cell systems in toxicity testing, *ATLA,* 15, 193, 1988.
26. **Clothier, R. H., Hulme, L. M., Smith, M., and Balls, M.,** Comparison of the *in vitro* cytotoxicities and acute *in vivo* toxicities of 59 chemicals, *Mol. Toxicol.,* 1, 571, 1989.
27. **Hulme, L. M., Reeves, H. L., Clothier, R. H., Smith, M., and Balls, M.,** Assessment of two alternative methods for predicting the *in vivo* toxicities of metallic compounds, *Mol. Toxicology,* 1, 589, 1989.
28. **Fry, J. R., Garle, M. J., Hammond, A. H., and Hatfield, A.,** Correlation of acute lethal potency with *in vitro* cytotoxicity, *Toxicol. in Vitro,* 4, 175, 1990.
29. **Fry, J. R., Garle, M. J., and Hammond, A. H.,** Choice of acute toxicity measures for comparison of *in vivo/in vitro* toxicity, *ATLA,* 16, 175, 1988.
30. **Hellberg, S., Eriksson, L., Jonsson, J., Lindgren, F., Sjöström, M., Wold, S., Ekwall, B., Gómez-Lechón, M. J., Clothier, R., Accomando, N. J., Grimes, A., Barile, F. A., Nordin, M., Tyson, C. A., Dierickx, P., Shrivastava, R. S., Tingsleff-Skaanild, M., Garza-Ocañas, L., and Fiskesjö, G.,** Analogy models for prediction of human toxicity, *ATLA,* 18, 103, 1990.
31. **Halle, W., Baeger, I., Ekwall, B., and Spielmann, H.,** Correlation between *in vitro* cytotoxicity and octanol/water partition coefficient of 29 substances from the MEIC programme, *ATLA,* 19, 338, 1991.
32. **Babich, H. and Borenfreund, E.,** Structure-activity relationship (SAR) models established *in vitro* with the neutral red cytotoxicity assay, *Toxicol. in Vitro,* 1, 3, 1987.

33. **Halle, W. and Spielmann, H.,** Two procedures for the prediction of acute toxicity (LD50) from cytotoxicity data, *ATLA,* 19, 20, 40, 1992.
34. **Balls, M., Atkinson, K. A., and Gordon, V. C.,** Complementation in the development, validation and use of non-animal test batteries, with particular reference to ocular irritancy, *ATLA,* 19, 429, 1991.
35. **Frazier, J. M.,** Alternatives to acute ocular and dermal toxicity tests in animals, *Dermato-toxicology,* 4th ed., Marzulli, F. N. and Maibach, H. I., Eds., Hemisphere, New York, 1991, 817.
36. **Gordon, V. C. and Bergman, H. C.,** EYTEX™, an *in vitro* method for evaluation of ocular irritancy, *Alternative Methods in Toxicology,* Vol. 5, Goldberg, A. M., Ed., Mary Ann Liebert, New York, 1987, 293.
37. **Borenfreund, E. and Puerner, J. A.,** Toxicity determined *in vitro* by morphological alterations and neutral red absorption, *Toxicol. Lett.,* 24, 119, 1985.
38. **Luepke, N. P.,** Hen's egg chorio-allantoic membrane test for irritation potential, *Food Chem. Toxicol.,* 23, 287, 1985.
39. **Burton, A. B. G., York, M., and Lawrence, R. S.,** The *in vitro* assessment of severe eye irritants, *Food Cosmet. Toxicol.,* 19, 471, 1981.
40. **Fry, J. R., Garle, M., and Hammond, A. H.,** Competing pathways in metabolism-mediated cytotoxicity *in vitro, Toxicol. in Vitro,* 4, 467, 1990.
41. **Shrivastava, R., John, G. W., Rispat, G., Chevalier, A., and Massingham, R.,** Can the *in vivo* maximum tolerated dose be predicted using *in vitro* techniques?, A working hypothesis, *ATLA,* 19, 393, 1991.
42. **Balls, M. and Clothier, R.,** Validation of alternative toxicity test systems: lessons learned and to be learned, *Mol. Toxicol.,* 1, 547, 1989.
43. **Purchase, I. F. H.,** An international reference chemical data bank would accelerate the development, validation and regulatory acceptance of alternative toxicology tests, *ATLA,* 18, 345, 1990.
44. **Balls, M., Botham, P., Cordier, A., Fumero, S., Kayser, D., Koëter, H., Koundakjian, P., Lindquist, N. G., Meyer, O., Pioda, L., Reinhardt, C., Rozemond, H., Smyrniotis, T., Spielmann, H., Van Looy, H., van der Venne, M.-T., and Walum, E.,** Report and recommendations of an international workshop on promotion of the regulatory acceptance of validated non-animal toxicity test procedures, *ATLA,* 18, 339, 1990.

Chapter 5

MODULATION BY DRUGS AND MEASUREMENT OF NATURAL KILLER CELL ACTIVITY

Guan-jie Chen, Steve Wood, and Ronald R. Watson

TABLE OF CONTENTS

I. INTRODUCTION

Since the early 1970s, it was recognized that a subpopulation of lymphocytes from normal humans or mice could kill cultured tumor cell lines;[1-8] these were therefore labeled "natural killer cells" (NK cells). NK cells have some unique characteristics which differ from other killer cells: (1) ability to kill without prior sensitization; (2) no MHC (major histocompatibility complex) recognition;[9-12] (3) ability to lyse culture cells in a short-term assay; and (4) possession of a pattern of specificity against target tumor cells.[13] NK cells have been shown to react with a wide variety of *in vitro* passaged cells as well as *in vivo* transplanted or explanted tumor cells. They can destroy autologous or syngeneic as well as allogeneic tumor cells.[14]

It is not clear whether NK cells make up a unique cell population or members of several distinct cell lineages. NK cells may be early or prethymus T cells[15,16] and may be closely related to the myeloid series. They appear to expressed by cell types of different lineage at various stages of differentiation.[15] NK cells are a distinct population of cells with lymphoid morphological features in humans,[17] mice,[18] and rats.[19] The feature of large azurophilic granules has ellicited the term "large granule lymphocyte" (LGL) as a means of identifying these cells. LGLs comprise about 5% of peripheral blood lymphocytes. These cells can be enriched on Percoll density gradient so that up to 80% are NK cells.[20-22] The peripheral blood and spleen are the major sources of NK cells with 6 to 7 and 3 to 4% of the lymphocytes being NK cells, respectively.[23] The NK cells are found in the red pulp of the spleen, while T cell recirculation is localized in the white pulp.

In the past, NK cells have been identified in a negative way as those cells that are not T cells, B cells, or macrophages. However, due to the development of the monoclonal antibody technique, some unique NK cell markers have been found. For human NK cells, there are B73.1 and 3G8 which recognize the F_{CR} (receptor for fragment C of IgG),[24-26] while others recognize $Cr_3(C_{3bi})$[27] and HNK-1 (Leu-7) which were produced by immunizing with purified LGL.[28] For mice, NK cells are identified by NK 1-1[29] and asialo GM which was proven to relate to the function of NK cells.[30] Kay and co-workers[31] found that only 50% of NK cells have SRBC receptors. No one surface marker for NK cells has been found, and NK cells also contain markers of T cells and monocytes. Therefore many but not all LGL are NK cells.

The mechanism of NK cell cytotoxicity shares similarities to cytotoxic T lymphocyte (CTL). The currently accepted hypothesis includes five steps:[32] (1) binding to the target cell through a NK cell receptor which recognizes particular structures on target cells; (2) triggering and activating of intercellular processes in the NK cells;[33] (3) release of some granules which contain substances like NK cytotoxic factor (NKCF);[34] (4) cytolysin molecules, for example, NKCF, bind to the target cell; and (5) lysis of target cell.

NK cell activity plays an important role in tumor surveillance, as lower activity is related to higher incidence of tumor.[35] NK cell activity is related to the antitumor host defenses during primary tumor growth[36-38] and metastatic growth[39,40] as well as to spontaneous tumor metastasis.[41,42] Besides the antitumor activity, NK cells show resistance to microbial pathogens. Some viruses are sensitive to NK cell activity[43,44] while other viruses are NK cell resistant.[45,46] Although direct NK cell attack on parasites is not an important mechanism, Fugui and Allison found both an increase in spleen cell number and NK cell activity in mice inoculated with babesia or malaria parasites.[47] NK cells may play a role in early resistance against parasites by limiting the degree of parasiemia before the development of the necessary T cell immunity.[48,49] Parasite infection results in an early, substantial elevation of NK cell activity in the spleen and peritoneal space. There is a strong possibility that the activated NK cells might be very effective against the invading parasites, if they could function in collaboration with a specific antibody, in the antibody-dependent cellular cytotoxicity (ADCC) model.[49] NK cells can also destroy some bacteria by direct lysis as well as by ADCC.[50-52] Although macrophages play an important role against fungal infection, NK cells also have a potential role in defense against fungi.[53-55]

NK cells, like other T cells, function in the intercellular reaction network. They have been shown to be involved in the regulation of immunoglobulin secretion and differentiation of B cells.[56,57] Also these cells produce soluble mediators, cytokines, to affect the function and differention of other cells.[56] NK cells influence immunoglobulin secretion.[57] Several kinds of cytokine can be produced by NK cells, including interferons (IFNs),[58] interleukin-1 (IL-1),[59] interleukin-2 (IL-2),[58,60] B cell growth factor (BCGF), now called IL-4,[61] colony-stimulating factor (CSF),[58] and NKCF.[62] Also NK cells can respond to various agents including cytokines, microbial challenges, and other environmental agents. IFNs have been related to increased NK cell activity[63,64] as well as to virus (RNA and DNA virus) infection.[65] Gidlund and co-workers[66] reported that the effect of viral infection on NK cell activity is mediated through the increase of gamma-IFN. IFNs have two major effects in viral-infected animals: (1) increasing NK cell activity to lyse virus-infected cells; and (2) protecting uninfected cells.[67-70] Ullberg et al.[71] have reported that IFN-α increases NK cell recruitment from a pre-NK cell precursor pool as well as lytic activity per cell or recycling capacity. However, others found that IFN-α added *in vitro* with 48 h incubation of T cells decreased the percentage of F^{+}_{CR} cells and E-rossetting cells, and caused no change in EAC-rossetting cells.[72] Thus IFN-α may decrease the expression of NK cell phenotypes. Another cytokine, IL-2, has been shown to increase NK cell activity.[73-75] Prostaglandin E_2 (PGE_2) has been shown to inhibit NK cell activity in cells treated with interferon.[76]

In addition, NK cell activity can be modulated by different drugs, such as morphine, cocaine, and alcohol. However, there are conflicting results of the effects of those drugs on NK cell activity and results are difficult to interpret. In human studies, NK cells incubated with β-endorphin, which is endogeous morphine, presented an increase in the cytolytic activity.[77-80] However, others found that human cells incubated with β-endorphin reduced the NK cell activity by half.[81] They also found opioid-mediated suppression of τ-IFN production by cultured peripheral blood mononuclear cells which is a strong NK cell activity stimulus.[82] This result supports the decreasing effect of morphine on NK cell activity. In animal studies, conflicting results are also noted. Shavit and co-workers[83,84] found that *in vivo* administration of morphine for 4 days reduced the spleen NK cell activity which could be blocked by the opioid antagonist naltrexone. However, Kraut[85] found morphine increased NK cell activity of splenocytes. Cocaine significantly decreased NK cell activity in human cultured lymphocytes, but only at a high dose (500 times greater than physiological achievable levels). *In vivo* a single dose of cocaine injection (0.6 mg/ml) significantly stimulated NK cell activity and total number.[86] Ethanol can increase NK cell activity in humans;[87-89] however, decreased NK cell activities have been associated with alcohol consumption.[90,91] Ethanol-induced changes on NK cell activity may occur via the neural system.[92] Due to the important role of NK cells in the immune system, reliable assays *in vitro* to detect NK cell activity have been developed and improved recently.

II. METHODS OF *IN VITRO* NK CELL ASSAYS

A. SUMMARY OF ASSAY

NK cell cytotoxic activity is assessed by its action upon target tumor cells (human K562 and murine YAC-1). K562 cells were derived from a patient who was in blastic crisis of leukemia. YAC-1 cells are a lineage of Moloney virus-induced lymphoma. The target cell is prelabeled with radioisotope (^{51}Cr) or fluorochrome (2′,7′-bis(carboxyethyl)-5,6-

carboxyfluorescein, "BCECF"); then various proportions of NK effector cells and target cells are mixed and incubated. During the incubation, as the NK cells destroy the target cells, radioisotope or fluorescence, which labeled the target cells before, is released into the supernatant. The amount of radioisotope (actually the counts of cpm in the supernatant), or the concentration of the fluorescence remaining in the target cells, is quantified and reflects NK cell activity.

B. CLASSICAL 4-h ^{51}Cr RELEASE ASSAY[93]

1. Materials and Equipment

Cell lines: K562 or YAC-1 (ATCC)
Cell culture flasks (Falcon)
HBSS solution (Gibco)
Fetal calf serum (Hyclone)
RPMI 1640 medium with L-glutamine (Gibco)
Sodium chromate (NEN, 1.0 mCi/ml, 37.0 MBq/ml)
Microtiter plate, U-bottom 96-wells (Falcon 3077)
37°C CO_2 incubator with 5% CO_2 (VWR)
37°C water bath (VWR)
Gamma counter
Centrifuge (Beckman TJ-R)
Multichannel pipetters (Costar 8-channel fixed volume)
Luminar flow hood (Labconco, Class II)
Microliter pipette tips (Rainin)
Microscope (Reichert-Jung)
Hemacytometer chamber (Baxter)
1% NP-40 (Sigma)
Trypan blue dye (Sigma)
LSM lymphocyte separation medium (Drganon Teknika)
0.01 *M* PBS
Petri dish (Falcon 3002)
Ether
Scissors
Forceps
70% ethanol (v/v)
Pasteur pipette (VWR)
Lysing butter (ammonium chloride, Tris-buffer)
15-ml and 50-ml centrifuge tubes (Falcon 2095, and VWR)
Blood collection tubes (Becton Dickinson)

2. Procedure

a. NK Cell Collection

NK cells from different tissue sources may be used as NK effector cells. Here we describe the procedures of collection of NK effector cells from human peripheral blood monocytes separated by using separation medium and from mouse splenocyte single-cell suspension.

i. Separation of Human Peripheral Blood Monocytes

a. Coat plastic petri dishes with fetal calf serum overnight.

b. Take blood sample from vein into blood-collecting tube which contained sodium heparin (Becton Dickinson). Dilute blood with equal amount of PBS.
c. Layer diluted blood carefully on top of LSM lymphocyte separation medium. The ratio is 2:3 (separation medium:diluted blood)
d. Centrifuge the sample at 700 g for 20 min. The monocyte band is removed by first carefully aspirating down to within 2 to 3 mm above the band and throwing the top layer away; then aspirate the band plus half of the fluid below the band. Place the monocytes into a 50-ml centrifuge tube and add equal volume of PBS. Mix gently by inversion and centrifuge at 400 g for 10 min.
e. The cells are washed again with PBS and resuspended in appropriate volume of RPMI 1640 medium (containing 10% of fetal calf serum) and distributed on the petri dishes which were precoated with fetal calf serum.
f. Nonadherent cells are removed from coated petri dish after 1 h of incubation.
g. Nonadherent cells are counted under microscope using Trypan blue dye exclusion and adjusted to desired concentration.

ii. Preparation of Murine Single Splenocyte Suspension

a. Sacrifice the mice by bleeding from axillar vein under ether anesthesia.
b. Place the spleen in the petri dish which contains RPMI 1640 medium.
c. Gently tearing the spleen with sterile forceps in petri dish, make single-cell suspension in a sterile hood.
d. Collect the suspension into a 15-ml centrifuge tube; centrifuge the tube at 180 g for 10 min.
e. Discard the supernatant and resuspend the cells in ammonium chloride lysing buffer for 2 min.
f. Centrifuge the cell again at 180 g for 10 min. Resuspend the cells in 5 ml RPMI 1640 medium containing 10% fetal calf serum; centrifuge again at 180 g for 10 min.
g. Discard the supernatant and resuspend the cells in 3 ml of RPMI 1640 medium plus 10% of fetal calf serum.
h. Count the cells under the microscope using Trypan blue dye exclusion and adjust to desired concentration.

b. Labeling the Target Cells

i. K562 or YAC-1 cells cultured in RPMI 1640 medium containing 10% of fetal calf serum in cell culture flask in 37°C, 5% CO_2 incubator.
ii. Before labeling, check the cells under the microscope. The cells should be in good condition (at least 90% viable), healthy and round shape.
iii. Spin the cells at 180 g for 10 min and resuspend in appropriate volume of medium.
iv. Count the cells under microscope using Trypan blue dye and adjust the cell number to 1×10^7/ml.
v. Take 1 ml of cell suspension (10^7 cells) in a 15-ml centrifuge tube and add 100 μl of sodium chromate (^{51}Cr) (100 μCi), mix well, and keep in 37°C water bath or 37°C incubator for 1 h, mixing gently every 15 min.
vi. Then add 10 ml of prewarmed HBSS.
vii. Centrifuge the tube at 180 g for 10 min, discard the supernatant into radioactive biohazard waste container, and transfer the cells into a 50-ml centrifuge tube which contains 50 ml of prewarmed HBSS. Use the HBSS solution to wash the tube several times and be sure to transfer all cells into the 50-ml tube.

viii. Then incubate the cells in 37°C incubator for at least $^1/_2$ h.
ix. Centrifuge the tube again at 180 g for 10 min, discard the supernatant, and resuspend the cells in 10 ml of medium.
x. Count the cell number under the microscope and adjust to 1×10^5/ml.

c. *Coincubation of NK Effector Cells and Target Cells for 4 h*

i. Distribute 0.1 ml of labeled target cell suspension (1×10^5/ml) into each well of 96-well microtiter plate (Falcon 3077).
ii. Put another 0.1 ml of different concentration of NK effector cell suspension into each well: for human peripheral blood NK effector cells usually use 1.25×10^6/ml, 2.5×10^6/ml, and 5×10^6/ml, representing 1:12.5, 1:25, and 1:50 (target cell:effector cell); for murine splenocyte NK effector cells usually use 2.5×10^6/ml, 5×10^6/ml, and 1×10^7/ml, representing 1:25, 1:50, and 1:100 (target cell:effector cell).
iii. Every concentration of each sample is triplicated. At the same time, instead of 0.1 ml effector cell suspension, put another 0.1 ml of medium alone or 0.1 ml of 1% NP-40 in two sets of 6-wells which serve as spontaneous release and maximum release controls.
iv. Centrifuge the plate at 180 g for 2 min to facilitate the reaction between effector cells and target cells.
v. Incubate the plate in 37°C, 5% CO_2 incubator for 4 h.
vi. After incubation, spin the plate at 180 g for 10 min and take 100 μl of supernatants from each well for counting the cpm on gamma counter.

d. *Calculation of Cytotoxic Index (CI) for NK Cell Activity*

$$\text{CI} = \frac{\text{Mean of test release cpm} - \text{mean of spontaneous release cpm}}{\text{Mean of maximum release cpm} - \text{mean of spontaneous release cpm}} \times 100\%$$

C. FLUORESCENCE METHOD FOR NK CELL ACTIVITY

1. Materials and Equipment

Cell line: K562 or YAC-1 (ATCC)
Cell culture flasks (Falcon)
BCECF-AM (Molecular Probes, Inc., Eugene, OR)
DMSO (dimethyl sulfoxide, Sigma)
NaN_3 (sodium azide, Sigma)
Fetal calf serum (Hyclone)
RPMI 1640 medium with L-glutamine (Gibco)
0.01 *M* PBS
37°C CO_2 incubator with 5% CO_2 (VMR)
Centrifuge (Beckman TJ-R)
Multichannel pipetters (Costar 8-channel fixed volume)
Luminar hood (Labconco, class II)
Microliter pipette tips (Rainin)
Microscope (Reichert-Jung)
Hemacytometer chamber (Baxter)
Trypan blue (Sigma)
LSM lymphocyte separation medium (Drganon Teknika)
Petri dish (Falcon 3002)

Ether
Scissors
Forceps
70% ethanol (v/v)
Pasteur pipette (VWR)
Lysing buffer (ammonium chloride, Tris-buffer)
15-ml and 50-ml centrifuge tubes (Falcon 2095 and VWR)
Blood collection tubes (Becton Dickinson)
96-well plate (Falcon 3077)
2% NP-40 (Sigma)
Fluoricon polystyrene assay particle (ϕ 3.1 μm, Baxter)
Pandex harvesting plate (Idexx, Portland, ME)
FAC analyzer (Baxter)

2. Procedure

a. NK Cell Collection

Same as in section II.B.

b. Labeling the Target Cells

i. K652 or YAC-1 cells cultured in flasks in RPMI 1640 medium containing 10% fetal calf serum in 37°C, 5% CO_2 incubator.
ii. Before labeling, check the cell condition as in ^{51}Cr assay. Wash the cells with PBS twice (180 g for 10 min) and resuspend cells in RPMI 1640 without fetal calf serum.
iii. Count the cells using Trypan blue exclusion method and adjust to 1×10^6/ml.
iv. Prepare BCECF-AM stock solution by adding 10 μl of DMSO to 50 μg of BCECF-AM in vials (5 mg/ml).
v. Take 2.5 ml of target cell suspension in a 15-ml centrifuge tube (1×10^6/ml) (* in RPMI without fetal calf serum) and add 5 μl of BCECF-AM stock solution, then incubate in 37°C, 5% CO_2 incubator for 30 min with cap loosened.
vi. After incubation, add 10 ml of PBS and centrifuge at 180 g for 10 min; then remove the supernatant and wash the cells once with PBS.
vii. Resuspend the cells in RPMI 1640 with 10% fetal calf serum.
viii. Count and adjust the cells to 5×10^4/ml.

c. Coincubation of NK Effector Cells and Target Cells

i. Adjust effector cell concentration to 2.5×10^6/ml, 1.25×10^6, and 6.25×10^5 for effector cell:target cell ratio of 50:1, 25:1, and 12.5:1 respectively.
ii. Preparation of mock effector cells or spontaneous release of target cells. Take 1 ml aliquot of each concentration of effector cell suspension mentioned in (i), resuspend the cells in 5 ml of PBS containing 0.1% NaN_3, and incubate at 37°C for 30 min. Wash the cells with PBS and resuspend in 1 ml of RPMI 1640 with 10% fetal calf serum. Place 50 μl of target cells in wells designated as spontaneous release in 96-well plate.
iii. Add 0.1 ml of different concentrations of effector cells to each well of 96-well plate with triplication and put same volume of *Mock cell* or 2% NP-40 in another set of tripication wells for maximum release.
iv. Add 0.1 ml of target cells to all wells except those designated for spontaneous release.
v. Spin the plate at 150 g for 3 min to facilitate cell contact.
vi. Incubate the plate in 37°C, 5% CO_2 incubator for 2 h.

d. Termination and Collection

i. Prepare bead suspension: Fluoricon polystyrene assay particles (ϕ 3.1 μm) are diluted to 1% (w/v) with PBS.
ii. At the end of the incubation period, add 50 μl of above bead suspension to each assay well.
iii. Mix the contents of each well by repeat pipetting 100 μl five times.
iv. One 50 μl aliquot is taken from each well and transferred to wells in a Pandex harvesting plate. After transfer of all assay wells the remaining empty wells of the Pandex harvesting plate are filled with 100 μl of PBS.

e. FCA Reading

i. Set signal channel to 485/535 nm wavelengths and set reference channel to 590/620 nm. Prime washing mechanism, washing reservoir which contains PBS.
ii. Set vacuum to 5 in. Hg.
iii. Set the gain of the instrument. A gain of 10 is usually optimal when using 10,000 target per incubation well (5000 targets per well in the harvesting plate). The gain is adjusted such that the maximum retention well gives between 60,000 and 80,000 RFU. The gain may need to be reset after initial reading of the plate. RFU from maximal retention wells for the lower E:T ratio will always be higher than that obtained for the higher E:T ratios due to effector quenching effects.
iv. Using the reference plate, set optical contrasts and run plate-centering program. This is done at least once a day, usually during the assay incubation period.
v. Make sure the printer is on-line and ready to receive data.
vi. Place Pandex harvesting plate in Pandex FCA.
vii. Start vacuum.
viii. When wells are completely emptied of fluid, wash wells once with vacuum remaining on.
ix. After washing wells once with PBS, when wells are completely evacuated, run read program and collect data.
x. Because we do not yet know at this point whether we need to reread the plate at a different gain we will assume that we do. When data are printing out, vacuum will shut off. The vacuum must be on when reading the plate; therefore it must be turned back on immediately after it is shut off. The gain can then be reread. If a second reading at an adjusted gain is not necessary, turn the vacuum off.
xi. Remove assay plate and discard. Turn lamp off. Store wash bottle in the refrigerator.

f. Calculation of Cytotoxic Index for NK Cell Activity

$$\%\ \text{CI} = \frac{\text{Spontaneous release fluorescence} - \text{test release fluorescence}}{\text{Spontaneous release fluorescence} - \text{maximum release fluorescence}} \times 100$$

D. RELATED TECHNICAL ASPECTS

In vivo assays for NK activity on animal models were created and improved by several groups of investigators.[94-96] In those assays, usually target tumor cells, which are sensitive to NK cells, were labeled with radioisotopes and were injected into animals intravenously. At different time points after injection of the target cells, animals were killed and radioactivity in organs (spleen, liver, and lungs) was measured. The difference in recovery of radioactivity reflects the NK activity of those organs. Others measured NK activity by measuring the survival time and tumor growth as end points after challenges by target tumor cell.

However, the major limitation of most *in vivo* studies is their reliability,[97] because the correlations seen in those experiments cannot be taken as evidence for an exclusive role of NK cells in *in vivo* destruction of target tumor cells. A very complex situation underlies the results obtained in those experiments, since not only NK cells, but also macrophages, T cells, and NC (natural cytotoxic) cells could contribute. Another limitation is that the contact between target cells is not as close as in an *in vitro* assay, so some uncorroborated results were obtained in *in vivo* assays, especially from spleen.[94] Compared to *in vivo* assays for NK activity, *in vitro* assay is more reliable, economical, and simpler. However, when a large number of target cells have been lysed in *in vitro* assay, nonlinear rate of ^{51}Cr release will be attributed. So an optimal ratio of target and effect cells should be carefully chosen (usual effect: target = 10:1 to 100:1).[98]

Since mycoplasma infection can increase *in vitro* NK activity and prolonged incubation time may obscure results from cytotoxicity of other kinds of killers, mycoplasma infection should be avoided and time restricted to 4 hours.

Since NK cell activity tends to be higher in the male and increases with age, it is necessary to exercise care in matching the sex and age in experimental and control groups. Cell preparation must be performed appropriately, because monocyte population and PMNs may suppress NK cell cytotoxic activity, and erythrocyte contamination may enhance the cytotoxicity.

ACKNOWLEDGMENT

The research in this review was stimulated by grants DA04827 and AA08037.

REFERENCES

1. **Takasugi, M., Micgey, M. R., and Terasaki, P. I.,** Reactivity of lymphocytes from normal persons on cultured tumor cells, *Cancer Res.*, 33, 2898, 1973.
2. **Rosenberg, E. B., McCoy, J. L., Green, S. S., Donelly, F. C., Siwarski, D. F., Levine, P. H., and Herberman, R. B.,** Destruction of human lymphoid tissue-culture cell lines by human peripheral lymphocyte in ^{51}Cr-release cellular cytotoxic assays, *J. Natl. Cancer Inst.*, 52, 345, 1974.
3. **Pross, H. F. and Jonal, M.,** Cytotoxic lymphocytes from normal donors. A functional marker of human non-T-lymphocytes, *Clin. Exp. Immunol.*, 21, 226, 1975.
4. **Peter, H. H., Pavie-Fisher, J., Fridman, W. H., Aubert, C., Cesarini, J. P., Rougin, R., and Kourilsky, K. M.,** Cell-mediated cytotoxicity *in vitro* of human lymphocytes against a tissue culture melanoma cell line (IGR3), *J. Immunol.*, 115, 539, 1975.
5. **Matthews, N. and MacLaurin, P. B.,** Spontaneous cytotoxic activity as a test of human lymphocyte function, *Lancet*, 1, 581, 1975.
6. **Kiessling, R., Klein, E., Pross, H., and Wigzell, H.,** Natural killer cells in the mouse. I. Cytotoxic cells with specificity for mouse Moloney Leukemia cells. Specificity and distribution according to genotype, *Eur. J. Immunol.*, 5, 112, 1975.
7. **Kiessling, R., Klein, E., Pross, H., and Wigzell, H.,** Natural killer cells in the mouse. II. Cytotoxic cell with specificity for mouse Moloney Leukemia cells. Characteristic of the killer cell, *Eur. J. Immunol.*, 5, 117, 1975.
8. **Herberman, R. B., Nunn, M. E., and Lavrin, D. H.,** Natural cytotoxic reactivity of mouse lymphoid cells against syngeneic and allogeneic tumors. I. Distribution of reactivity and specificity. II. Characterization of effector cells, *Int. J. Cancer*, 16, 216-229 & 230-239, 1975.
9. **Kaphan, J. and Callewaert, D. M.,** Are natural killer cells germ-line V-gene-encoded prothymocytes specific for self and nonself histocompatibility antigens? in *Natural Cells-mediated Immunity Against Tumors*, Herberman, R. B., Ed., Academic Press, New York, 1980, 893.

10. **Seeley, J. K. and Golub, S. H.,** Studies on cytotoxicity generated in human mixed lymphocyte culture. I. Time course and target spectrum of several distinct concomitant cytotoxic activities, *J. Immunol.*, 120, 1415, 1978.
11. **Ortaldo, J. R., Oldham, R. K., Cannon, G. C., and Herberman, R. B.,** Specificity of natural cytotoxic reactivity of normal human lymphocyte against a myeloid leukemia cell line, *J. Natl. Cancer Inst.*, 59, 77, 1977.
12. **Ortaldo, J. R., Bonnard, G. D., Kind, P. D., and Herberman, R. B.,** Cytotoxicity by cultured human lymphocytes: characteristics of effector cells and specificity of cytotoxicity, *J. Immunol.*, 122, 1489, 1979.
13. **Ortaldo, J. R. and Herberman, R. B.,** Specificity of NK cells, in *Human Cancer Immunology,* Vol. 4, Serron, B., Rosenfeld, C., and Herberman, R. B., Eds., Elsevier Biomedical Press, Amsterdam, 1982, 17.
14. **Ortaldo, J. R. and Herberman, R. B.,** Specificity of NK cells, in *Natural Killer Cell,* Serrou, B., Rosenfeld, C., and Herberman, R. B., Eds., Elsevier Biomedical Press, Amsterdam, 1982, 17.
15. **Pollack, S. B.,** Phenotype, functional heterogeneity and lineage of natural killer cells, in *Immunobiology of Natural Killer Cells,* Evalotzova, and Herberman, R. B., Eds., CRC Press, Boca Raton, FL, 1986, 98.
16. **Brooks, C. G., Kuribayashi, K., Sale, G., and Henney, C. S.,** Characterization of five cloned murine cell line showing high cytolytic activity against YAC-1 cells, *J. Immunol.*, 128, 2326, 1982.
17. **Timonen, T., Ortaldo, J. R., and Herberman, R. B.,** Characteristics of human large granular lymphocytes and relationship to natural killer and K cells, *J. Exp. Med.*, 153, 569, 1981.
18. **Luini, W., Boraschi, D., Alberti, S., Aleotti, A., and Tagliabue, A.,** Morphological characterization of a cell population responsible for natural killer activity, *Immunology,* 43, 663, 1981.
19. **Reynolds, C. W., Timonen, T., and Herberman, R. B.,** Natural killer (NK cells) cell activity in the rat. I. Isolation and characterization of the effector cells, *J. Immunol.*, 127, 282, 1981.
20. **Timonen, T. and Saksela, E.,** Isolation of human killer cells by density gradient centrifugation, *J. Immunol. Meth.*, 36, 285, 1980.
21. **Timonen, T., Ortaldo, J. R., and Herberman, R. B.,** Characteristics of human large granular lymphocytes and relationship to natural killer and K cells, *J. Exp. Med.*, 153, 569, 1981.
22. **Timonen, T., Ortaldo, J. R., and Herberman, R. B.,** Analysis by a single cell cytotoxicity assay of natural killer (NK cells) cell frequencies among human large granular lymphocytes and of the effects of interferon on their activity, *J. Immunol.*, 128, 2514, 1982.
23. **Reynalds, C. W. and Ward, J. M.,** Tissue and organ distribution of NK cells, in *Immunology of Natural Killer Cells,* Vol. 1, Lotzova, E. and Herberman, R. B., Eds., CRC Press, Boca Raton, FL, 1986, 64.
24. **Fleit, H. B., Wright, S. D., and Unkeless, J. C.,** Human neutrophil Fcr receptor distribution and structure, *Proc. Natl. Acad. Sci. U.S.A.*, 79, 3275, 1982.
25. **Perussia, B., Starr, S., Abraham, S., Fanning, V., and Trinchieri, G.,** Human natural killer cells analyzed by B73.1, a monoclonal antibody blocking Fc receptor functions. I. Characterization of the lymphocyte subset reactive with B73.1, *J. Immunol.*, 130, 2133, 1983.
26. **Perussia, B., Acuto, O., Terhorst, C., Faust, J., Lazarus, R., Fanning, V., and Trinchieri, G.,** Human natural killer cells analyzed by B73.1, a monoclonal antibody blocking Fc receptor functions. II. Studies of B73.1 antibody-antigen interaction on the lymphocyte membrane, *J. Immunol.*, 130, 2142, 1983.
27. **Kay, H. D. and Horwitz, D. A.,** Evidence by reactivity with hybridoma antibodies for a probable myeloid origin of peripheral blood cells active in natural cytotoxicity and antibody-dependent cell mediated cytotoxicity, *J. Clin. Invest.*, 66, 847, 1980.
28. **Abo, T., Cooper, M. D., and Balch, C. M.,** Characterization of HNK cells-1$^+$ (Leu-7) human lymphocytes. I. Two distinct phenotypes of human NK cells with different cytotoxic capability, *J. Immunol.*, 129, 1752, 1982.
29. **Tam, M. R., Emmon, S. L., and Pollack, S. B.,** Analysis and enrichment of murine natural killer cells with the fluorescence-activated cell sorter, *J. Immunol.*, 124, 650, 1980.
30. **Reynolds, C. W., Sharrow, S. O., Ortaldo, J. R., and Herberman, R. B.,** Natural killer activity in the rat. II. Analysis of surface antigen on LGL by flow cytometry, *J. Immunol.*, 127, 2204, 1981.
31. **Kay, H. D., Bonnard, G. D., West, W. H., and Herberman, R. B.,** A functional comparison of human Fc-receptor bearing lymphocytes active in natural cytotoxicity and antibody-dependent cellular cytotoxicity, *J. Immunol.*, 118, 2058, 1977.
32. **Herberman, R. B.,** Introduction, in *Mechanisms of Cytotoxicity of NK Cells,* Herberman, R. B and Callewaert, D. M., Eds., Academic Press, Orlando, 1985, 1.
33. **Saksela, E., Carpen, O., and Virtanen, I.,** Cellular secretion associated with human natural killer cell activity, in *NK Cells and Other Natural Effector Cells,* Herberman, R. B., Ed., Academic Press, 1982, 983.
34. **Wright, S. C. and Bonavida, B.,** Selective lysis of NK cells-sensitive target cells by a soluble mediator released from murine spleen cells and human peripheral blood lymphocytes, *J. Immunol.*, 126, 1516, 1981.

35. **Strayer, D. R., Cartar, W. A., Mayberry, S. D., Pequignot, E., and Brodsky, I.,** Low natural cytotoxicity of peripheral blood mononuclear cells in individual with high familial incidences of cancer, *Cancer Res.*, 44, 370, 1984.
36. **Riesenfeld, I., Orn, A., Gidlund, M., Axberg, I., Alm, G. V., and Wigzell, H.,** Positive correlation between *in vitro* NK cells activity and *in vivo* resistance toward AKR lymphoma cells, *Int. J. Cancer,* 25, 399, 1980.
37. **Herberman, R. B. and Holden, H. T.,** Natural cell-mediated immunity, *Adv. Cancer Res.*, 27, 305, 1978.
38. **Kiessling, R. and Wigzell, H.,** An analysis of the murine NK cells as to structure function and biological relevance, *Immunol. Rev.*, 44, 165, 1979.
39. **Gorelik, E., Wiltrout, R., Okumura, K., Habu, S., and Herberman, R. B.,** Role of NK cells in the control of metastatic spread and growth of tumor cells in mice, *Int. J. Cancer,* 30, 107, 1982.
40. **Hanna, N. and Fidler, I. J.,** Expression of metastatic potential of allogeneic circulating and xenogeneic neoplasma in young nude mice, *Cancer Res.*, 41, 438, 1981.
41. **Talmadge, J. E., Meyers, K. M., Prieur, D. J., and Starkey, J. R.,** Role of NK cells in tumor growth and metastasis in beige mice, *Nature,* 284, 622, 1980.
42. **Hanna, N.,** Role of natural killer cells in control of cancer metastasis, *Cancer Metastasis Rev.*, 1, 45, 1982.
43. **Bukowski, J. F., Woda, B. A., and Welsh, R. M.,** Pathogenesis of murine cytomegalovirus infection in normal killer cell-depleted mice, *J. Virol.*, 52, 119, 1984.
44. **Ebihara, K. and Minamiskima, Y.,** Protective effect of biological response modifiers on murine cytomegalovirus infection, *J. Virol.*, 51, 117, 1984.
45. **Welsh, R. M., Biron, C. A., Bukowski, J. F., McIntyre, K. W., and Yang, H.,** Role of natural killer cells in virus infection of mice, *Surv. Synth. Pathol. Res.*, 3, 409, 1984.
46. **Welsh, R. M. and Kiessling, R. W.,** Natural killer cell response to lymphocytic chroiomenigitis virus in beige mice, *Scan. J. Immunol.*, 11, 363, 1980.
47. **Eugui, E. M. and Allison, A. C.,** Differences in susceptibility of various mouse strains to haemoprotozoan infections: possible correlation with natural killer activity, *Parasit. Immunol.*, 2, 277, 1980.
48. **Clark, I. A. and Allison, A. C.,** Babesia microt and *Plasmodium berghei yoeli* infection in nude mice, *Nature,* 252, 328, 1974.
49. **Hunter, K. W., Jr., Folks, T. M., Sayler, P. C., and Strickland, G. T.,** Early enhancement followed by suppression of NK cells activity during murine malarial infection, *Immunol. Lett.*, 2, 209, 1981.
50. **Nencioni, L., Villa, L., Boraschi, D., Berti, B., and Tagliabue, A.,** Natural and antibody-dependent cell-mediated activity against *Salmonella typhimurium* by peripheral and intestinal lymphoid cells in mice, *J. Immunol.*, 130, 903, 1983.
51. **Tagiabue, L., Nencioni, L., Villa, L., Keren, D. F., Lowell, G. H., and Boraschi, D.,** Antibody-dependent cell-mediated antibacterial activity of intestinal lymphocytes with secretory IgA, *Nature,* 306, 184, 1983.
52. **Tarkkanen, J., Saksela, E., and Lanier, L. L.,** Bacterial activation of human killer cells, characteristics of the activation process and identification of the effector cells, *J. Immunol.*, 137, 2418, 1986.
53. **Murphy, J. W. and McDaniel, D. O.,** *In vitro* reaction of natural killer (NK cells) cells against *Cryptococcus neoformans, J. Immunol.*, 128, 1577, 1982.
54. **Hidore, M. R. and Murphy, J. W.,** Correlation of natural killer cell activity and clearance of *Cryptococcus neoferemans* from mice after adoptive transfer of splenic nylon wool-nonadherent cells, *Infect. Immunol.*, 51, 547, 1986.
55. **Lotzova, E.,** NK cell role in regulation of the growth and functions of hemopoietic and lymphoid cells, in *Immunobiology of Natural Killer Cell,* Vol. 2, Lotzova, E. and Herberman, R. B., Eds., CRC Press, Boca Raton, FL, 1986, 89.
56. **Abrruzo, L. V. and Rowley, D. A.,** Homeostasis of the antibody response: immunoregulation by NK cells, *Science,* 222, 581, 1983.
57. **Arai, S., Yamamoto, H., Itoh, K., and Kumagar, K.,** Suppressive effect of human natural killer cells on pokeweed mitogen-induced B cell differentiation, *J. Immunol.*, 131, 651, 1983.
58. **Kasahara, T., Djeu, J. Y., Dougherty, S. F., and Oppenheim, J. J.,** Capacity of human large granular lymphocyte (LGL) to produce lymphokines: interleukin-2, interferon and colony stimulating factor, *J. Immunol.*, 131, 2379, 1983.
59. **Scala, G., Allave, P., Djeu, J. Y., Kasahara, T., Ortaho, J. R., Herberman, R. B., and Oppenheim, J. J.,** Human large granular lymphocytes are potential inducers of interleukin-1, *Nature,* 309, 56, 1984.
60. **Domzig, W. and Stadler, B. M.,** The relation between natural killer cells and interleukin-2, in *NK Cells and Other Natural Effect Cells,* Herberman, R. B., Ed., Academic Press, New York, 1982, 409.
61. **Herberman, R. B.,** in *Proc. Int. Symp.: Natural Killer Activity and Its Regulation,* Excerpta Medica, Tokyo, 1983.

62. **Wrights, S. C. and Bonarida, B.,** Studies on the mechanism of natural killer cell-mediated cytotoxicity (CMC). I. Release of cytotoxic factors specific for NK cells-sensitive target cells (NK cellsCF) during co-culture of NK cells effector cell with NK cells target cells, *J. Immunol.,* 129, 433, 1982.
63. **Herberman, R. B., Nunn, M. E., Holden, H. T., Staal, S., and Djeu, J. Y.,** Augmentation of natural cytotoxic reactivity of mouse lymphoid cells against syngeneic and allogeneic target cells, *Int. J. Cancer,* 19, 555, 1977.
64. **Welsh, R. M. and Zinkernagel, R. M.,** Heterospecific cytotoxic cell activity induced during the first three days of acute lymphocytic choriomeningitis virus infection in mice, *Nature,* 268, 646, 1977.
65. **Welsh, R. M.,** Natural cell-mediated immunity during viral infections, in *Natural Resistance to Tumor and Viruses,* Haller, O., Ed., Springer-Verlag, Berlin, 1981, 83.
66. **Gidlund, M., Orn, A., Wigzell, H., Senik, A., and Gesser, I.,** Enhanced NK cells activity in mice infected with interferon interferon-inducer, *Nature,* 273, 759, 1978.
67. **Trinchieri, B. G. and Santoli, D.,** Anti-viral activity induced by culturing lymphocytes with tumor derived or virus-transformed cells. Enhancement of human natural killer cell activity by interferon and antagonistic inhibition of susceptibility of target cells to lysis, *J. Exp. Med.,* 147, 1314, 1978.
68. **Trinchieri, G., Santoli, D., Granato, D., and Perussia, B.,** Antagonistic effects of interferons on the cytotoxicity mediated by natural killer cells, *Fed. Proc. Fed. Am. Soc. Exp. Biol.,* 40, 2705, 1981.
69. **Weish, R. M., Karre, K., Hamsson, M., Kunkel, L. A., and Kiessling, R. W.,** Interferon-mediated protection of normal and tumor target cells against lysis by mouse natural killer cells, *J. Immunol.,* 126, 219, 1981.
70. **Moore, M., White, W. J., and Potter, M. R.,** Modulation of target cell susceptibility to human natural killer cells by interferon, *Int. J. Cancer,* 25, 565, 1980.
71. **Ullberg, M., Merrill, J., and Jondal, M.,** Interferon-induced NK cells augmentation in human: an analysis of target recognition, effector cell recruitment and effector cell recycling, *Scan. J. Immunol.,* 14, 285, 1981.
72. **Fridman, W. H., Gresser, I., Bandu, M. T., Aguet, M., and Neauport-Sautes, C.,** Interferon enhances the expression of Fcr receptor, *J. Immunol.,* 124, 2436, 1980.
73. **Ortaldo, J. R., Mason, A. T., Gerard, J. P., Henderson, L. E., Farrar, W., Hopkins, R. F., III, Herberman, R. B., and Rabin, H.,** Effects of natural and recombinant IL-2 on regulation of τ-IFN production and natural killer activity: lack of involvement of the TAC antigen for these immunoregulatory effects, *J. Immunol.,* 133, 779, 1984.
74. **Weigert, D. A., Stutman, G. J., and Johnson, H. M.,** Interleukin-2 enhances natural killer cell activity through induction of gamma interferon, *Infect. Immunol.,* 41, 992, 1983.
75. **Lattime, E. C., Pecoraro, G. A., and Stutman, O.,** The activity of natural cytotoxic cells is augmented by interleukin-2 and interleukin-3, *J. Exp. Med.,* 157, 1070, 1983.
76. **Leung, K. H. and Koren, H. S.,** Regulation of human natural killing. II. Protective effect of interferon on NK cells from suppression by PEG_2, *J. Immunol.,* 129, 1742, 1982.
77. **Mettews, P. M., Froelich, C. J., Sibbitt, W. L., Jr., and Bankurst, A. D.,** Enhancement of natural cytotoxicity by β-endorphin, *J. Immunol.,* 130, 1658, 1983.
78. **Froelich, C. J. and Bankurst, A. D.,** The effect of β-endorphin on natural cytotoxicity and antibody dependent cellular cytotoxicity, *Life Sci.,* 35, 261, 1984.
79. **Mandler, R. N., Biddison, W. E., Mandler, R., and Serrate, S. A.,** β-Endorphin augments the cytolytic activity and interferon production of natural killer cells, *J. Immunol.,* 136, 934, 1986.
80. **Kay, N., Worley, J. E., and Van Ree, J. M.,** Enhancement of human lymphocyte natural killing function by non-opioid fragments of β-endorphin, *Life Sci.,* 40, 1083, 1987.
81. **Prete, P., Levin, E. R., and Pedram, A.,** The *in vitro* effects of endogenous opiates on natural killer cells, antigen-specific cytolytic T cells and T-cell subsets, *Exp. Neurol.,* 92, 349, 1986.
82. **Peterson, P. K., Sharp, B., Gekker, G., Brummitt, C., and William, F. K.,** Opioid-mediated suppression of interferon-gamma production by cultured peripheral blood mononuclear cells, *J. Clin. Invest.,* 80, 824, 1987.
83. **Shavit, Y., Lewis, J. W., Terman, G. W., Gale, R. P., and Liebskind, J. D.,** Opioid peptides mediate the suppressive effect of stress on natural killer cell cytotoxicity, *Science,* 223, 188, 1984.
84. **Shavit, Y., Terman, G. M., Lewis, J. W., Rane, C. J., Gale, R. P., and Liebskind, J. D.,** Effect of footshock stress and morphine on natural killer lymphocytes in rats: studies of tolerance and cross-tolerance, *Brain Res.,* 372, 382, 1986.
85. **Kraut, R. P. and Greenbery, A. H.,** Effects of endogenous and exogenous opioids on splenic natural killer cell activity, *Nat. Immun. Cell Growth Regul.,* 5, 28, 1986.
86. **Dyke, C. V., Stesin, A., Jones, R., Chuntharapai, A., and Seaman, W.,** Cocaine increases natural killer cell activity, *J. Clin. Invest.,* 77, 1387, 1986.
87. **Saxena, Q. B., Mezey, E., and Adler, W. H.,** Regulation of natural killer activity *in vitro:* the effect of alcohol consumption on human peritoneal blood natural killer activity, *Int. J. Cancer,* 26, 413, 1980.

88. **Mutif, S. I., Darban, H. R., and Watson, R. R.,** Alcohol, cancer and immunomodulation, *Crit. Rev. Oncol./Hematol.*, 9, 243, 1989.
89. **Rice, C., Hudig, D., Lad, P., and Mendelsohn, J.,** Ethanol activation of human natural cytotoxicity, *Immunopharmacology,* 6, 303, 1983.
90. **Ristow, S. S., Starkey, J. R., Hass, G. M.,** Inhibition of natural killer cell activity *in vitro* by alcohols, *Biochem. Biophys. Res. Commun.*, 105, 1315, 1982.
91. **Nair, M. P. N., Sehwartz, S. A., Kronfol, Z. A., Heimen, E. P., Pottahil, R., and Greden, J. F.,** Immunoregulatory effects of alcohol on lymphocyte responses to human immunodeficiency virus proteins, in *Alcohol, Immunomodulation and AIDS,* Alan R. Liss, 1989, 221.
92. **Petitto, J. M., McIntyre, T. D., McRac, B. L., Skolnick, P., and Arora, P. K.,** Differential immune responsiveness in mouse lines sensitively bred for high and low sensitivity to alcohol, *Behavior and Immunity,* 4, 39, 1990.
93. **Rosenberg, E. B., McCoy, J. L., Green, S. S., Donnelly, F. C., Siwarski, D. F., Levine, P. H., and Herberman, R. B.,** *J. Natl. Cancer Inst.*, 52, 345, 1974.
94. **Riccardi, C., Puccetti, P., Santoni, A., and Herberman, R. B.,** Rapid *in vivo* assay of mouse natural killer cell activity, *J. Natl. Cancer Inst.*, 63, 1041, 1979.
95. **Djeu, J. Y., Huang, K. Y., and Herberman, R. B.,** Augmentation of mouse natural killer activity and induction of interferon by tumor cell *in vivo, J. Exp. Med.*, 151, 781, 1980.
96. **Riccardi, C., Santoni, A., Barlozzari, T., Puccetti, P., and Herberman, R. B.,** *In vivo* natural reactivity of mouse against tumor cells, *Int. J. Cancer,* 25, 475, 1980.
97. **Riccardi, C., Santoni, A., Barlozzari, T., and Herberman, R. B.,** Role of NK cells in rapid *in vivo* clearance of radiolabeled tumor cells, in *Natural Cell-Mediated Immunity Against Tumor,* Herberman, R. B., Ed., Academic Press, New York, 1980, 1121.
98. **Callewaert, D. M.,** Quantitation of human natural and antibody-dependent cytotoxicity, in *Natural Cell-Mediated Immunity Against Tumors,* Herberman, R. B., Ed., Academic Press, New York, 1980, 295.

Chapter 6

IN VITRO MEASURES OF MONONUCLEAR PHAGOCYTE FUNCTIONS

Guan-jie Chen, Bernhard Watzl, Dennis S. Huang, Katsuyasu Tachibana, Dennis Way, and Ronald R. Watson

TABLE OF CONTENTS

I. INTRODUCTION

Research in toxicology and pharmacology is in the process of developing *in vitro* methods to reduce the number of animals used for drug testing. With the explosion of information and understanding of the immune system over the past decade, the *in vitro* measurement of cellular immune functions became an important target of research in toxicology and pharmacology.[1-2] Immunotoxicology and immunopharmacology measurements are critical to assess risk/benefits of compounds to all aspects of the host defense system. Immune cells undergo rapid proliferation, which makes the immune system a very sensitive target for toxic compounds. Since the immune system is very interconnected, even minor reductions of single immune functions may result in reduced host resistance.

The immune system represents an important target organ for studying toxicology and pharmacology for the following reasons: (1) immune cells are required for host resistance and so exposure to immunotoxicants can modify susceptibility to infectious diseases and growth of cancer; (2) immunocompetent cells require continued proliferation and differentiation for self-renewal and are sensitive to agents that affect proliferation; and (3) the cellular and molecular biology of the immune system is better understood than many other organ systems; therefore, the mechanisms by which agents are immunoalterative can be determined. Advantages of *in vitro* tests include the isolation of whole organism influences, rapid drug response, measurement of direct effect on cells (dose-response studies), use of genetically stable cell material, and a testing environment that can easily be controlled.[3-5]

Mononuclear phagocytes are derived from myeloid progenitors in the bone marrow. Because of their convenient isolation and ability to be cultured and activated *in vitro,* they are ideal target cells to study toxicological and pharmacological effects of drugs *in vitro*. After proliferation and differentiation, the mononuclear cell normally leaves the bone marrow within 24 h.[6] Promonocytes from the bone marrow differentiate to blood monocytes that are delivered to and circulate for a brief period in the blood stream as immature cells.[7] They migrate from the blood into organs and tissues where they differentiate further into mononuclear phagocytes, which include circulating blood monocytes, free macrophages (peritoneal macrophages), and fixed macrophages in connective tissue (Kupffer cells) or on the endothelial layer of the blood capillaries (microglia and alveolar macrophages) with limited proliferative capacity. Differentiation into macrophages is accompanied by morphological, biochemical, and functional changes. Since macrophages in various tissues exhibit differences in morphological, biochemical, and functional activities,[8] there could be a number of developmentally distinct lineages. In other words, the difference between these macrophages may be enforced by restricted factors which are existing in those tissues, or may be the preselected lineages that will lead them to the home of those particular sites. Specific bone marrow clones may be the precursors of those subclasses of macrophages, and they may have individual unique tissue destination and different capacities for differentiation.[7] However, others believe that both types of heterogenicity—developmental basis and phenotypical induction—probably exist.[9]

The differentiation and proliferation of monocytes is under the influence of soluble mediators.[10] IL-3 (interleukin-3) promotes granulopoiesis and lymphopoiesis; IL-6 (interleukin-6) may cause the further differentiation of macrophages.[10,11] GM-CSF (granulocyte-monocyte colony-stimulating factor) stimulates the proliferation of GM-precursors but not other hemopoietic cells. GM-CSF can enforce GM-precursors from the G_0 phase into the S phase, and the effect is dose-dependent[12] such as higher concentrations of GM-CSF will cause the formation of granulocytic progeny, but lower concentrations will induce the formation of macrophage progeny.[13] Recently, it has been shown that GM-CSF stimulates the proliferation of macrophages via the activation of Na^+/H^+ antiport.[14] There are a series of substances that can modulate the level of GM-CSF including serum lipoproteins,[15] chalones,[16] prostaglandin E_2,[17,18] and environmental factors such as LPS (lipopolysacchride) that can change GM-CSF levels as well.[19,20] Moreover, receptors for these cytokines are found ont he surface of macrophages[21] such as receptors of CSF-1 (colony-stimulating factor -1).[22]

Macrophages play a central role in the host immune response. They participate in humoral and cell-mediated immunity by antigen presentation and by secretion of soluble mediators that can regulate the functions of T and B lymphocytes. Macrophages are very important in the host defense system by chemotaxis, phagocytosis, and cytotoxicity as part of immune survillance.[23] For instance, macrophages have been shown to have cytotoxic functions against bacteria,[24,25] protozoa,[26-28] viruses,[29,30] fungi,[31] and neoplastic cells.[32-35]

Macrophages have also been shown to have extensively biosynthetic capabilities resulting in the secretion of complement components, a wide range of enzymes, interferons, prostaglandins, and numerous other biologically active factors.[36] These factors are able to modulate the activities of the other lymphoreticular cells. Macrophages are critical to the development and regulation of the immune responses as accessory cells to facilitate or as suppressor cells to limit host responses to a stimulus.

The prerequisite of a macrophage function is activation which can be readily measured *in vitro*. Characteristics of macrophage activation include the alteration of metabolic level, enzyme synthesis, and the expression of surface markers.[37] To differentiate, the variation of functional macrophages is often dependent upon the accompaniment of the expression of different surface antigens.[38] It has been shown that Ia (mouse major histocompatibility complex class II) antigen is not involved in the initial binding with antigens, but it is essential in the antigen presenting process.[39] Activated macrophages express Ia, Fc receptors ($Fc_\tau RI$, $Fc_\tau RII$, and $Fc_\tau RIII$)[40], and C3b receptors (CR1 and CR3).[41,42] The expression of different surface antigens is necessary at different anatomical sites or at specific stages of macrophage differentiation. Thus C3b receptors may mediate special function of its maturation.[43,44] Cytokines mediate activation of macrophages including interferons (IFN-α,β, and τ),[45] GM-CSF,[46,47] IL-2 (interleukin-2),[48] IL-3 (interleukin-3),[49,50] IL-4 (interleukin-4),[51,52] MIF (macrophage migration inhibition factor),[53] LAIF (leukocyte adherence inhibition factor),[54] and LPS,[55] as well as autocrine or paracrine IL-1 (interleukin-1).[56-58] IFN-τ is the most effective and versatile activator.[45] It is able not only to stimulate macrophages to increase the expression of MHC class II antigen during 10 min to 4 h, but also the activity of protein kinase C and the concentration of intracellular Ca^{2+} during 4 to 12 h. It also increases the synthesis of several enzymes in macrophages.[59] Different factors may modulate the activation of macrophages in different ways such as via altering the patterns of the expression of macrophage proteins.[60-62] Also, activated macrophages secrete different products to meet the needs of cell functions in different organs or tissues. For example, resident macrophages secrete prostaglandin E_2, hydrogen peroxide,[63] plasminogen activator, or collagenase.[64] There are also many factors that suppress the activation of macrophage, including prostaglandin E_2,[65-68] α_2-macroglobulin protease complexes (α_2MP), transforming growth factor-β (TGF-β),[69] and IFN-α and -β. However, IFN-α and -β have both stimulating and suppressing effects.[59,70]

Many drugs such as cocaine, morphine, and ethanol affect functions and numbers of macrophages. A low dose of cocaine has the tendency toward increasing the number of macrophages, while a high dose induces a decrease tendency.[71] By 24-h post-cocaine injection, phagocytic activity had decreased to 75%.[72] We also observed the different effects on the production of tumor necrosis factor (TNF) by the treatment of cocaine to murine macrophages *in vitro*. Our data indicated that a low dose of cocaine stimulates the TNF production by alveolar macrophages but not by peritoneal macrophages. However, higher doses of cocaine decrease the TNF production by peritoneal macrophage but causes no change in alveolar macrophage.[73] Morphine inhibits the phagocytic activity of peritoneal macrophages.[74] Morphine-pellet implantation attenuates the tumorcidal activity of BCG-elicited peritoneal macrophages.[75] However, the suppression of the tumorcidal activity can be restored by adding IFN-τ *in vitro*. This effect has been proven because of the suppression of IFN-τ production during the morphine-pellet implantation *in vivo*.[76] Ethanol decreases the host resistance to *Pneumonia klebsiella* by reducing TNF production of macrophages[77] and reduces endotoxin-induced serum TNF.[78] Ethanol has also been shown to suppress the functions of macrophages including the inhibition of macrophage migration to lung,[79] the decrease of macrophage adherence, phagocytosis, antibacterial activity, and Fc receptor function *in vitro*,[80-84] and the reduction of bacterial clearance by peritoneal macrophages *in vivo*.[85] For instance, rats fed ethanol for 3 weeks showed reduced clearance and killing of perfused bacteria.[86] Clearly, macrophages play a central role in host immunity.[23-32,35] Therefore, the *in vitro* methodology becomes extremely important to investigate the activities and to evaluate the role of macrophages in the host defense system in physiology, pathology, toxicology, and immunopharmacology.

II. *IN VITRO* METHODS

A. COLLECTION, SEPARATION, AND IDENTIFICATION

1. Collection and Separation

Macrophages can be collected from different tissues and organs.

a. Macrophages from murine peritoneal cavity — Resident or elicited (thioglycollate) macrophages can be collected from the peritoneal cavity. For collection of thioglycollate-elicited macrophages, mice are injected with 1 ml per mouse of thioglycollate medium (2.98 g/100 ml, autoclaved, and stored in the dark for 1 week at room temperature before use) intraperitoneally 5 days before sacrifice. Anesthetized mice are fixed with needles on a board. Blood can be collected from the axillar vein and the skin is opened to expose the abdomen without damaging the abdominal membrane. Five ml of sterile saline containing 10 μ/ml of heparin sodium is injected into the peritoneal cavity by using a 21-gauge needle without sticking the viscera. Gently shake the mouse or press its abdominal wall; then slowly withdraw the exudate from the peritoneal cavity using a 21-gauge needle. Collect the exudate in a 50-ml sterile centrifuge tube which is kept on ice. The procedures of injection and withdrawing are repeated several times until 25 to 30 ml of exudate are obtained. The tubes are centrifuged at 180 g for 10 min, washed, and resuspended with the cells in RPMI-1640 containing 10% of fetal calf serum (FCS). The viability of the cells is checked with trypan blue dye exclusion. Count the cell number in a 1:1 dilution with 4% acetic acid on a hemacytometer, and identify the macrophages by morphological criteria. The cells are distributed into a petri dish and incubated in a 5% CO_2 incubator at 37°C for 2 h. Wash the cells with prewarmed saline (kept in a 37°C water bath) 3 times in order to remove the nonadherent cells. The cells are recollected by using a cell scraper or trypsin solution.

b. Macrophages from murine alveolar lavage — Mice are anesthetized intramuscularly with 0.1 ml per mouse of sodium phenylbarbiturate (1.3 mg/ml). Mice are fixed on a board and the skin around the neck of the mice is sterilized with 70% ethanol. Expose the bronchus and lung by carefully cutting off the tissue, and make a small cut on the upper side of the bronchus which is large enough to insert the sterile silicon rubber tube, which is connected with the open end of the butterfly. Then cut off the needle side of the butterfly (Vacutainer, Becton-Dickinson Co.). Fasten the silicon rubber tube and bronchus connection by using surgical thread. Connect a syringe (1 ml) filled with sterile saline to the open end of the butterfly. Slowly inject 1 ml of saline into the lung. Injecting and aspirating saline into and out of the lung is repeated several times; then the lavage is collected into a 50-ml centrifuge tube which is kept on ice. The procedures of the injection are repeated and lavage is harvested several times until at least 10 ml of the lavage per mouse are collected. The lavage is centrifuged (180 g × 10 min) and the cells are resuspended with RPMI-1640 medium containing 10% FCS and counted. Viability of the cells is measured in the same procedure shown in peritoneal macrophage purification. Normally, more than 90% of the cells in the lavage are macrophages. In the case of infected mice, macrophages may need to be purified by using petri dish adherent procedures to remove lymphocytes which may be present at that condition, as shown in the procedures for peritoneal macrophages.

c. Modified isolation method — A simple improved isolation method was developed and described elsewhere.[87] Briefly, an overnight FCS-coated petri dish is capable of selectively binding macrophages. Mouse macrophages effectively attach after 15 min on a FCS-coated petri dish at 37°C. The adherent cells are easily removed by PBS (0.01 *M* PB, 0.145 *M* NaCl, pH 7.4) containing 0.2% EDTA and 5% FCS (EDTA-FCS). Longer incubation times (40 min) are required to detach mouse macrophages at 4°C.

d. Others — Adherence to glass bead columns or to collagen monolayers.[88]

2. Identification of Macrophages

a. Morphological identification — Macrophages can be identified morphologically under the light microscope, as has been described elsewhere.[89]

b. Cytochemical identification — Macrophages can be identified by using nonspecific esterase-staining methods. Macrophages express positive results on red or reddish-brown staining granules pattern.[90]

Reagents

- Solution A: add 1 g of hexazonium pararochloride (Sigma) in 20 ml of distilled water to 5 ml of prewarmed HCl (12 *N*, kept in 50 to 60°C water bath), which is cooled down, mixed, and then filtered through filter paper; the solution can be stored at 4°C for 3 mo.
- Solution B: 4% sodium nitrite (w/v, Sigma) in distilled water (prepare before use; can be kept at 4°C for only 2 days).
- Solution C: mix an equal volume of A and B solutions, and then adjust pH to 5.0 with 1 *N* NaOH.
- Solution D: 0.1 *M* sodium acetate (Sigma); adjust pH to 5.0 with 2 *M* acetic acid.
- Solution E: mix 10 ml solution D with 1 ml solution C.
- Solution F: 9.5 ml of 1/15 *M* PB (pH 6.3) plus 0.5 ml of solution E.
- Solution G: 10 mg of α-naphthyl butyrate (Sigma) in 0.5 ml of ethylene glycol monoethyl ether (Sigma).
- Solution H: mix F and G, then filter through filter paper (Whatman).

A smear or monolayer slide of macrophages is fixed with 2.5% glutaraldehyde (in PBS or saline, pH 7.2) at 4°C for 20 min. Wash the slide with PBS or saline three times. Then add 15 mg of NaF to 10 ml of solution H; add 2 to 3 drops of this solution to the slide. Incubate the slide for 10 min to 3 h at room temperature. During this period check the color under the microscope. After the color appears, wash the slide three times with PBS, and add 2% methyl green (Sigma). After 5 min, dehydrate the sample with 50%, 80%, and then 100% ethanol. Add xylene, and then use balsam to seal sample with coverslip.

B. FUNCTIONAL ASSAYS

1. Phagocytosis

Interest in immune function and dysfunction has resulted in numerous mononuclear cell phagocytic assays designed to quantify both particulate ingestion and killing. Many assays, however, suffer serious limitations, including low observation numbers when using operator-interactive methodologies. Therefore, flow cytometry (FCM) has risen to the forefront as the method of choice allowing accurate, objective analysis of thousands of cellular events.[91,104,105] Additionally, FCM allows both physical and statistical separation of specific cell types based on their surface, internal, and phagocytic markers.[92] Activation or suppression of phagocytic function and killing *in vivo* and *in vitro* using routine FCM has been well documented.[93] Thus, FCM represents a new technology capable of precise simultaneous measurements of multiple parameters on thousands of cells in seconds, making *in vitro* analysis of toxicological and pharmacological agents simple, accurate, and repeatable.[94,95]

Procedure — Suspensions or whole tissue aggregates $\approx$ 1 mm^3 containing known or suspected phagocytes are adjusted to 1×10^6 phagocytes per ml in a buffered (preferably containing 20 m*M* HEPES) complete medium of pH 7.2. Since FCM allows gating for any definable population, little attention is given to contaminating cell types during preparation. Test particles (i.e., fluorescent microspheres, 1.34 μm diameter, Polyscience, Inc.) are added to the milieu at 1×10^2 to 1×10^4 particles per phagocyte, a level calculated to exceed the maximum per cell phagocytic potential. Incubation times vary from 30 to over 120 min. Using two time points, one typically early and one later, cellular phagocytic transit times can be calculated as a mean fluorescence of all phagocytic cells ($X_{Ft2} - X_{Ft1} / t_2 - t_1 = R_{phagocytosis}$). Polypropylene reaction tubes are incubated ideally in a horizontal position in a 37°C shaking water bath, achieving maximal mixing between particles and cells. Excess beads are removed by layering the reaction mixture over a medium containing 2% BSA (w/v) and centrifuged at 150 × g for 10 min. The supernatant with free beads is aspirated, and the cells are typically washed a second time by centrifugation and resuspended in a FBS-containing complete medium with 10% DMSO and frozen unprotected at −20°C. FCM analysis involves quick-thawing samples at 37°C and staining with 50 μl/ml propidium iodide (PI). Samples are routinely held in this staining milieu overnight at 4°C prior to analysis. The particle (typically GREEN fluorescence) voltage and threshold are set on a pure particle sample, while the size (FALS), smoothness (90° light scatter), and DNA (RED fluorescence) are set from a control cell population. The particle fluorescence voltage settings remain unchanged throughout the collection process, while the cellular parameters may need adjustment if several tissue types or populations are tested consecutively. For determination of population involvement in phagocytosis, ungated collection of all nucleated cells is taken and analyzed for percentage of cells containing one or more beads. In rate determinations, a second gated collection is taken where only cells containing beads are stored for analysis. Using this approach it is possible to determine the frequency of phagocytosis in any given population as well as the rate of phagocytosis and recruitment to the phagocytic process. Thus it is possible to accurately evaluate *in vitro* and *in vivo* alterations to the phagocytic process.

2. Antibody-Dependent Cellular Cytotoxicity (ADCC)

Macrophages have Fc receptors on their surface which enable them to recognize and destroy the target cells by binding to specific antibodies on the surface of target cells. The method for measuring ADCC has been described elsewhere in detail.[96] Briefly, the target cells used for ADCC assay can be erythrocytes or tumor cells lines, and they are usually labeled with isotopes (^{51}Cr, ^{125}I); the effector cells are mononuclear cells and are suspended in RPMI-1640 medium with 5% FCS to a final concentration of 1×10^6 monocytes per ml. The ratio of effector and target cell is 1:1 for erythrocyte target cells and 5 to 25:1 for tumor target cells. Briefly, a mixture of cell suspension with a suitable ratio of target and effector cells containing the appropriate diluted specific antibody against the target cells is incubated for 20 hours. Meanwhile, mix sets for spontaneous release by adding the target cells and specific antibody without effector cells and for maximum release by adding target cells with 1% of NP-40. After incubation, the same amount of supernatants is taken from experimental, spontaneous, and maximum release groups, and radioactivities are measured. Calculate the activity of ADCC according to the formula:

$$\% \text{ Cytotoxicity} = (\text{experimental release} - \text{spontaneous release})/(\text{maximum release} - \text{spontaneous release}) \times 100$$

3. Chemotaxis Assay

Macrophages respond to some soluble mediators that may be secreted by other cells and then migrate toward the attractant in the inflammatory area. The *in vitro* method for measuring chemotaxis has been well documented elsewhere (see References 97 and 98 for details).

4. Nonspecific Cytotoxicity against Microorganisms

Besides natural killer cells, macrophages accomplish natural cytotoxicity to microorganisms as well. Several *in vitro* assays have been set up well to detect nonspecific cytotoxicity.[99] The nonspecific cytotoxicity assay is designed to investigate the lytic effect directly via the release of radioactivity from isotope-prelabeled target microorganisms. The radioactive compounds include ^{51}Cr, ^{111}In, [^{3}H] thymidine, [^{3}H] proline, and [^{125}I] iododeoxyuridine.

Procedures — The isolation of microorganisms as well as peritoneal mononuclear phagocytes and isotope-labeling [^{3}H]TdR of microorganisms is as described in detail previously.[99] Briefly, different concentrations of effector cells are coincubated with labeled target cells in 96 U-bottom plates (Falcon) for 48 h at 37°C. At the end of the incubation period, supernatant is collected after centrifugation of the plates. The spontaneous release is determined by adding the targets without effector cells in the well. The maximum release is measured by adding the labeled targets with 0.1 ml 10% sodiumdodecylsulfate (SDS). The percentage of lysis is calculated:

$$\% \text{ Cytotoxicity} = (\text{cpm of samples} - \text{cpm of spontaneous release})/(\text{cpm of maximum release} - \text{cpm of spontaneous release}) \times 100$$

5. Macrophage-Mediated Tumor Cytotoxicity

Macrophage-mediated tumor cytotoxicity *in vitro* was studied by a radioactive release assay detailed elsewhere.[100] Mononuclear phagocytes are collected from either normal or experimental (test) groups. Target cells in the exponential growth phase are labeled with [^{125}I] iododeoxyuridine (Amersham International Ltd., Bucks, England) for 24 h. After harvesting the target cells, they are counted and adjusted to the desired cell concentration. After purification, a series of suspensions of effector cells in different concentrations are prepared as well. Labeled target cells are then coincubated with different concentrations of effector cells for 72 h at 37°C. Finally, the adherent cells are lyzed by adding to each well 0.1 ml of 0.5 *N* NaOH. The cytotoxic activity is calculated by measuring the radioactivity of the lysate as follows:

$$\% \text{ Cytotoxicity} = (\text{cpm in target cells cultured with normal mononuclear phagocytes} - \text{cpm in target cells cultured with test mononuclear phagocytes})/(\text{cpm in target cells cultured with mononuclear phagocytes}) \times 100$$

6. Production and Quantitation of Cytokines

Macrophages are capable of being cultured *in vitro* and stimulated by mitogen to produce cytokines, including IL-1, IL-6, TNF, and interferon α and β (IFN-α/β). For instance, cultured murine peritoneal macrophages are stimulated with LPS for the production of TNF. The level of TNF in culture supernatants will be measured by using enzyme-linked immunosorbent assay (ELISA):

a. Macrophage culture — Collect the macrophages as described before and count the macrophage cell number according to their morphological criteria or nonspecific esterase staining. Adjust the cell number to 1×10^6/ml and then add 200 μl of cell suspension to individual wells of a 96-well plate (Falcon 3072). The plate is incubated at 37°C, 5% CO_2 incubator for 1 to 2 h. Wash the plate with prewarmed saline or PBS (kept in 37°C water bath) 3 times (add saline or PBS, then aspirate the supernatant), and then add 100 μl of complete RPMI-1640 medium (containing 10% FCS, 100 μ/ml of penicillin and 100 μg/ml of streptomycin, 2 m*M* of glutamine) to the cells. LPS in RPMI-1640 is added to the cell suspension. Final concentration of LPS for murine peritoneal macrophage is 0.1 to 1.0 μg/ml. Incubate the plate at 37°C, 5% CO_2 incubator for 24 h. Centrifuge the plate at 180 g for 10 min, and transfer the supernatant to microtubes on the rack (Bio-Rad, 1 ml capacity, size: 8.8 × 45 mm) by using multichannel pipettes (Costar, 100 μl fixed volume). Keep the samples at −70°C until measuring. Recently, an improved method for culturing murine splenic macrophages has been described.[101]

b. Determination of TNF in macrophage culture supernatant by using an ELISA method — Coat the 96-well ELISA plate (Dynatech Immulon 2) with 50 μl of hamster anti-murine TNF monoclonal antibody (Genzyme, diluted 1:500 in carbonate buffer, pH 9.6) and store at 4°C overnight. Wash once with PBS-Tween (0.01 *M* PBS containing 0.145 *M* of NaCl and 0.05% Tween), then dry the plate, add 100 μl of BSA (bovine serum albumin, 1% w/v in 0.01 *M* PBS) to each well, and incubate the plate at 37°C for 2 h. Add 50 μl of standards (series dilution of recombinant murine TNF [Genzyme] diluted in complete RPMI-1640 medium), or macrophage supernatant samples to 96-well plate. Incubate the plate at 37°C for 1 h. Wash and dry the plate, then add 50 μl of rabbit antimurine TNF polyclonal antibody (obtained from Genzyme and diluted 1:125 in PBS-Tween) to each well and incubate at 37°C for 1 h. Wash and dry the plate as before, then add 50 μl of goat anti-rabbit IgG horseradish peroxidase conjugate (American Qualex, diluted in 1:5000 in PBS-Tween) to each well, and incubate the plate at 37°C for 1 h. Wash the plate with PBS-Tween 3 times and once with PBS. After carefully drying the plate, 100 μl of ABTS (0.54 g of 2,2-azino-bis-[3-ethylbenzthiazoline]-6-sulfonic acid, Sigma, and 21.0 g of citric acid monohydrate, in 1 liter of water, pH 4.2, with final concentration of 0.03% H_2O_2) is added to each well. Incubate the plate at room temperature for 30 min. The optical density is measured by spectophotometry (Titertek Multiskan Plus) at 405 nm. Detection limit: 10 pg per well (0.2 ng/ml).

7. Production and Quantitation of Prostaglandins

Prostaglandins are important regulatory factors of the function of macrophages. The methods for quantitation of prostaglandins are well documented[102] and several commercial kits are available.

III. EVALUATION OF *IN VITRO* CULTURE OF MACROPHAGES TO REPRESENT *IN VIVO* FUNCTION

Mononuclear phagocytes are available in large numbers from various tissues to study their functions *in vitro*, especially if one recognizes the problems of isolation, purification, and cell-cell interactions. While primary murine mononuclear phagocytes grow readily in short-term culture, they are unable to replicate under *in vitro* conditions except under special circumstances.[103] The content of the serum supplements markedly affects macrophage functions which include antibody, hormone, and lipid content as well as the variation with respect to contamination by bacterial endotoxin or other growth or toxic factors among different batches of serum. Although the attachment can be useful for macrophage enrichment by washing away nonadherent cells, the progress in detachment of macrophages may cause cell membrane damage or loss. If this is critical, one can use these cells cultured initially,[103] isolated (mixed cells), or a macrophage cell line. Furthermore, macrophages are very sensitive to environmental changes. For example, macrophages carry out endocytosis toward serum components and plastic culture surfaces because the cell culture on plastic in a medium with FCS is a different environment than that of *in vivo*.[88] The longer these cells are in culture, the less they resemble their *in vivo* counterparts.[103] Nevertheless, macrophages can be recovered in high yield after adherence and subsequently show high ability (80 to 100%) to readhere, as well as phagocytosis, and to secrete cytokines. To use these responsive cells to study and interpret the host immunocompetency, the time of *in vitro* maintenance and culture-induced morphologic, functional, and biochemical changes need to be carefully evaluated.

However, mononuclear phagocytes are easily distinguished by the red or reddish-brown staining granules pattern after nonspecific esterase staining; the granules of esterase reaction product may also be found in T lymphocytes and null cells.[87] Therefore, the most efficiency in the cell determination is utilized by the combination of several techniques to characterize the criteria of mononuclear phagocyte populations.

ACKNOWLEDGMENT

This work was supported by NIH research grants AA 08037 and DA 04827.

REFERENCES

1. **Luster, M. L., Munson, A. E., Thomas, P. T., Holsapple, M. P., Fenters, J. D., White, K. L., Lauer, L. D., Germolec, D. R., and Dean, J. H.,** Development of a testing battery to assess chemical-induced immunotoxicity: National Toxicology Program's guidelines for immunotoxicity evaluation in mice, *Fund. Appl. Toxicol.*, 10, 2, 1988.
2. **Luster, M. L., Ackermann, M. F., Germolec, D. R., and Rosenthal, G. J.,** Perturbations of the immune system by xenobiotics, *Environ. Health Perspect.*, 81, 157, 1989.
3. **Stengerg, K.,** Cellular methods for measuring drug toxicity *in vitro, TIPS,* June, 218, 1986.
4. **Flamm, W. G. and Lorentzen, R. J.,** The use of *in vitro* methods in safety evaluation, *In Vitro Toxicol.*, 1, 1, 1987.
5. **Norbury, K. C. and Thomas, P. T.,** Assessment of immunotoxicity, in *Handbook of In Vivo Toxicity,* Arnold, D. L., Grice, H. C., and Krewski, D. K., Eds., Academic Press, New York, 1990, 409.
6. **Furth, R. V.,** Phagocytic cells, in *Inflammation, Basic Principles, and Clinical Correlations,* Gallin, J., Goldstein, I., and Snyderman, R., Eds., Raven Press, New York, 1988.
7. **Silverstein, S. C.,** Membrane receptors and the regulation of mononuclear phagocyte effector functions, in *Macrophages and Natural Killer Cells,* Norman, S. J. and Sorkin, E., Eds., Plenum Press, New York, 1982, 21.
8. **Happner, G. H. and Fulton, A. M.,** Macrophage heterogeneity, in *Macrophages and Cancer,* Happner, G. H. and Fulton, A. M., Eds., CRC Press, Boca Raton, FL, 1988, 2.
9. **Metcalf, D.,** Macrophage heterogeneity, in *Mononuclear Phagocyte Biology,* Volkman, A., Marcel Dekker, New York, 1984, 489.

10. **Sachs, L., Lotem, J., and Shabo, Y.,** The molecular regulations of macrophage and granulocyte development — Role of MG I-2/IL-6, *Ann. N.Y. Acad. Sci.*, 557, 417, 1989.
11. **Van-Snick, J.,** Interleukin-6: an overview, *Annu. Rev. Immunol.*, 8, 253, 1990.
12. **Burgess, A. W. and Metcalf, D.,** Colony-stimulating factor and the differentiation of granulocytes and macrophages, in *Experimental Hematology Today*, Baum, S. J. and Ledney, G. D., Eds., Springer Verlag, Heidelberg, 1977, 135.
13. **Metcalf, D.,** Clonal analysis of proliferation and differentiation of paired daughter cells: action of granulocyte-macrophage colony-stimulating factor on granulocyte-macrophage precursors, *Proc. Natl. Acad. Sci. U.S.A.*, 77, 5327, 1980.
14. **Vallance, S. J., Dowers, C. P., Cragoe, E. J., and Whetton, A. D.,** Granulocyte-macrophage colony-stimulating factor can stimulate macrophage proliferation via persistent activation of Na+/H+ antiport. Evidence for two distinct role for Na+/H+ antiport activation, *Biochem. J.*, 265, 359, 1990.
15. **Metcalf, D. and Rusell, S.,** Inhibition by mouse serum of hemopoietic colony formation *in vitro, Exp. Hematol.*, 4, 339, 1976.
16. **Paukorits, W. R. and Hinterberger, W.,** Molecular weight and some chemical properties of the granulocyte chalone, *Blut*, 37, 7, 1978.
17. **Williams, N.,** Preferential inhibition of murine macrophages colony formation by prostaglandin E, *Blood*, 53, 1089, 1979.
18. **Pelus, L. M., Broxmeyer, H. E., Kurland, J. I., and Moore, M. A. S.,** Regulation of macrophage and granulocyte proliferation: specificities of prostaglandin E and Lactoferrin, *J. Exp. Med.*, 150, 277, 1979.
19. **Kurland, J. I., Broxmeyer, H. E., Pelus, L. M., Bockman, R. S., and Moore, A. S.,** Role of monocyte-macrophage derived colony-stimulating factor and prostaglandin E in the positive and negative feedback control of myeloid stem cell proliferation, *Blood*, 52, 388, 1978.
20. **Corradin, B. and Mauel, J.,** Phagocytosis of leishmania enhances macrophage activation by IFN-τ and lipopolysaccharide, *J. Immunol.*, 146, 279, 1991.
21. **Gorden, S., Perry, V. H., Rabinowitz, S., Chung, L.-P., and Rosen, H.,** Plasma membrane receptors of the mononuclear phagocyte system, in *Macrophage Plasma Membrane Receptors*, Gorden, S., Ed., Company of Biologists, Cambridge, 1988, 1.
22. **Rettenmier, C. N., Roussel, M. F., and Sheer, C. J.,** The colony-stimulating factor-1 (CSF-1) receptor and its ligand, in *Macrophage Plasma Membrane Receptors*, Gorden, S., Ed., Company of Biologists, Cambridge, 1988, 27.
23. **Gjoen, T., Seljelid, R., and Kolset, S. O.,** Binding of metastatic colon carcinoma cells to liver macrophage, *J. Leukocyte Biol.*, 45, 362, 1988.
24. **North, R. J.,** in *Mechanisms of Cell-mediated Immunity*, McClusky, R. J. and Cohen, S., Eds., John Wiley & Sons, New York, 1974, 185.
25. **Rook, G. A.,** The role of activated macrophage in protection and immunopathology in tuberculosis, *Res. Microbiol.*, 14, 253, 1990.
26. **Murray, H. W., Juangbhanich, C. W., Nathan, C. F., and Cohn, Z. A.,** Macrophage oxygen-dependent antimicrobial activity. II. The role of oxygen intermediates, *J. Exp. Med.*, 150, 950, 1979.
27. **Wegueira, N., Kaplan, G., and Cohn, Z. A.,** in *The Mononuclear Phagocyte*, Furth, R. V., Ed., Martinus Nijhoff, The Hague, 1980, 1587.
28. **Gattegno, L., Staffar, L., and Vaysse, J.,** Inhibition by monoclonal antibody anticomplement type 1 on interaction between senescent human red blood cells and monocytic-macrophagic cell, *J. Leucocyte Biol.*, 45, 422, 1989.
29. **Lemerle, S.,** Macrophage activation syndrome linked to Epstein-Barr virus, *Ann. Pediatr. (Paris)*, 36, 539, 1989.
30. **Lucchiari, M. A. and Pereira, C. A.,** A major role of macrophage activation by interferon-gamma during mouse hepatitis virus type 3 infection: genetically dependent resistance, *Immunobiology*, 180, 12, 1989.
31. **Flesch, I. E., Schwamberger, G., and Kaufmann, S. H. E.,** Fungicidal activity of IFN-gamma-activated macrophage: extracellular killing of cryptococcus neofermans, *J. Immunol.*, 142, 3219, 1989.
32. **Nathan, C. F., Silverstein, S. C., Brukner, L. H., and Cohn, Z. A.,** Extracellular cytolysis by activated macrophages and granulocytes: hydrogen peroxide as a mediator of cytotoxicity, *J. Exp. Med.*, 149, 100, 1979.
33. **Nathan, C. F., Nogueir, N., Juangbhanich, C., Ellis, J., and Cohn, Z. A.,** Activation of macrophage *in vitro:* correlation between hydrogen peroxide release and killing of *Trypanosoma cruzi, J. Exp. Med.*, 149, 1056, 1979.
34. **Fidler, I. J.,** Eradication of cancer metastasis by tumoricidal macrophages, *Adv. Exp. Med. Biol.*, 233, 415, 1988.
35. **Bielat, K. L., Halpern, J., Simich, J., Huben, R. P., and Ambrus, J. L.,** A morphological analysis of an *in vitro* model of cytotoxic antitumor activity, *Cancer Detect. Prev.*, 12, 1, 1988.

36. **Decker, K.,** Biological active products of stimulated liver macrophages (Kupffer cells), *Eur. J. Biochem.*, 192, 245, 1990.
37. **Reichard, S. and Kojima, M.,** Section V. Surface and receptors of mononuclear phagocytes, in *Macrophage Biology*, Reichard, S. and Kojima, M., Eds., Alan R. Liss, New York, 1985, 407.
38. **Becker, S. and Takiguchi, M.,** Enhanced Ia density induced by interferon-gamma results in enhanced accessory function by human monocytes, in *Macrophage Biology*, Reichard S. and Kojima, M., Eds., Alan R. Liss, New York, 1985, 455.
39. **Ziegler, K. and Unanue, E. R.,** Identification of a macrophage antigen-processing event required for I-region-restricted antigen presentation to T lymphocytes, *J. Immunol.*, 127, 1869, 1981.
40. **Mellman, I.,** Structure and function of Fc receptors on macrophages and lymphocytes, *J. Cell. Sci. Suppl.*, 9, 45, 1988.
41. **Law, S. K. A.,** C_3 receptor on macrophages, in *Macrophage Plasma Membrane Receptor*, Gorden, S., Ed., Company of Biologists, Cambridge, 1988, 67.
42. **Law, S. K.,** C_3 receptors on macrophages, *J. Cell. Sci. Suppl.*, 9, 67, 1988.
43. **Griffin, F. M. and Mullinax, R. J.,** Augmentation of macrophage complement receptor function in vitro. III. C_3b receptors that promote phagocytosis migrate within the plane of the macrophage plasma membrane, *J. Exp. Med.*, 154, 291, 1981.
44. **Wright, S. D. and Silverstein, S. C.,** Complement receptor modulation and function in cultured human monocytes, *J. Cell Biol.*, 91, 255a, 1981.
45. **Fuchs, H. J., Czarniecki, C. W., Chiu, H. H., Sniezek, M., and Shellito, J. E.,** Interferon-gamma increases alveolar macrophage Ia antigen expression despite oral administration of dexamethasone to rats, *Am. J. Respir. Cell. Mol. Biol.*, 1, 525, 1989.
46. **Smith, P. D., Lamerson, C. L., Banks, S. M., Saini, S. S., Wahl, L. M., Calderone, R. A., and Wahl, S. M.,** Granulocyte-macrophage colony-stimulating factor augments human monocyte fungicidal activity for *Candida albicans*, *J. Infect. Dis.*, 161, 999, 1990.
47. **Ho, J. L., Reed, S. G., Wick, E. A., and Giordano, M.,** Granulocyte-macrophage and macrophage-colony-stimulating factor activate intramacrophage killing of *Leishmania mexicana amazonasis*, *J. Infect. Dis.*, 162, 224, 1990.
48. **Kos, F. J.,** Augmentation of recombinant interleukin-2-dependent murine macrophage-mediated tumor cytotoxicity by recombinant tumor necrosis factor-alpha, *Immunol. Cell. Biol.*, 67 (Pt):433, 1989.
49. **Frendl, G. and Beller, D. I.,** Regulation of macrophage activation by IL-3. I. IL-3 functions as a macrophage-activating factor with unique properties, including Ia and lymphocyte function-associated antigen-1, but not cytotoxicity, *J. Immunol.*, 144, 3392, 1990.
50. **Frendl, G. and Beller, D. I.,** Regulation of macrophage by interleukin-3. Interleukin-3 and lipopolysaccharide act synergistically in the regulation of interleukin-1 expression, *J. Immunol.*, 144, 3400, 1990.
51. **Phillips, W. A., Croatto, M., and Hamilton, J. A.,** Priming the macrophage respiratory burst with interleukin-4:enhancement with TNF-alpha but inhibition by IFN-gamma, *Immunology*, 70, 498, 1990.
52. **Flesch, I. E. A. and Kaufmann, S. H. E.,** Activation of tuberculostatic macrophage functions by gamma-interferon, IL-4 and tumor necrosis factor, *Infect. Immunol.*, 58, 2675, 1990.
53. **Chess, L., Rocklin, R. E., MacDermott, R. P., David, J. R., and Schlossman, S. F.,** Leukocyte inhibition factor (LIF):production by purified human T and B lymphocytes, *J. Immunol.*, 115, 315, 1975.
54. **Powell, A. E., Sloss, A. M., and Smith, R. N.,** Leukocyte-adherence inhibition: a specific assay of cell-mediated immunity dependent on lymphokine-mediated collaboration between T lymphocytes, *J. Immunol.*, 120, 1957, 1978.
55. **Isogai, E.,** Macrophage activation by leptospiral lipopolysaccharide, *Int. J. Med. Microbiol.*, 273, 200, 1990.
56. **Fieren, M. W. J. A., Van den Bend, G. J. C. M., and Bonta, I. L.,** Increased *in vitro* release of interleukin-1 by LPS stimulated peritoneal macrophage obtained from patients on continuous ambulatory peritoneal dialysis (CAPD) during an infectious peritonitis, *Agents Actions*, 29, 30, 1990.
57. **Jacobs, R. F., Tabor, D. R., Burks, A. W., and Campbell, G. D.,** Elevated interleukin-1 release by human alveolar macrophage during the adult respiratory distress syndrome, *Am. Rev. Respir. Dis.*, 140, 1686, 1989.
58. **Bowers, W. E., Ruhoff, M. S., and Goodell, E. M.,** Conditioned medium from activated rat macrophage and the recombinant factors, IL-1 beta and GM-CSF, enhance the accessory activity of dentritic cells, *Immunobiology*, 180, 362, 1990.
59. **Adams, D. O.,** Molecular interaction in macrophage activation, *Immunol. Today*, 10, 33, 1989.
60. **Largen, M. T. and Tannenbaum, C. S.,** LPS regulation of specific protein synthesis in murine peritoneal macrophages, *J. Immunol.*, 136, 988, 1986.
61. **Tannenbaum, C. S., McKernan, L. N., and Largen, M. T.,** Differential protein synthesis by murine peritoneal macrophage elicited by various stimuli, *J. Leukocyte Biol.*, 41, 527, 1987.

62. **MacKay, R. J., Pace, J. L., Jappe, M. A., and Ruseell, S. W.,** Macrophage activation-associated proteins: characterization of stimuli and conditions needed for expression of proteins 47 b, 71/73, and 120, *J. Immunol.*, 142, 1639, 1989.
63. **Nathan, C. F., Brukner, L. H., Silverstein, S. C., and Cohn, Z. A.,** Extracellular cytolysis by activated macrophages and granulocytes. I. Pharmacologic triggering of effector cells and the release of hydrogen peroxide, *J. Exp. Med.*, 149, 84, 1979.
64. **Gordon, S.,** in *The Mononuclear Phagocyte*, Furth, R. V., Ed., Martinus Nijhoff, The Hague, 1980, 1273.
65. **Wahl, L. M., Olsen, C. E., Sandberg, A. L., and Mergenhagen, S. E.,** Prostaglandin regulation of macrophage collagenase production, *Proc. Natl. Acad. Sci. U.S.A.*, 74, 4955, 1977.
66. **Znilling, B. S. and Justement, L. B.,** Prostaglandin regulation of macrophage function, in *Macrophage and Cancer*, Heppner, G. H. and Hulton, A. M., Eds., CRC Press, Boca Raton, FL, 1988, 61.
67. **Kozlov, V., Poveshchenko, A., and Gromykhina, N.,** Some mechanisms involved in the prostaglandin E_2 immunosuppressive effect in (CBA × C57 BL) F1 mice *in vivo*, *Cell. Immunol.*, 128, 242, 1990.
68. **Parhar, R. S. and Lala, P. K.,** Prostaglandin E_2-mediated inactivation of various killer lineage cells by tumor-bearing host macrophages, *J. Leukocyte Biol.*, 44, 474, 1989.
69. **Tsunawaski, S., Sporn, M., and Nathan, C.,** Comparison of transforming growth factor-beta and a macrophage-deactivating polypeptides from tumor cells. Differences in antigeniecity and mechanism of action, *J. Immunol.*, 142, 3462, 1989.
70. **Kato, T., Kitaura, M., Inaba, K., Watanabe, Y., Kawade, Y., and Muramatsu, S.,** Supression of macrophage Ia expression by endogenous interferon-alpha/beta, *J. Interferon Res.*, 9, 393, 1989.
71. **Bagasra, O. and Forman, L.,** Functional analysis of lymphocytes subpopulations in experimental cocaine abuse I. Dose-dependent activation of lymphcyte subsets, *Clin. Exp. Immunol.*, 77, 289, 1989.
72. **Ou, D. W., Shen, M.-L., and Luo, Y.-D.,** Effects of cocaine on the immune system of BALB/C mice, *Clin. Immunol. Immunopathol.*, 52, 305, 1989.
73. **Chen, G.-J., Tachibana, K., Huang, D. S., and Watson, R. R.,** Cocaine modulation of tumor necrosis factor by macrophages from retrovirally infected mice, submitted for publication.
74. **Casellas, A. M., Guardiola, H., and Renard, F. L.,** Inhibition by opioids of phagocytosis in peritoneal macrophages, *Neuropeptides*, 18, 35, 1991.
75. **Bryant, H. U., Yoburn, B. C., Inturrisi, C. E., Bernton, E.W., and Holaday, J. W.,** Morphine-induced immunomodulation is not related to serum morphine concentration, *Eur. J. Pharmacol.*, 149, 165, 1988.
76. **Hung, C. Y., Lefkowitz, S. S., and Geber, W. F.,** Interferon inhibition by narcotic analysis, *Proc. Soc. Exp. Biol. Med.*, 142, 106, 1973.
77. **Nelson, S., Bagby, G. J., and Summer, W. R.,** Alcohol-induced suppression of tumor necrosis factor — a potential risk factor for secondary infection in the acquired immunodeficiency syndrome, in *Alcohol, Immunomodulation and AIDS*, Alan R. Liss, New York, 1990, 211.
78. **D'Souza, N. B., Bagby, G. J., Nelson, S., Lang, H. C., and Spitzer, J. J.,** Acute alcohol infusion suppresses endotoxin-induced serum tumor necrosis factor, *Alcoholism Clin. Exp. Res.*, 13, 295, 1989.
79. **Guarneri, J. J. and Laurenzi, G. A.,** Effect of ethanol on the mobilization of alveolar macrophages, *J. Lab. Clin. Med.*, 72, 40, 1968.
80. **Rimland, D. and Hand, W. L.,** The effect of ethanol on adherence and phagocytosis by rabbit alveolar macrophages, *J. Lab. Clin. Med.*, 95, 918, 1980.
81. **Rimland, D.,** Mechanisms of ethanol-induced defeats of alveolar macrophage function, *Alcoholism*, 8, 73, 1983.
82. **Bagasra, O., Howeedy, A., and Kajdacsy-Balla, A.,** Macrophage function in chronic experimental alcoholism. I. Modulation of surface receptors and phagocytosis, *Immunology*, 65, 405, 1988.
83. **Mirland, B. and Mirland, J.,** Reduced Fc receptor function in human monocytes exposed to ethanol *in vitro*, *Alcohol Alcoholism*, 19, 211, 1984.
84. **Gilhus, N. E. and Matre, R.,** *In vitro* effects of ethanol on subpopulations of human blood mononuclear cells, *Int. Arch. Allergy Appl. Immunol.*, 68, 382, 1982.
85. **Louria, D. B.,** Susceptibility to infection during experimental alcoholic intoxication, *Trans. Assoc. Am. Physicians*, 76, 102, 1963.
86. **Galente, D., Andreans, A., and Perna, P.,** Decreased phagocytic and bactericidal activity of the hepatic reticuloendothelial system during chronic ethanol treatment and its restoration by levamisole, *J. Reticuloendothel. Soc.*, 32, 179, 1982.
87. **Miller, G. A. and Morahan, P. S.,** Use of nonspecific esterase stain, in *Methods for Studying Mononuclear Phagocytes*, Adams, D. O., Edelson, P. J., and Koren, H. S., Eds., Academic Press, New York, 1981, 367.
88. **Hester, R. B. and Walker, W. S.,** Separation of murine mononuclear phagocytes by density gradients of percoll, in *Methods for Studying Mononuclear Phagocytes*, Adams, D. O., Edelson, P. J., and Koren, H. S., Eds., Academic Press, New York, 1981, 195.

89. **Carr, I.,** Morphological identification of macrophages, in *Manual of Macrophage Methodology,* Herscowitz, H. B., Holden, H. T., Bellanti, J. A., and Ghaffar, A., Eds., Marcel Dekker, New York, 1974, 187.
90. **Stadnyk, A. W., Befus, A. D., and Gauldie, J.,** Characterization of nonspecific esterase activity in macrophages and intestinal epithelium of the rat, *J. Histochem. Cytochem.,* 381, 1, 1990.
91. **Bjerknes, R., Bassoc, C., Sjursen, H., Laerum, O., and Solberg, C.,** Flow cytometry for the study of phagocyte function, *Rev. Infect. Dis.,* II, 16, 1989.
92. **Doolittle, M., Bohman, R., Durstenfeld, A. and Cascarano, J.,** Identification and characterization of liver nonparenchymal cells by flow cytometry, *Hepatology,* 7, 696, 1987.
93. **Cummings, N. P., Pabst, M. J., and Johnston, R. B.,** Activation of macrophages for enhanced release of superoxide anion and greater killing of *Candida albicans* by injection of muramyl dipeptide, *J. Exp. Med.,* 152, 1659, 1980.
94. **Steinkamp, J. A., Wilson, J. S., Saunders, G. C., and Stewart, C. C.,** Phagocytosis: flow cytometric quantitation with fluorescent microspheres, *Science,* 215, 64, 1982.
95. **Stewart, C. C., Lehnert, B. E., and Steinkamp, J. A.,** *In vitro* and *in vivo* measurement of phagocytosis by flow cytometry, *Meth. Enzymol.,* 132, 183, 1986.
96. **Koren, H. S.,** Antibody-dependent cellular cytotoxicity — lysis of hapten-modified target cells, in *Manual of Macrophage Methodology,* Herscowitz, H. B., Holden, H. T., Bellanti, J. A., and Ghaffar, A., Eds., Marcel Dekker, New York, 1981, 315.
97. **Boyden, S.,** The chemotactic effect of mixture of antibody and antigen on polymorphonuclear leucocytes, *J. Exp. Med.,* 115, 453, 1962.
98. **Lohr, K. M. and Snyderman, R.,** *In vitro* methods for the study of macrophage chemotaxis, in *Manual of Macrophage Methodology,* Herscowitz, H. B., Holden, H. T., Bellanti, J. A., and Ghaffar, A., Eds., Marcel Dekker, New York, 1981, 303.
99. **Landolfo, S., Giovanna, M., and Martinetto, P.,** Macrophage natural cytotoxicity against *Trichomonas vaginalis,* in *Manual of Macrophage Methodology,* Herscowitz, H. B., Holden, H. T., Bellanti, J. A., and Ghaffar, A., Eds., Marcel Dekker, New York, 1981, 297.
100. **Tachibana, K., Sone, D., Tsubura, E., and Kishino, Y.,** Stimulatory effect of vitamin A on tumoricidal activity of rat alveolar macrophages, *Br. J. Cancer,* 49, 343, 1984.
101. **Crocker, P. R., Hill, M., and Gorden, S.,** Regulation of a murine macrophage haemaggulutinin (sheep erythrocyte receptors) by a species-restricted serum factor, *Immunology,* 65, 515, 1988.
102. **Wahl, L. M.,** Production and quantitation of prostaglandins, in *Manual of Macrophage Methodology,* Herscowitz, H. B., Holden, H. T., Bellanti, J. A., and Ghaffar, A., Eds., Marcel Dekker, New York, 1981, 423.
103. **Meltzer, M. S.,** Peritoneal mononuclear phagocytes from small animals, in *Methods for Studying Mononuclear Phagocytes,* Adams, D. O., Edelson, P. J., and Koren, H. S., Eds., Academic Press, New York, 1981, 63.
104. **Case, T., Way, D., Witte, M., Larson, D., Witte, C., and Copeland, J.,** *In vitro* phagocytosis of fluorescent microspheres by coronary vascular endothelial cell lines from human heart transplant recipients, *Clin. Res.,* 39, 146A, 1991.
105. **Ramirez, G., Case, T. C., Borgs, P., Way, D. L., and Whitte, M. H.,** *In vitro* phagocytosis by endothelial cell lines of different origins, *Clin. Res.,* 39, 274A, 1991.

Chapter 7

AN *IN VITRO* NEPHROTOXICITY ASSAY IN RENAL PROXIMAL TUBULES

J. F. Sina and M. O. Bradley

TABLE OF CONTENTS

I. INTRODUCTION

The kidney is a major site of xenobiotic-induced toxicity, due to such factors as the large volume of blood it filters and the organ's reabsorption characteristics. Whole animal studies rely upon such endpoints as measurement of enzyme (BUN/creatinine) elevations in the serum or morphological evaluation (in terminal experiments) to indicate whether a compound is toxic. However, for mechanistic studies or more precise definition of the toxic insult, it would be valuable to have an *in vitro* model which is well characterized and effectively mimics specific nephron segments. Such a method would complement the animal work by providing a system where one has better control of experimental variables such as extrarenal influences (hormonal, physiological), animal-to-animal variation, etc.

In vitro studies of renal toxicity (as well as physiology, pharmacology, biochemistry) have been performed using a number of tissue preparations ranging from whole perfused organ[1,2] to slices[3,4] to tubule segments[5] to cells,[6] and such methods have been the subject of some recent reviews.[7-9] As an example of how *in vitro* nephrotoxicity methods can complement animal studies, this chapter will focus on the utility and limitations of renal tubule suspensions in toxicology. We will attempt to emphasize various points to consider in applying the *in vitro* model to studies of nephrotoxicity.

II. TUBULE ISOLATION

To develop an appropriate *in vitro* system, one needs to consider (1) the most effective means of isolating the tissue, and (2) how closely the model chosen mimics the *in vivo* situation. There are a number of techniques by which renal proximal tubules may be obtained, and the most appropriate method depends upon the ultimate use of the final preparation.

A. MICRODISSECTION

Where precise identification of the proximal tubule segment is required, microdissection of individual tubules may provide the most appropriate target material. Particularly for studies of kidney physiology, single perfused tubules provide a good model.[10] The advantages afforded by precise identification of the target material, however, must be balanced against the disadvantages of low yields and prolonged isolation times.

The microdissection technique is quite straightforward, simply requiring microscopic identification of the target segments and development of dexterity with microsurgical instruments. Tubules can be teased free from either cortex that has been partially digested with collagenase[11,12] or from undigested tissue.[13,14] The potential damage to the basement membrane of the tubules from the collagenase treatment must be weighed against the relative difficulty of performing the dissection on undigested material and the potential for membrane damage due to the mechanical tearing of the connective tissue of the nephron.

For purposes of *in vitro* toxicology, we have found the microdissection techniques somewhat limiting, since it is difficult to isolate large quantities of tubule segments in a reasonable time period. This limits the number of parameters or test agents which can be analyzed in a single experiment, hindering relatively large screening projects. Additionally, very sensitive biochemical methods must be developed since the amount of tissue sample is very limited. This tends to restrict the types of endpoints that can be measured. Thus, although microdissection has been used for physiological studies,[11,15] its use for toxicology studies is somewhat limited.

B. ENZYMATIC METHODS

To obtain greater yields of tubule segments, most investigators follow a protocol in which kidney cortex is isolated and the nephron components are separated either mechanically or enzymatically. In our own laboratory, we use a method employing mild enzymatic digestion followed by mechanical disruption. The method has been presented in detail elsewhere,[7] but will be briefly described here.

Since the original purpose for our investigations was to examine toxicity due to antibiotic exposure, we chose to use a sensitive species, the rabbit, as the source of tubules. We have found, however, that this isolation procedure requires only minor modifications when other species are used. Normally, we use female New Zealand rabbits (approximately 2.5 to 3 kg weight, or 3 mo age), since older animals appear to have more connective tissue in the kidney, resulting in more difficult digestion and less satisfactory yields. The animals are sacrificed, and kidneys are removed aseptically, without *in situ* perfusion (a step which we have found unnecessary for our purposes). In a sterile environment (tissue culture hood), kidneys are rinsed with buffer (Hanks' balanced salt solution, GIBCO), split longitudinally, and decapsulated. An approximately 1-mm thick slice is cut from the outer cortex of each kidney half using a Stadie-Riggs tissue slicer. Slices are rinsed in buffer, minced finely, then rinsed again. The final rinse is decanted and replaced with 100 ml collagenase solution (45 U/ml DMEM containing 20 m*M* HEPES) per 2 kidneys.

After a 1-h digestion at 30°C in a rotary water bath, the collagenase is replaced with cold (4°C) medium. At this point, the nephron structure is still intact, though some of the connective tissue has been removed. The mincate is then passed through a 19-gauge needle to mechanically disrupt the nephron and separate proximal tubules from other nephron components. After filtration through a 500 μ mesh to remove large clumps, the preparation is settled for 15 min at room temperature. A large amount of cell debris and single cells remains in the medium and can be drawn off and discarded. Settled tubules are resuspended in culture medium, and layered onto a Percoll (Pharmacia) gradient. (Centrifugation of a 35% solution of Percoll at 29,000 $\times$ g for 45 min forms a continuous 20 to 50% gradient.) The loaded gradients are centrifuged at 130 $\times$ g for 15 min to separate proximal tubules (which band near the bottom of the gradient) from glomeruli, cell debris, and distal tubules (which tend to remain near the top). The proximal tubule band is then collected, washed by centrifugation in culture medium, and diluted in a manner appropriate for the specific experimental design.

We have found that this procedure routinely yields tubule suspensions in which approximately 95% of the tubular structures are proximal and have good viability and function (see below). With minor variations,[7] one can obtain tubules from a variety of species, including human, for comparative studies or extrapolation.

C. MECHANICAL SEPARATION

Where there is a concern over the use of digestive enzymes, nonenzymatic procedures may be used to isolate proximal tubules. These techniques are generally modifications of those developed by Meezan et al.[16] and Carlson et al.[17] The methods rely on perfusion of the kidneys *in situ* with buffer (to clear thc blood), then with iron oxide particles of a size which will lodge in the capillary bed of the glomeruli. Following perfusion, the cortex is removed, minced, and homogenized in a Potter-Elvehjem tissue grinder with a loose-fitting pestle. The homogenate, containing disrupted nephron components, is passed through a series of sieves to separate the glomeruli and proximal tubules from chunks of tissue and cell debris. The tubules and glomeruli are separated by stirring the sample with a magnetic stir bar. The glomeruli are attracted to the stir bar and can be physically removed.

Our experience has been that this method produces a greater yield of proximal tubules, but of less purity than can be attained using enzymatic digestion and separation on a Percoll gradient. Since the enzymatic/mechanical isolation was satisfactory for our purposes, we made only limited attempts at further purification. Some investigators have reported that the mechanical disruption of the nephron causes less damage to the membrane than does enzymatic digestion. For instance, Hjelle et al.[18] found that membrane-associated enzymatic activities (γ-glutamyl transpeptidase, amino-peptidase M, alkaline phosphatase, etc.) could be preserved with a mechanical digestion procedure (though no direct comparison was made to tubules isolated enzymatically in this study). A recent comparative study of an enzymatic and a mechanical isolation procedure[19] pointed out some similarities and differences in the resultant preparations. They found that in enzymatically isolated tubules, basal oxygen consumption was higher and tubular morphology was retained for a shorter period of time, and they concluded that both events were caused by membrane damage due to enzymatic treatment. However, other biochemical parameters (LDH retention, lipid peroxidation, nystatin-stimulated O_2 consumption) were quite similar in tubules isolated by either procedure.

It is probable that some damage is done to the proximal tubule basement membrane by the physical trauma of mechanically tearing the connective tissue of the nephron and as well as by enzymatic digestion; it may simply be a matter of degree of damage. Thus, whichever method of isolation is chosen, the viability and functional integrity of the tubules needs to be assessed to make certain that the preparation is suitable for the intended purpose of the study.

III. CHARACTERIZATION

One key to developing an appropriate *in vitro* model is examining the resultant preparation for various markers of specificity, viability, and/or function. For proximal tubules, these parameters should be reflective of normal kidney function and correlate with the endpoint(s) to be ultimately measured in the system.

One way to identify the isolated tubules as being proximal is to process the preparation with periodic acid Schiff (PAS) which stains the mucoproteins of the glycocalyx of the brush border. Since only the proximal tubules have a lumenal brush border, this is a very specific, easily visualized marker. Morphological methods are generally quite time-consuming and labor intensive, and thus are not a measurement that one would routinely perform. However, in the early stages of development of the isolation techniques, histochemistry can be invaluable providing a positive visual identification, confirming that the tissue of interest is indeed present.

As an alternative (or in addition to histochemistry), one can measure the activity of various segment specific enzymes, as described by Toutain et al.[20] These investigators measured alkaline phosphatase and alanine aminopeptidase (brush border markers) which are specific for proximal tubules compared with hexokinase as a marker of distal tubules. Since enzyme assays are generally relatively quickly and easily performed, they allow one to easily monitor the purity of the preparation through the various steps of the isolation procedure.

Hormone responsiveness can also be used as an indicator of whether isolated tubules are proximal or distal. For instance, vasopressin and calcitonin act predominantly on distal tubules, while parathyroid hormone stimulates cAMP production mainly in proximal tubules.[12,21,22] This hormonal responsiveness has been used to characterize preparations by a number of investigators.[23,24]

The next question, after identifying the preparation as being predominantly proximal tubules, concerns their viability. Most of the standard cytotoxicity assays (MTT, leucine incorporation, LDH leakage) can be used as a quick indicator. We have found, however, that staining with vital dyes can be misleading. For instance, freshly isolated tubules incubated with trypan blue will show virtually every cell taking up the dye, normally an indication of dead cells. In this case, the presence of the dye indicates the functioning of the active transport system.

This ability of proximal tubules to transport certain substances can be used as a measure of both tubule viability and functionality. For instance, it is well known that tubules concentrate certain sugars against a concentration gradient.[25] Sina et al.[23] analyzed this transport in proximal tubule segments, showing that 3-*O*-methylglucose (which enters the cells by facilitated diffusion) rapidly equilibrates across the membranes while α-methylglucose (α-methyl D-glucopyranoside) is actively transported and concentrated intracellularly. Other substances such as divalent anions,[26] organic anions and cations such as para-aminohippurate (PAH) and tetraethylammonium (TEA),[15,27] and various amino acids[28] are also actively transported and can serve as markers.

IV. UTILITY

Isolated tubule suspensions have been used in many applications for toxicology, pharmacology, and physiology. In this section we will focus mainly on ways in which these suspensions can be used to complement animal studies and reduce the number of animals used. Before getting to specific examples, however, we need to stress two points. First, before use, the tubule preparation must be adequately characterized to be sure that it mimics the desired *in vivo* parameter(s). And second, one needs to determine whether the model is appropriate for the question being addressed. If either point is ignored, there is a risk of generating artifactual data which will confuse, rather than inform.

A. SCREENING

Our primary reason for developing the isolated tubule methodology in our laboratory was to investigate the relative nephrotoxic potential of new chemical entities. By using the *in vitro* approach we could quickly identify an appropriate candidate to bring forward into full safety testing, while reducing the number of animals and amount of compound required for prescreening. The techniques used have been described elsewhere,[5,7] but will be briefly summarized here.

Tubules are prepared as described above from one or two rabbits and plated into 6-well plates (35-mm wells) in a 0.5 ml volume. The material from one rabbit is sufficient to obtain 40 wells with approximately 800 μg protein per well. Test material is prepared in an appropriate solvent such that twice the final concentration is contained in 0.5 ml. The solution is filter sterilized and 0.5 ml is added to appropriate wells for a final volume of 1-ml containing tubules and 1X test compound. The plates are incubated at 37°C on a rocker platform oscillating at 3 oscillations per min. At an appropriate time (usually 20 h), we pulse with ^{3}H-leucine for 3 h, then harvest by freezing at −70°C. Protein is later extracted by solubilization in 0.2 *N* NaOH and precipitation with 10% trichloroacetic acid, with extensive washing. Samples of the final solubilized pellet are analyzed for protein determination by the Lowry method[29] and for incorporation of radiolabel into protein by scintillation counting. The data are expressed as percent change in incorporation relative to control and usually are presented graphically in order to compare the shapes of the dose-response curves.

We evaluated this method for our purposes (screening antibiotic candidates) by comparing the relative toxicity of a series of cephalosporins. This was designed to determine whether the method was capable of distinguishing among structurally related analogs. The results[5] showed that in most cases, the *in vitro* ranking of the compounds correlated with the *in vivo* observations, although cephalothin was an exception. While cephalothin is only slightly toxic in rabbit, we found it to be very cytotoxic in our assay. Further investigation showed that this antibiotic is cleared from the kidney *in vivo* much more rapidly than the other cephalosporins with which we were working. In the *in vitro* assay, there is no mechanism for clearance of the compound, and this results in exaggerated toxicity. Thus, to make satisfactory comparisons among test materials, it is important to know whether the pharmacokinetic parameters are similar. This is based on the idea that toxicity is a function of the inherent toxicity of a compound as well as on the effective exposure of the target organ to the material. The *in vitro* assay is generally able to give an indication of only the inherent cytotoxicity, not account for pharmacokinetic differences.

In a practical application, we tested a series of analogs of thienamycin. Eleven compounds with the core carbapenem structure were analyzed *in vitro* against the marketed product, imipenem (the antibiotic component of Primaxin). In this series of experiments we ran a dose-response curve for both the test material and imipenem in the same assay, and asked whether the test compound was more, less, or equitoxic with the reference compound. In 10 of 11 cases, the *in vitro* assay was predictive of the relative toxicity determined *in vivo.* In the one discrepant case, there was some ambiguity in the *in vivo* study.

This is just one example of how this methodology can be used for comparative screening. A cautionary note is that we have done this type of study with a limited number of compounds from only five classes of chemicals, cephalosporins, thienamycins, aminoglycosides, angiotensin-converting enzyme inhibitors, and cyclosporins. The possibility exists that the assay will not be adequate for some chemical classes. Further, while the method is very useful for rank ordering compounds based on toxicity, in most cases, we have been unable to reliably predict an actual *in vivo* nephrotoxic dose from the *in vitro* data, even when pharmacokinetic data are taken into account. For some compounds the prediction of dose is quite good; however, for others, even within the same chemical class, the reliability is poor.

B. MECHANISTIC STUDIES

A well-characterized tubule suspension model can be appropriate for various mechanistic studies. For instance, Guder[30] used this system to examine the interaction of angiotensin II (AII) on the proximal tubule. Taking advantage of the fact that culture conditions can be easily manipulated, he was able to examine the effects of various peptides and ions on gluconeogenesis stimulated by AII. This allowed the author to infer the mechanism by which AII exerts some of its effects, hypothesizing that potassium, but not calcium, influences the mechanism of AII action.

In the area of toxicology, Rush and Ponsler[31] used isolated tubule suspensions to explore mechanisms of cephaloridine nephrotoxicity. Examining parameters of mitochondrial and peroxidative damage, as well as various conditions of thiol depletion, they suggested that lipid peroxidation is a likely mechanism of cephaloridine toxicity, and that altered thiol status may play a role, at least *in vitro.* The authors also point out that some discrepancies exist between data generated *in vitro* and the results that would be expected based on *in vivo* observations, and are careful not to over interpret the *in vitro* data. This is an important point. While *in vitro* studies can complement animal studies and sometimes provide data which is difficult to generate *in vivo,* one always needs to be aware of the limitations of indiscriminate extrapolation of *in vitro* data to the intact animal.

In our own lab, we have examined the mechanism of toxicity of a number of pharmaceuticals. Our work with an angiotensin converting enzyme (ACE) inhibitor will illustrate this point. Enalapril is a generally well tolerated and effective antihypertensive. However, in dogs (though not monkeys or rats) high doses of the compound cause proximal tubule degeneration. As detailed elsewhere,[7] we first showed that the *in vitro* system was appropriate for addressing questions relating to this drug. This was done by mimicking in the *in vitro* model various *in vivo* observations (such as metabolism of the prodrug to the active form, enalaprilat, and demonstration of the differential toxicity of these two materials as observed *in vivo.*)

At this point, we were able to ask a number of questions in an attempt to focus on a potential mechanism of toxicity. For instance, could the toxicity be related to the pharmacologic action? We tested the toxicity of the pharmacologically inactive enantiomer against enalapril and found that the inactive material was approximately 2.5-fold more toxic. This confirmed *in vivo* observations which had suggested that the ACE inhibitory action was not responsible for the toxicity.

We were able to examine the salt form of the material and found that the presence or absence of a maleate salt did not explain the toxicity. We also compared the toxicity of other ACE inhibitors in this assay and found similar dose-response curves for many of the materials. Closer examination revealed that each of the inhibitors that contained an ester moiety showed similar kinetics and levels of toxicity to enalapril. Thus we were able to use the *in vitro* work to suggest the involvement of this ester group in the mechanism of toxicity, and this has been the focus of our continuing efforts.

In short, any pharmacological, biochemical, or toxicological parameters that can be examined at the cellular level can be studied in this type of *in vitro* system. In some cases tubules, which retain the 3-dimensional structure and thus more normal cell-to-cell interactions, may provide a better system than monolayer cultures. For instance, we have found that sugar transport is more effectively maintained in tubules, even after 24 h, than in confluent primary cultures.[23] Of course if exposures exceed 24 to 36 h, the tubule architecture breaks down, and monolayer cultures result. Again, the extent of utility of this system depends upon the questions that must be addressed.

C. SPECIES SPECIFICITY

During toxicology studies, questions often arise concerning the suitability of a particular species for the experimental purpose or regarding extrapolation of results among species. Tubule suspensions can be useful to address such issues. Relatively slight variations in the protocol are required to obtain tubule suspensions from a variety of species,[7] thus allowing comparisons to be made *in vitro*. For instance, our laboratory has investigated whether the differences in species susceptibility to the nephrotoxic antibiotic cephaloridine can be reproduced *in vitro*.

It is known that rabbits are very sensitive to the nephrotoxic effects of this compound, followed by monkey, dog, rat, and mouse in order of decreasing sensitivity. The difference in sensitivity *in vivo* between rabbit and mouse is estimated to be approximately 34-fold. In the *in vitro* assay we found that the cephaloridine D_{37} (i.e., dose-reducing leucine incorporation to 37% of control) ranged from 0.7 m*M* for rabbit, to 1.4 m*M* for human, to 1.7 m*M* in dog, 2.3 m*M* in rat, and 3.0 m*M* in mouse. The order of toxicity among species was maintained *in vitro;* however, the degree of sensitivity was compressed dramatically. This result is most likely due to pharmacokinetics. We know, for instance, that the T1/2 for cephaloridine clearance from rabbit kidney is approximately 3 h, while in mouse the T1/2 is only 20 min, resulting in a large difference in effective exposure time between these two species. *In vitro,* however, the tubules were exposed to drug for a standard 23 h regardless of species of origin. These results suggest that the inherent toxicity of the compound as measured in the *in vitro* toxicity assay is only part of the reason for species susceptibility. In this case, it appears that the pharmacokinetic considerations may be more important in determining species differences.

This work does point out, however, the strength of this method as well as a weakness. It would be a tedious (and in humans unethical) task to perform whole-animal nephrotoxicity assays in many different species, whereas *in vitro* it is a relatively simple task. In the case of cephaloridine, however, one needs to account for the pharmacokinetics rather than simply the inherent toxicity. While this may not be the case for other chemical classes, it is definitely a point to be addressed in interpretation of *in vitro* data.

D. MARKERS OF TOXICITY

An important question that arises in using *in vitro* systems is what parameter(s) is an appropriate measure of toxicity. Some investigators have attempted to answer this question experimentally,[32] but the answer really depends upon the question being asked. The actual decision must be based on whether one is simply measuring general cell death, or needs a more specific (and perhaps more sensitive) early indication of loss of cell or tissue function.

Various measurements of cell death are common to *in vitro* studies: trypan blue dye exclusion, uptake of radiolabeled precursors, enzyme release (usually LDH[33,34]), mitochondrial dye reduction (MTT[35,36]), ATP content,[37] total protein,[38] etc. Each parameter has advantages and disadvantages, and one needs to understand when to use and when not to use each. For instance, trypan blue is actively transported by kidney tubule fragments, suggesting that the tubules are nonviable, when in fact they are functioning as expected (as discussed above). The utility of the endpoints can also be dependent upon the mechanism of toxicity of the test material. In general, if one is unsure of the mechanism, a general indicator of toxicity, such as leucine incorporation into protein, is the wiser choice of endpoints. For instance, even though many investigators use lactate dehydrogenase (LDH) leakage as a sensitive indicator of cell death, we found with the cephalosporin antibiotics that no LDH leakage into the medium was seen over the 24-h time course of our experiments, even up to the limit of solubility of the test agents.

Since we wanted to use the tubule assay for screening analogs of drug candidates, the ability to rank related compounds in order of toxic potential was very important. We examined three different endpoints (leucine incorporation, LDH leakage, ATP content) in proximal tubule suspensions to determine which parameter would be more reliable in predicting the *in vivo* toxicity of cephalosporins. The data indicated that leucine incorporation was the best parameter to measure. LDH gave no response (as mentioned above), and ATP levels decreased only at concentrations of drug approximately 3 to 4 times those doses needed to see a response with leucine incorporation. Again, the point to be remembered is that this situation may be different with compounds which exert their toxic action by other mechanisms; so, it is important for the investigator to examine different parameters in his or her own lab.

We also measured toxicity in this system as a loss of function, specifically the ability of the tubules to concentrate α-methyl glucose.[23] We found that this measure of tubule function was as sensitive as leucine incorporation, but required much more effort, and was thus not amenable to extensive screening experiments. However, if one is addressing issues related to mechanisms of toxicity, such parameters as concentration of sugars, organic ion transport, etc. (i.e., those parameters used to characterize the preparation in the first place) may be more appropriate.

Additionally, toxicity endpoints may suggest a mechanism of toxicity. For instance, reduction of the tetrazolium dye (MTT) occurs only in functional mitochondria; so, a decrease in MTT dye reduction is indicative of damage to the functioning of this organelle. Similarly, neutral red is taken up into intact lysosomes; thus a decrease in neutral red uptake can indicate deficiencies in transport or storage, giving a clue to the way in which the compound exerts its toxicity. It is important, therefore, in setting up a model system, to measure multiple endpoints, not only to determine which parameter is most sensitive and appropriate, but also to gain additional knowledge as to mechanisms of toxicity.

V. LIMITATIONS

As with any assay or method, one needs to be aware of the limitations and potential artifacts. As stressed above, it is important that the tubule preparation be well characterized so that it closely mimics the *in vivo* situation. It is also important to understand something about the *in vivo* situation. For instance, nephrotoxicity may result through many mechanisms such as altered glomerular filtration rate (as in the case of cyclosporins) or glomerular toxicity, renal papillary necrosis (caused by nonsteroidal anti-inflammatory agents), prerenal insult such as mechanical blockage, as well as direct toxicity to the proximal tubule cells. It is therefore necessary to ask whether the *in vitro* model is reasonable in light of the problem to be addressed.

Also, as illustrated above, pharmacokinetic factors are not accounted for in the standard *in vitro* assay, but must be considered in extrapolating the results to predict toxicity in the whole animal. For purposes of comparing related materials as to toxicity, one needs to assume that pharmacokinetics will not be substantially different among the test agents. However, one must bear in mind that the *in vitro* data simply reflect inherent cellular toxicity, i.e., the consequences resulting from a particular concentration of the chemical coming into direct contact with the cell.

Another potential limitation is that the tubules can be maintained in their three-dimensional state for only 24 to 36 h; then the cells begin to spread over the culture dish to form a monolayer. Thus, the tubule fragments themselves are useful for acute, rather than chronic exposures. Chronic exposures would have to be done either on monolayers of proximal kidney tubule cells, or by using an *in vivo*/*in vitro* protocol where the animal is dosed chronically and then the tubules are isolated and assayed.

Cryopreservation of tubule fragments is somewhat difficult, so that material must be freshly isolated for each study. While this may not be a serious problem with rodents and rabbits, with other species such as dog, monkey, and human, where tissue availability may be limiting, one needs to make the most efficient use possible of the tissue. For instance, while the kidneys of one rabbit yield enough material for 40 different experimental aliquots, a dog or human kidney will yield substantially more material. If the tubules cannot be used in a single experiment, they need to be either cultured as cells or discarded. An acceptable cryopreservation system would allow more complete use to be made of these preparations. Even with this limitation, many more samples can be tested in the *in vitro* assay, greatly reducing the need for whole animal studies.

VI. CONCLUSIONS

We have described an *in vitro* system for testing nephrotoxic potential of various chemicals in proximal tubule segments. This method has the advantage of being a simpler, more easily manipulated model than whole animals, allowing experiments which would be difficult to approach or interpret *in vivo*. The system also allows comparative *in vitro* studies with tissue from different species, including human, in a relatively simple, straightforward manner, enabling one to gain perspective for extrapolation among species. Thus, this *in vitro* model effectively complements work in whole animals.

The caveats have also been discussed, including the fact that pharmacokinetic parameters are not necessarily accounted for, that tubule fragments can be kept intact for only a relatively short time, and that this model cannot mimic every interaction which might be involved at the organ level in the toxicity of a test material. However, if used with these limitations in mind, proximal tubule fragments can contribute in many ways to the assessment of chemical toxicity.

REFERENCES

1. **Ross, B. D.,** The isolated perfused rat kidney, *Clin. Sci. Mol. Med.*, 55, 513, 1978.
2. **Maack, T.,** Physiological evaluation of the isolated perfused kidney, *Am. J. Physiol.*, 238, F71, 1980.
3. **Kacew, S. and Hirsch, G. H.,** Evaluation of nephrotoxicity of various compounds by means of *in vitro* techniques and comparison to *in vivo* methods, in *Toxicology of the Kidney*, Hook, J. B., Ed., Raven Press, New York, 1981, 77.
4. **Ruegg, C. E., Gandolfi, A. J., Nagle, R. B., Krumdieck, C. L., and Brendel, K.,** Preparation of positional renal slices for study of cell-specific toxicity, *J. Pharmacol. Meth.*, 17, 111, 1987.
5. **Sina, J. F., Bean, C. L., Noble, C., and Bradley, M. O.,** An *in vitro* assay for cytotoxicity to proximal tubule suspensions from rabbit kidney, *In Vitro Toxicol.*, 1, 13, 1986.
6. **Boogaard, P. J., Mulder, G. J., and Nagelkerke, J. F.,** Isolated proximal tubular cells from rat kidney as an *in vitro* model for studies on nephrotoxicity, *Toxicol. Appl. Pharmacol.*, 101, 144, 1989.
7. **Sina, J. F., Noble, C., Bean, C. L., and Bradley, M. O.,** Renal tubules *in vitro* as a model for nephrotoxicity, in *In Vitro Toxicology: Model Systems and Methods*, McQueen, C. A., Ed., Telford Press, Caldwell, NJ, 1989, 263.
8. **Boogaard, P. J., Nagelkerke, J. F., and Mulder, G. J.,** Renal proximal tubular cells in suspension or in primary culture as *in vitro* models to study nephrotoxicity, *Chem.-Biol. Interact.*, 76, 251, 1990.
9. **Handler, J. S.,** Studies of kidney cells in culture, *Kidney Int.*, 30, 208, 1986.
10. **Burg, M. B.,** Introduction: background and development of microperfusion technique, *Kidney Int.*, 22, 417, 1982.
11. **Burg, M. B. and Orloff, J.,** Oxygen consumption and active transport in separated renal tubules, *Am. J. Physiol.*, 203, 327, 1962.
12. **Imbert, M., Chabardes, D., Montegut, M., Clinque, A., and Morel, F.,** Adenylate cyclase activity along the rabbit nephron as measured in single isolated segments, *Pflügers Arch.*, 354, 213, 1975.
13. **Wilson, P. D., Anderson, R. J., Breckon, R. D., Nathrath, W., and Schrier, R. W.,** Retention of differentiated characteristics by cultures of defined rabbit kidney epithelia, *J. Cell. Physiol.*, 130, 245, 1987.
14. **Kaufman, J. S. and Hamburger, R. J.,** Potassium transport in the isolated proximal convoluted tubule, *Am. J. Physiol.*, 244, F409, 1983.
15. **Tarloff, J. B. and Brand, P. H.,** Active tetraethylammonium uptake across the basolateral membrane of rabbit proximal tubule, *Am. J. Physiol.*, 251, F141, 1986.
16. **Meezan, E., Brendel, K., Ulreich, J., and Carlson, E. C.,** Properties of pure metabolically active glomerular preparation from rat kidneys. I. Isolation, *J. Pharmacol. Exp. Ther.*, 187, 332, 1973.
17. **Carlson, E. C., Brendel, K., Hjelle, J. T., and Meezan, E.,** Ultrastructural and biochemical analyses of isolated basement membranes from kidney glomeruli and tubules and brain and retinal microvessels, *J. Ultrastruct. Res.*, 62, 26, 1978.
18. **Hjelle, J. T., Morin, J.-P., and Trouet, A.,** Analytical cell fractionation of isolated rabbit renal proximal tubules, *Kidney Int.*, 20, 71, 1981.
19. **Rodeheaver, D. P., Aleo, M. D., and Schnellmann, R. G.,** Differences in enzymatic and mechanical isolated rabbit renal proximal tubules: comparison in long-term incubation, *In Vitro Cell. Dev. Biol.*, 26, 898, 1990.
20. **Toutain, H., Vauclin-Jaques, N., Fillastre, J.-P., and Morin, J.-P.,** Isolation of a pure suspension of proximal tubule cells from the rabbit kidney: morphological, biochemical and metabolic assessment, *Cell Biol. Int. Rep.*, 13, 701, 1989.
21. **Morel, F.,** Sites of hormone action in the mammalian nephron, *Am. J. Physiol.*, 240, F159, 1981.
22. **Scholer, D. W. and Edelman, I. S.,** Isolation of rat kidney cortical tubules enriched in proximal and distal segments, *Am. J. Physiol.*, 237, F350, 1979.
23. **Sina, J. F., Bean, C. L., Noble, C., and Bradley, M. O.,** Isolation and characterization of proximal tubule suspensions from rabbit for *in vitro* studies, *In Vitro Toxicol.*, 1, 5, 1986.
24. **Chen, T. C., Curthoys, N. P., Lagenaur, C. F., and Puschett, J. B.,** Characterization of primary cell cultures derived from rat renal proximal tubules, *In Vitro*, 25, 714, 1989.
25. **Mullin, J. M., Weibel, J., Diamond, L., and Kleinzeller, A.,** Sugar transport in the LLC-PK_1 renal epithelial cell line: similarity to mammalian kidney and the influence of cell density, *J. Cell. Physiol.*, 104, 375, 1980.
26. **Dennis, V. W. and Brazy, P. C.,** Divalent anion transport in isolated renal tubules, *Kidney Int.*, 22, 498, 1982.
27. **Grantham, J. J.,** Studies of organic anion and cation transport in isolated segments of proximal tubules, *Kidney Int.*, 22, 519, 1982.

28. **Hillman, R. E., Albrecht, I., and Rosenberg, L. E.,** Transport of amino acids by isolated rabbit renal tubules, *Biochim. Biophys. Acta,* 150, 528, 1968.
29. **Lowry, O. H., Rosebrough, N. J., Farr, A. L., and Randall, R. J.,** Protein measurement with the folin phenol reagent, *J. Biol. Chem.,* 193, 265, 1951.
30. **Guder, W. G.,** Stimulation of renal gluconeogenesis by angiotensin II, *Biochim. Biophys. Acta,* 584, 507, 1979.
31. **Rush, G. F. and Ponsler, G. D.,** Cephaloridine-induced biochemical changes and cytotoxicity in suspensions of rabbit isolated proximal tubules, *Toxicol. Appl. Pharmacol.,* 109, 314, 1991.
32. **Garrett, N. E. and Lewtas, J.,** Cellular toxicity in Chinese hamster ovary cell cultures, *Environ. Res.,* 32, 455, 1983.
33. **Anuforo, D. C., Acosta, D., and Smith, R. V.,** Hepatotoxicity studies with primary cultures of rat liver cells, *In Vitro,* 14, 981, 1978.
34. **Decker, T. and Lohmann-Matthes, M.,** A quick and simple method for the quantitation of lactate dehydrogenase release in measurements of cellular cytotoxicity and tumor necrosis factor (TNF) activity, *J. Immun. Meth.,* 15, 61, 1988.
35. **Mosmann, T.,** Rapid colorimetric assay for cellular growth and survival: application to proliferation and cytotoxicity assays, *J. Immun. Meth.,* 65, 55, 1983.
36. **Islet, M., Holtei, W., and Hilgard, P.,** The tetrazolium dye assay for rapid *in vitro* assessment of cytotoxicity, *Arzneim.-Forsch./Drug Res.,* 39(II), 747, 1989.
37. **Kemp, R. B., Cross, D. M., and Meredith, R. W. J.,** Adenosine triphosphate as an indicator of cellular toxicity *in vitro, Food. Chem. Toxicol.,* 24, 465, 1986.
38. **Shopsis, C. and Eng, B.,** Rapid cytotoxicity testing using a semi-automated protein determination on cultured cells, *Toxicol. Lett.,* 26, 1, 1985.

Chapter 8

CONTINUOUS RENAL CELL LINES AS *IN VITRO* TOOLS TO STUDY NEPHROTOXICITY

Gerhard Gstraunthaler and Walter Pfaller

TABLE OF CONTENTS

I. INTRODUCTION

The kidneys regulate the excretion and homeostasis of water and solutes. They are metabolically active organs and possess the ability to actively concentrate certain substances and the potential to metabolically activate or to bioconvert a variety of xenobiotic compounds. Therefore, the kidneys are frequent targets for toxins similar in chemical structure to physiologically handled substances.

Another characteristic of the kidney is its marked intraorgan heterogeneity in structure,[1] metabolism,[2] and function.[3,4] Besides the differences between the vascular (glomerular) and tubular structures, the functional unit, the nephron is composed by different segments, each consisting of distinct cell types.[5-7] (For the exact nomenclature of renal structures and tubular segments, respectively, the reader is referred to the "standard nomenclature for structures of the kidney".[8]) These epithelial cells, lining the nephron, are responsible for renal work — reabsorption and secretion of water and solutes.

These well-defined biochemical and physiological properties make renal tubular cells specifically susceptible to toxic (or ischemic) insults. As a consequence of renal heterogeneity, mechanisms of chemically induced or ischemic cell injury cannot be explored easily in whole organ studies, but must be evaluated at the level of the respective renal tissue region, nephron segment, or glomerular or tubular cell type, respectively. A number of examples have been described, in which exposure of kidneys, either *in vivo* or *in vitro,* to nephrotoxic xenobiotics or ischemia led to specific patterns of renal cell injury and functional impairment.[9-12]

The vulnerability of renal epithelial cells to toxic insults is largely due to the cell's capacity to transport, and thus to accumulate, toxic xenobiotics via normally existing transport systems[13-15] which may give rise to intracellular toxic concentrations. Thus, the toxicity of certain substances in nephron segment cells is largely determined by their transport characteristics.[16-18]

Due to the morphological and functional heterogeneity and complexity of the kidney, the assessment of normal and impaired organ function has traditionally been a "technique-oriented" field. In basic renal physiological and nephrological research, a set of methodologies has been developed, which offers a number of *in vitro* model systems applicable to renal physiology, pharmacology, and toxicology studies.[19] Among these, renal epithelial cells in tissue culture — primary cultures as well as continuous cell lines — have emerged as important tools to study *in vitro* toxic and/or ischemic renal cell injury.[20-24]

II. USE OF CULTURED RENAL CELLS IN THE *IN VITRO* ASSESSMENT OF XENOBIOTIC-INDUCED NEPHROTOXICITY

Research focused on renal cell culture virtually exploded within the last years. To a large extent this is due to improved methodologies for growing homogenous cultures of renal cells. Despite these advancements, however, certain limitations still exist in using cultured renal cells for research purposes. First, there are at least 15 to 20 cell types that resemble the kidney.[6,8] Second, there exists a considerable gap in available information with respect to markers, which may be used to unambiguously identify the respective *in situ* ancestor cell.[25] Third, the situation is even more complicated by the fact that cells tend to dedifferentiate during maintenance in culture for many passages. The use of new and more natural substrata may help to overcome this problem.[26-32] Despite these limitations, this area of research has attracted many investigators and has turned out to represent a reasonable alternative strategy in studying basic renal cellular functions and their modulation by experimental maneuvers.[33-35]

In general, modern cell and tissue culture techniques enable the cultivation of renal epithelial cells at a state of differentiation, comparable with the tissue *in vivo*. Due to the degree of epithelial differentiation, epithelial transport characteristics can be explored by culturing the cells on permeable supports, thereby separating the apical from the basolateral compartment by the cell monolayer.[36-40] For biochemical analysis, for the isolation of cell organelles or membrane vesicle preparations,[41] as well as for toxicological studies,[42] any amount of reasonably homogenous populations of cells can be raised in appropriate tissue culture vessels.

More recently renal cell culture gained importance for the exploration of the mode of action of potentially nephrotoxic xenobiotics and drugs. Depending on the retention of adequate renal cellular functions, which are known to interfere with xenobiotic or drug action,[43] renal cell cultures bear the advantage of providing an experimental system uninfluenced by higher order regulatory systems, which must be considered in whole body experiments and make interpretation of effects often extremely difficult or impossible.

For successful applications of cell and tissue cultures in combination with nephrotoxicology studies, some requirements must be met by the *in vitro* test systems:

1. Retention of the polar architecture of epithelia and expression and proper distribution of membrane enzyme and transport systems.[44-46]
2. Presence of vectorial solute and water transport, manifested by dome formation,[47-49] and generation of transepithelial electrical properties, i.e., spontaneous transepithelial potential difference, resulting from a certain transepithelial resistance and short circuit current.[50-52]
3. Cellular uptake routes for xenobiotics from either the apical or basolateral side as observed *in vivo et situ*.[14,15]
4. Expression of nephron segment-specific characteristics, i.e., distinct metabolic and transport properties, and hormone responsiveness, respectively.[25]

It should be mentioned at this point that virtually none of the continuous renal epithelial cell lines described fulfill all these criteria.[25,53]

Despite this disadvantage, tissue cultures per se offer a whole set of advantages useful for physiologic, pharmacologic, and toxicologic studies. Continuous cell lines, which by definition are capable of indefinite growth, can be maintained for as long as desired under defined and controlled environmental conditions. The ability to either biochemically or genetically modify cultured cells allows the selection and isolation of sublines, strains, clones, and mutants out of a parental cell population. Furthermore, the ability to change experimental parameters individually, or in combination, singly or sequentially in short- or long-term application, provides the possibility to investigate mechanistic aspects of cell injury and damage at the cellular and subcellular level.[21-24]

In the following sections, the most widely used continuous renal epithelial cell lines,[25] their specific properties retained in culture as well as their usefulness in nephrotoxicity studies, will be described.

The use of the intestinal carcinoma cell lines HT-29,[36] Caco-2,[54] and T_{84}[55] as model systems for intestinal transport and metabolism studies has been reviewed in detail elsewhere.

III. CONTINUOUS RENAL EPITHELIAL CELL LINES

A. INTRODUCTION

Several permanent (or continuous) cell lines (for definitions see References 56 and 57) of renal origin were established years ago. However, at that time the main goal for establishing

TABLE 1
Continuous Renal Epithelial Cell Lines

Cell line	Species	Proposed segmental origin
LLC-PK_1	Pig	Proximal tubule
OK	Opossum	Proximal tubule
JTC-12	Monkey	Proximal tubule
MDCK	Dog	Distal tubule/coll. duct
A6	*Xenopus laevis*	Distal tubule/coll. duct

renal epithelial lines was to get permanent growing epithelia for virus replication and for studies on virus-host cell relationships[58,59] or to obtain renal epithelia as a source for the production of plasminogen activators.[60] Another application was to obtain cells from organisms with an abnormal karyotype for chromosome research.[61,62] The use of permanent cell lines by renal and transport physiologists started in the early 1970s, when it was recognized that these cell lines retained a number of kidney-specific characteristics.

Most of the cell lines described (Table 1) are available from the American Type Culture Collection (ATCC), Rockville, MD. The differentiated characteristics of these cell lines have been summarized in detail elsewhere.[25]

1. LLC-PK_1 Cells (ATCC CRL 1392)

The LLC-PK_1 cell line was developed in 1958 by Hull et al.[60] from a mince of a whole kidney from a normal male Hampshire pig. The cells are epithelioid and nontumorigenic, form domes, and produce considerable amounts of plasminogen activators. LLC-PK_1 cells retained several features of the proximal tubule.[63-65] The cells express high activities of renal brush border membrane marker enzymes and Na^+-dependent apical transport of glucose, amino acids, and phosphate. A basolateral, secretory, transport of organic cations has recently been described.[43,66] Morphologically, the apical membrane domain is characterized by the presence of microvilli, which increase in number and size with culture age.[67] Cell-cell contacts are well developed. The junctional complexes are characterized by the occurrence of desmosomes and fairly shallow occluding junctions indicative for the low electrical tightness of the monolayer epithelium[68,69] (Figure 1).

This permanent type of cell line has lost, however, some features usually characteristic for proximal tubular cells. Transepithelial organic anion transport of *p*-aminohippurate could not be recovered in LLC-PK_1 epithelia.[66,68] Also the hormone responsiveness of LLC-PK_1 cells does not match the *in vivo* situation in the proximal nephron.[70] LLC-PK_1 cells do not respond to parathyroid hormone (PTH),[71] but express both hormone receptor subtypes for vasopressin V_1- and V_2-receptors[72-74] and responsiveness to calcitonin[75,76] and oxytocin.[77,78] Metabolically, LLC-PK_1 cells are unable to perform gluconeogenesis. Adaptation to more selective culture conditions, i.e., replacement of glucose by pyruvate or maintenance of cells in low glucose media can reestablish the expression of this pathway.[63,65] Furthermore, LLC-PK_1 cultures exhibit ammoniagenic response to metabolic acidosis under standard as well as rocked culture conditions.[79-82]

2. OK Cells (ATCC CRL 1840)

The OK cell line was initiated in 1975 by Koyama et al.[62] from a female opossum kidney. The line was originally characterized with respect to morphology and chromosome constitution.[61] More recently, the cells have been shown to be a useful model in the study of renal proximal tubule function.[83] The cell line possesses a number of different receptors

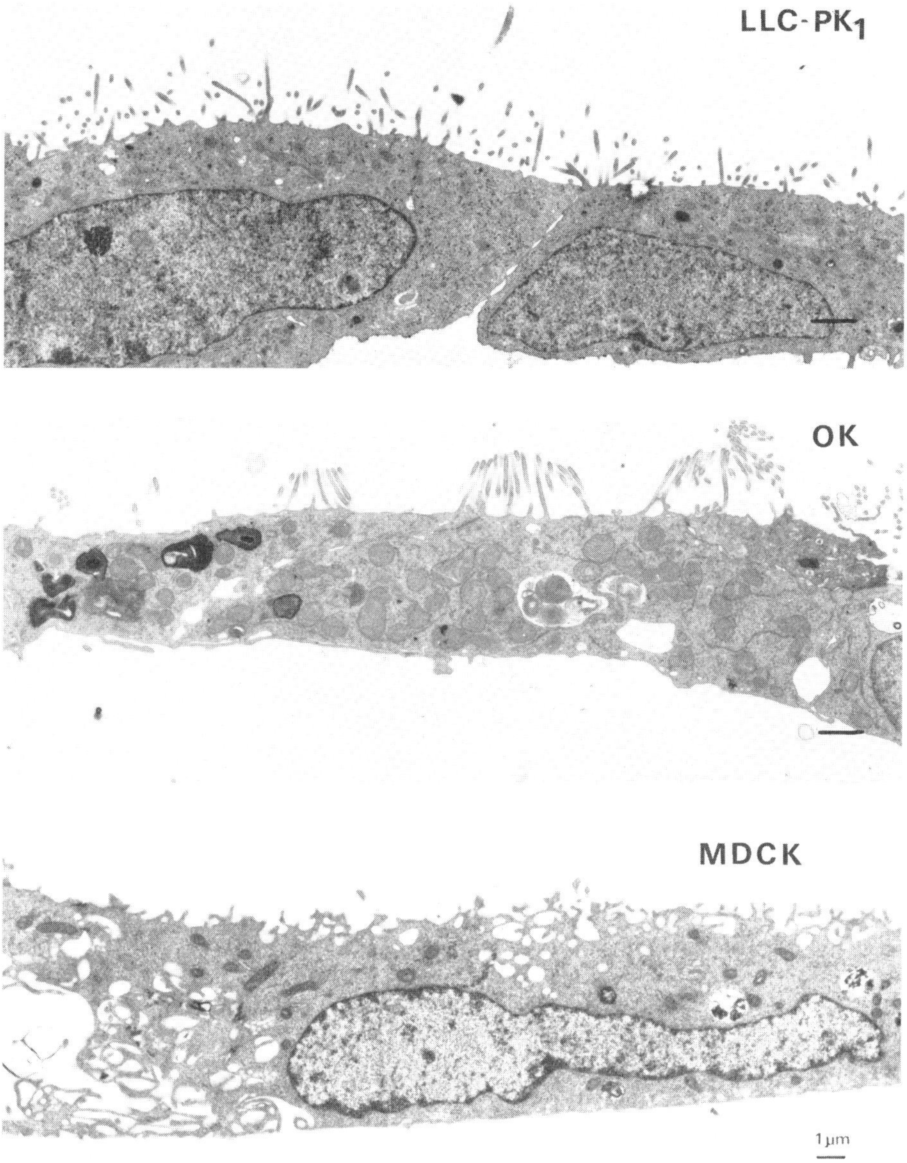

FIGURE 1. Electron micrographs of continuous renal epithelial cells on solid substrata (plastic tissue culture dishes). For morphological details see text.

including α-adrenergic receptors and receptors for insulin, serotonin, PTH, and atrial natriuretic factor. In particular, the PTH responsiveness of OK cells has been used to study the hormonal regulation of Na^+/P_i-transport and Na^+/H^+ exchange at the cellular level *in vitro*.[84-88] The internalization and catabolism of insulin, another characteristic function of proximal tubule cells, has been studied using OK cells.[89-91] In contrast to LLC-PK_1 cells, microvilli are assembled in patches. Furthermore, OK cells seem to contain larger amounts of mitochondria than other cell lines of proximal tubular origin (Figure 1).

3. JTC-12 Cells

JTC-12 cells were derived from the kidney cortex of a normal cynomolgus female monkey.[92] A subline (JTC-12.P3) has been adapted to grow in synthetic medium additionally supplemented with nonessential amino acids. Like LLC-PK_1 and OK cells, JTC-12 cells also retained differentiated properties characteristic of renal proximal epithelium: expression of renal brush border membrane enzyme activities and apical Na^+-dependent transports of hexose, amino acids, and inorganic phosphate.[93] PTH, isopropylnorepinephrine, and prostaglandin E_1 increase the cellular cAMP levels, indicating that receptors for these hormones are preserved. Calcitonin, vasopressin, and glucagon failed to raise intracellular cAMP.[94] Interestingly, although JTC-12 cells respond to PTH, Na^+/P_i transport is not affected.[71] Furthermore, JTC-12 cells respond to 1,25-dihydroxyvitamin D_3 by an enhanced conversion into $24,25(OH)_2D_3$.[95]

4. MDCK Cells (ATCC CCL 34)

The MDCK (Madin-Darby canine kidney) cell line was established in 1958 from the kidney of a female cocker spaniel. For many years, the cell line was primarily used for virus production.[58] The differentiated properties of MDCK cells have been examined extensively.[37,52,96,97] Although maintained in culture for almost 30 years, the cells retained the differentiated features of transporting epithelia.[51,98] The hormone responsiveness of MDCK cells points towards a distal tubular origin.[99] More recently, functional evidence for a collecting duct origin of MDCK cells has been established.[53,100-102]

So far there exist two functionally distinct cell strains: one with high (strain I) and one with low (strain II) transmonolayer resistance.[103,104] Cells of strain I are more columnar in appearance and display well-developed lateral cellular interdigitations,[46,105] whereas the low resistance cells are fairly flat (Figure 1). There exists no evidence for differences in the morphology of junctional complexes;[106] however, both MDCK strains differ considerably in their glycosphingolipid patterns.[107,108] In addition, differences in the lipid composition of the apical and basolateral membrane domains have been reported.[109-111] Since the MDCK wild type culture seems to be quite heterogeneous,[53] a number of additional MDCK clones have been isolated.[25,48]

When grown on solid supports, domes are formed. The cells are usually ciliated and bear a number of short microvilli.[112] Using semipermeable substrata, cell height and the formation of lateral cellular processes increase.[32] Furthermore, the occurrence of electron dense (dark) cells, similar to those found in the collecting duct *in vivo,* increase remarkably (Figure 2).

5. A6 Cells (ATCC CCL 102)

The A6 cell line was initiated in 1965 by K. A. Rafferty by primary cultivation of normal kidneys from *Xenopus laevis.*[50] Confluent A6 cultures resemble collecting duct epithelium.[113] They exhibit a high transepithelial electrical resistance and respond to aldosterone with an increase in short circuit current.[114,115] Interestingly, a complete response of A6 cells to vasopressin is only seen when the cells are grown on permeable supports[33] and thus are organized into a differentiated epithelium.[116,117]

B. CULTURE CONDITIONS FOR RENAL EPITHELIA IN NEPHROTOXICITY TESTING

Permanent renal epithelial cell lines do not exactly match the morphological appearance of their *in vivo et situ* ancestor cells. However, similarities with respect to gross morphology can be recognized.[118] Cell polarity is maintained, and junctional complexes at the apical cell pole are developed accordingly (Figures 1 and 2). However, cell size and shape depend on many conditions not yet very well understood.

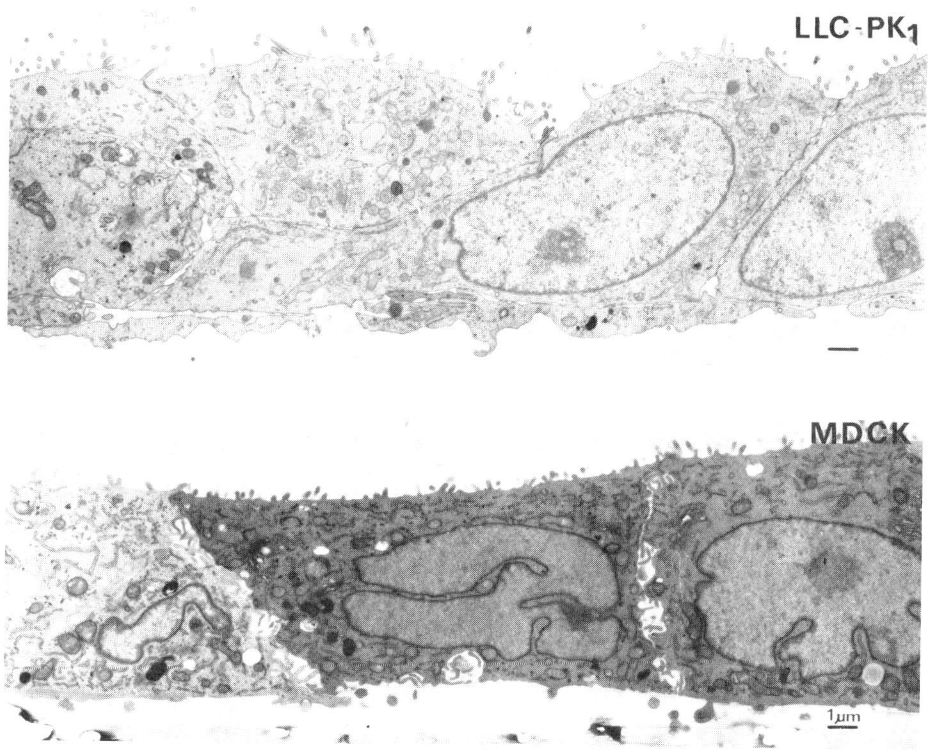

FIGURE 2. Electron micrographs of LLC-PK_1 and MDCK monolayers grown on collagen-coated cellulose ester filters (Millicell™ HA tissue culture inserts, Millipore Corp.).[131] For morphological details see text.

Tissue culture parameters, like media composition with respect to serum, hormone and growth factors, culture substrata, and extracellular matrix components, substantially influence the expression of specific morphological features and functions and thus the degree of cell differentiation. The expression of membrane enzymes and transport systems significantly varies with culture duration. It is therefore essential to precisely define the culture conditions for each cell line used and each functional parameter studied in physiological or toxicological experiments. The LLC-PK_1 epithelial cell line continuously increases in the expression of apical membrane enzyme activities and apically localized Na^+-dependent hexose transport during cell growth and differentiation into a mature epithelium,[119-123] which is accompanied by an increase in apical membrane surface area.[67] In contrast, however, apical Na^+-dependent phosphate transport has been shown to decrease in LLC-PK_1 cells with culture age,[41,124,125] whereas in OK cells, Na^+/P_i transport increases with culture duration.[41]

Another major factor influencing cell shape, size, and degree of differentiation seems to be the culture substratum, either the extracellular matrix itself on which the cultured epithelium rests[126-129] or the physical tissue culture support.[38,130] In a number of studies it has impressively been shown that the degree of morphological and functional differentiation of epithelial cells from different tissue origin considerably increases when the epithelia are cultured on permeable surfaces, thereby providing free access of tissue culture medium to the basolateral membrane surface[33,39,40,54,116,131-133] (Figure 2). Furthermore, this technique of culturing transporting epithelia represents the prerequisite for studying epithelial dysfunction in *in vitro* nephrotoxicity testing (see below).[22]

C. *IN VITRO* CELL FUNCTIONS WITH RESPECT TO NEPHROTOXICITY TESTING

A major route through which xenobiotic compounds are processed in the kidney for excretion is conjugation with glutathione, resulting in the formation of mercapturic acids.[134] However, renal biotransformation of chemicals does not only result in excretory metabolites, but may also be associated with the formation of highly reactive nephrotoxic compounds.[135,136] In particular *S*-glutathione and *S*-cysteine conjugates have been assumed to be potent nephrotoxins. The presumed site of *S*-cysteine conjugate toxicity is the proximal tubular epithelium. In several studies, *S*-cysteine conjugate transport and toxicity have been elaborated on LLC-PK_1 cultures.[137-141] LLC-PK_1 cells respond to toxic *S*-glutathione and *S*-cysteine conjugates and transform *S*-cysteine conjugates to toxic mercapturates.[137,141] Furthermore, these conjugates are taken up by a basolateral amino acid transport system.[138,140] Recently, mercapturic acid formation was also shown in OK cells.[142] Thus, cultured epithelial cells may also serve as model systems to study specific aspects of renal biotransformation and the resulting nephrotoxicity.

The recent observation of the expression of the multidrug transporter (*P*-glycoprotein)[143,144] in renal epithelial cell lines,[145,146] which is normally present in the apical membrane of the proximal tubule,[147,148] opens new ways to study multidrug resistance of renal cells and the elimination of chemotherapeutic agents by the kidney.

D. TECHNIQUES OF *IN VITRO* TOXICITY TESTING

Several strategies are currently followed to assess nephrotoxicity. The most common is histopathology, which at least in the intact organ ensures the localization of the various sites of damage within the kidney (glomerulus, the various nephron segments, interstitum, and vasculature). Another route of increasing importance is urine protein analysis, mainly based on the measurement of urinary enzyme activities excreted by renal epithelial cells.[149-151] Although this approach noninvasively detects renal epithelial injury, the monitoring of this event fails to detect subtle injury and changes in epithelial reabsorption and secretion. In addition, mechanisms of action of toxicants at the cellular level are difficult to be assessed with this approach.

Since nephrotoxicity represents a serious health risk, there exists increasing demand to develop screening procedures which rapidly and reliably detect adverse effects of xenobiotics. The design of such a new approach should be in a way that screening can be carried out efficiently, i.e., with low cost systems and simple experimental setups. In addition the possibility to compare test effects with a reference substance must be given.

Most of the criteria just listed are fulfilled by continuous renal epithelial cell cultures. In analogy to the above-mentioned nephrotoxicity tests, confluent epithelial monolayers grown in culture dishes can be monitored for maintenance of layer integrity following the administration of a toxic xenobiotic using light microscopy analogous to histopathology (Figure 3). The intactness of cells is easily determined by measuring the release of marker enzymes of various cellular compartments into the culture medium just like in urine analysis[22] (Figure 4). The most simple procedure is the determination of lactate dehydrogenase activity.[152,153] *N*-acetyl-glucosaminidase may be indicative for additional lysosomal damage. Glutamate dehydrogenase activity may be utilized to detect mitochondrial damage, and gamma-GT or alkaline phosphatase activity would be indicative for a release of apical membranes into the supernatant medium.[154] One should, however, keep in mind that the toxic compound studied may also inhibit one or the other marker enzyme.[20,42] Thus morphological and biochemical assay systems should always be applied in combination.

Another set of parameters, which can be used to ascertain the nephrotoxic action of xenobiotics, are those defining the integrity and transport function of the cultured epithelium.

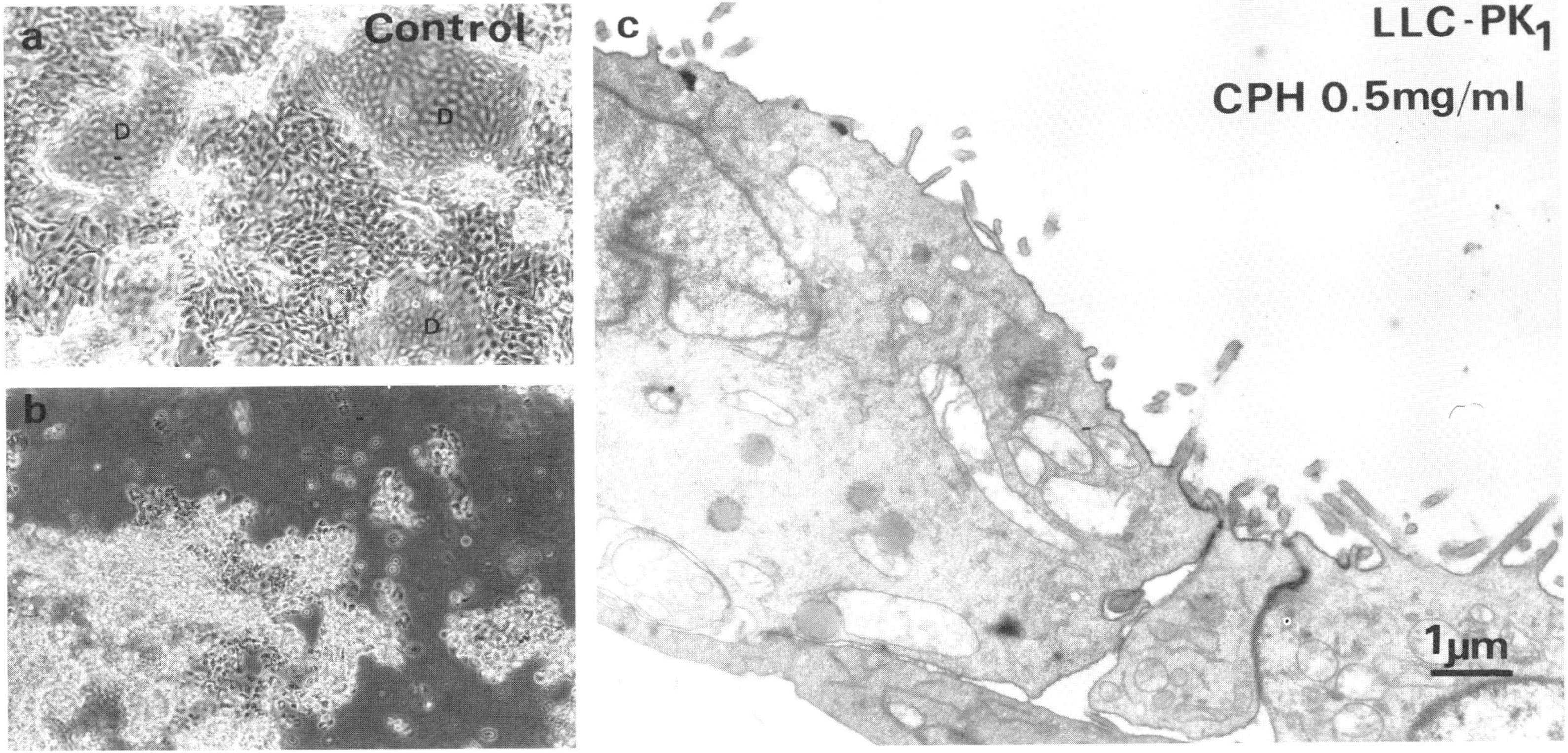

FIGURE 3. Cephalosporin-induced morphologic changes of LLC-PK_1 cells grown in plastic tissue culture dishes. Left panel: phase contrast micrographs of controls (a), and of LLC-PK_1 cultures after 24 h treatment with 0.5 mg/ml cephaloridine (CPH), (b). Right: electron micrograph of CPH-treated LLC-PK_1 cells (24 h, 0.5 mg/ml). CPH-induced mitochondrial damage, mitochondrial swelling, clarification of the mitochondrial matrix, and disruption of cristae membranes can be clearly recognized.

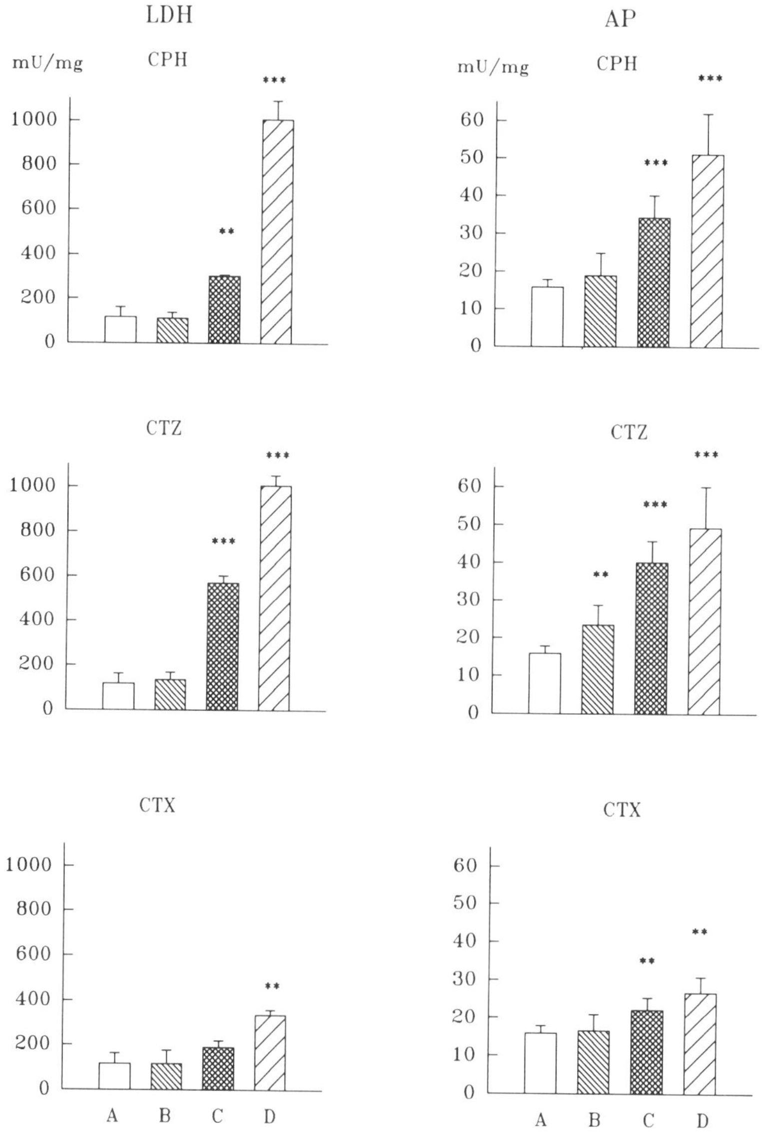

FIGURE 4. Cephalosporin-induced release of the cytosolic marker enzyme lactate dehydrogenase (LDH) and the apical membrane marker alkaline phosphatase (AP). LLC-PK_1 cultures in tissue culture dishes were incubated for 24 h with different concentrations of cephaloridine (CPH), ceftazidime (CTZ), and cefotaxime (CTX), and enzyme activities determined in the supernatant culture medium. A: controls; B: CPH 0.25, CTZ 0.75, and CTX 2.5 mg/ml; C: CPH 0.5, CTZ 1.5, and CTX 5.0 mg/ml; D: CPH 1.0, CTZ 3.0, and CTX 10.0 mg/ml. Values are given as specific activities and represent means ± SD (n = 6). Statistically significant differences to controls are indicated by asterisks. *: $p < 0.05$; **: $p < 0.01$, ***: $p < 0.001$.

These parameters include the microscopic observation of domes[101,155] (Figure 3a) and/or the monitoring of transepithelial electrophysiological parameters in Ussing-type chambers.[36,37,51,54,68,69] In particular, these latter parameters seem to provide the most sensitive measures of epithelial integrity and thus of the barrier function of the cultured epithelium.[47,156-159] In this respect, measurements of epithelial "leakage" of indicator compounds[160] should additionally be mentioned.

The influence of toxic xenobiotics upon dome formation may be utilized to judge gross disturbances of transepithelial water and solute transport. This approach, however, suffers from the fact that toxins can be administered only from the apical side of the epithelial monolayer.

Application of semipermeable culture substrata would overcome this problem, but these substrata prevent monolayers from dome formation. But, as already outlined above, this culture technique offers to use epithelial monolayers in Ussing chamber-like experimental setups. Observation of dome formation or disappearance can now be replaced by measurement of transepithelial electrochemical gradients induced by vectorial solute transports as measures for epithelial integrity. They include (1) the spontaneous transepithelial potential difference, (2) the transepithelial resistance, (3) the ion transport-generated short circuit current, and (4) the anion-to-cation permeability ratio as a measure of the shunt path permselectivity of the epithelium.[159] The latter parameter especially has been successfully applied for leaky epithelia, like the proximal nephron.[161] Due to the low transepithelial resistance (100 to 400 ohms·cm^2) of most of the cultured epithelia and the mammalian proximal tubule, accurate measurements of the transepithelial resistance are difficult to perform and are highly dependent on the geometry of the Ussing-chamber device and on the geometry and reproducibility of the electrode position, respectively.[51,162,163] Despite these facts, the differential effects of reactive oxidants on apical and basolateral membrane domains and epithelial conductance of MDCK monolayers, for example, have been studied by this approach.[164] The effects of phorbol ester tumor promoters on LLC-PK$_1$ epithelial tight junctions have also been studied using this experimental setup.[165]

In our laboratory, we recently determined the functional integrity of cephalosporin-treated LLC-PK$_1$ epithelia by measuring dilution potentials after imposing concentration gradients for both sodium and chloride across the cultured epithelium.[22] The application of dilution potentials offers the simplest way to assess monolayer cation-to-anion permeability ratios[47,68,162,163] and thus epithelial integrity and its affection by toxins. In this type of experiment, no major assumptions with respect to geometry of electrode position must be made. The only electrophysiological parameter to be monitored is the solute gradient-induced change in the spontaneous transepithelial potential difference, which can easily be monitored by calomel half cells connected to the bathing solutions by agar bridges.

Cephalosporines, for example, have long been known to dose dependently injure the kidney and lead to reduced glomerular filtration, glucosuria, and proteinuria. Histopathologically vast necroses of the proximal tubular S-2 segment occur. Application of cephaloridine, ceftazidime, and cefotaxime to monolayer cultures of LLC-PK$_1$ cells grown either on solid or semipermeable substrata represents a good example to validate the use of cell culture for nephrotoxicity testing. Although the doses applied are difficult to compare with those used in animal experiments or found to be nephrotoxic in man, the differences in cephalosporine concentrations triggering morphologic signs of injury (Figures 3b and c) and/or enzyme release (Figure 4) are of the same order of magnitude. The concentration necessary to induce injury by cephaloridine is three times lower than that of ceftazidime and ten times lower than that of cefotaxime, which is in line with studies on whole animals.[166] Electrophysiologic assessment of cephalosporine effects on the intactness of the epithelial barrier grown on filter inserts displays a completely comparable dose dependency but with a considerably higher sensitivity (Figure 5). These results are of particular interest, since LLC-PK$_1$ cells lack a basolateral organic anion transporter, which is assumed to substantially contribute to cephalosporine accumulation and nephrotoxicity. The latter aspect may illustrate the usefulness of continuous renal cell line in context with the clarification of mechanistic aspects of nephrotoxic cell injury.

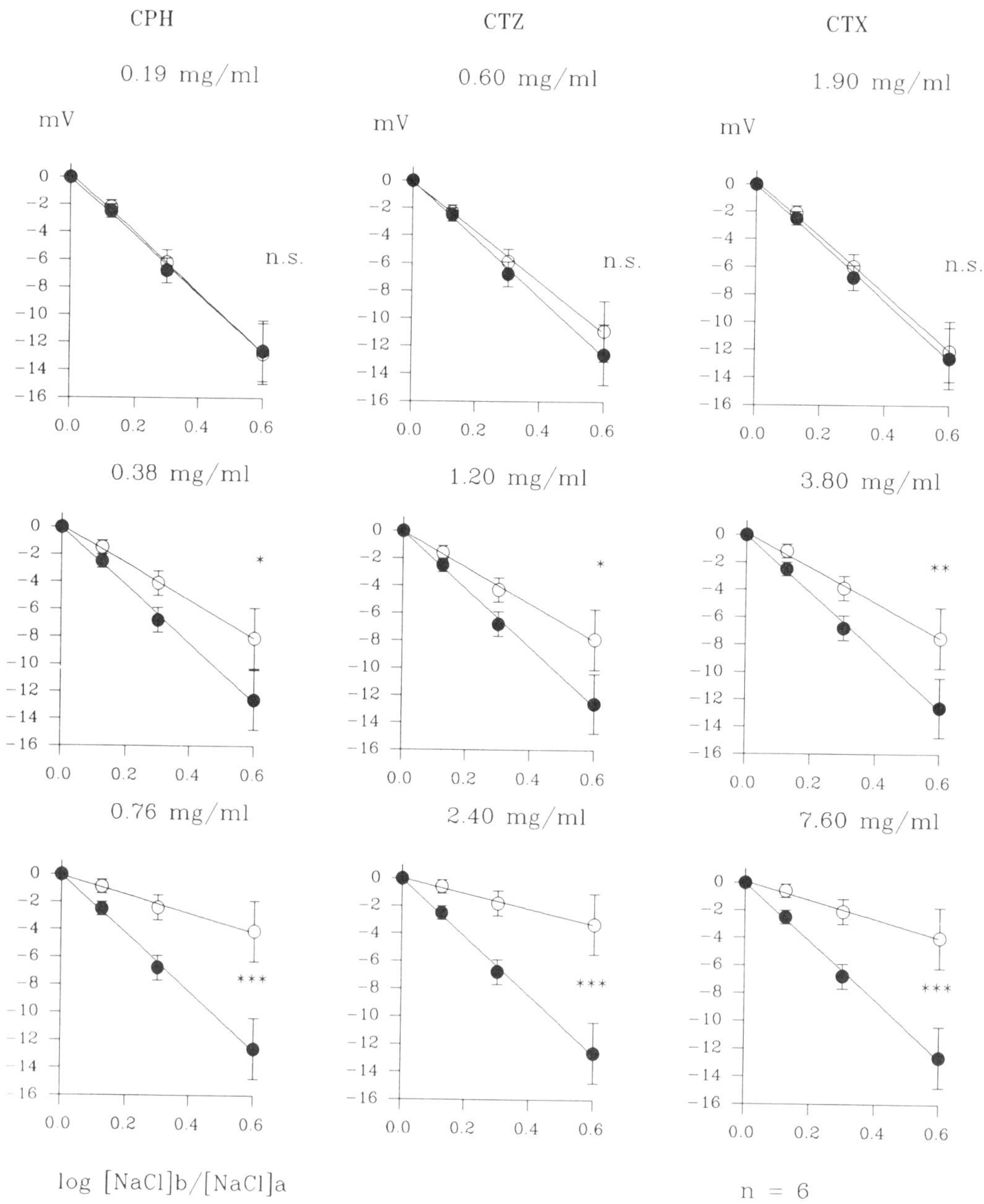

FIGURE 5. Effects of cephalosporin treatment on epithelial permeability of filter-grown LLC-PK_1 monolayer cultures. LLC-PK_1 epithelia were cultured on collagen-coated cellulose ester filter inserts (Millicell™ HA, Millipore Corp.)[131] for 10 to 14 days. Thereafter, LLC-PK_1 epithelia were incubated for 24 h with cephaloridine (CPH), ceftazidime (CTZ), and cefotaxime (CTX) at the concentrations indicated. Full circles are controls and empty circles are cephalosporin-treated monolayers. The functional integrity of cultured epithelia was determined by measuring dilution potentials after imposing concentration gradients for both sodium and chloride across control and cephalosporin-treated cultures, i.e., the anion-to-cation permeability ratio.[68,161-163] This was done by replacing the apical bathing solution (phosphate-buffered saline, PBS) with PBS, in which 25%, 50%, and 75%, respectively, of the NaCl content were replaced by isosmotic amounts of mannitol. The resulting changes in the spontaneous transepithelial potential difference (PD_{te}) were recorded with a high impedance microvoltmeter (Keithley 197 DMM) connected to the bathing solutions by calomel half cells with 3 *M* KCl/2% agar bridges.[68,162,163] The monitored changes in PD_{te} are displayed in the ordinate, and the abscissa gives the imposed transepithelial NaCl concentration ratio (log $[NaCl]_b/[NaCl]_a$). Values represent means ± SD; ns: no significant difference to control; *: $p < 0.05$; **: $p < 0.01$; ***: $p < 0.001$; (n = 6).

LLC-PK_1 cells also have been successfully used as a model system to study aminoglycoside nephrotoxicity.[154,167,168] In a number of comparative studies on the cytotoxicity of aminoglycoside antibiotics, continuous renal cell lines have been successfully applied.[152,153,169-171] Furthermore, the cellular mechanisms of *cis*-platinum[172] and heavy metal nephrotoxicity[173-175] have been explored in LLC-PK_1 cultures. Recently, the method of continuous recording of cell membrane potential with the use of intracellular microelectrodes[176] was applied to elucidate the mechanisms of cadmium, cobalt, and mercury toxicity in MDCK cells.[177-179]

Filter-grown monolayers in combination with electron microscopy and morphometry may be utilized to study transcytosis[43,105,180,181] and its alteration by toxic xenobiotics.[183] These latter techniques may gain importance for testing renal side effects of peptidic or other macromolecular drugs currently under development.

IV. CONCLUSION AND FUTURE OUTLOOK

The most important aspects for using cell culture techniques in testing of nephrotoxic side effects of xenobiotics are either screening of newly synthetized drugs or environmental contaminants, which are suspected to exert adverse effects to the kidney, or to investigate mechanistic aspects leading to renal cell injury. Especially with respect to the latter, renal epithelial cultures offer the possibility of easy access to the object of interest, the objects are provided in nearly unlimited amounts, and they match reasonably well their site of nephronal origin. In this context, continuous renal cell lines represent the experimental system of choice. They are easy to grow, maintain, and handle, they are largely commercially available (e.g., from the ATCC), and retain most of the basic functions of their ancestor cell, at least in cases of permanent proximal and collecting duct cells (LLC-PK_1, OK, JTC-12, MDCK, A6). The inevitable advantage, however, is that an enormous amount of information with regard to culture conditions, differentiated functions, like metabolism, transport, and hormone responsiveness, is available from the literature.[21,25,118] The disadvantage is the fact that they may suffer from the loss of one or the other *in vivo et situ* function as a result of prolonged cultivation. Under these circumstances, or in case one of the lost functions seem to be the predominant target for a nephrotoxic xenobiotic under investigation, the more laborious and difficult application of primary cultures must be put on. In addition one must keep in mind that some continuous cell lines are heterogenous, and multiple cell types might be present in an uncloned wild type culture.

Therefore methods should be developed to reexpress the ''lost functions'' or to tailor new cell lines more closely matching the cell type of origin in continuous cell lines. Such an enterprise may include several partially, all ready available cell biology techniques.

The most simple approach would be adaptation to culture conditions, which more closely resemble the *in vivo* environment of the respective cell type. As already mentioned, omission or drastic reduction of glucose and replacement against pyruvate in the media used for cultivation of LLC-PK_1 cells enables reexpression of gluconeogenesis.[63,65] Fusion of cells of continuous cell lines[34,183] stemming from the same *in vivo* ancestor cell of different species and with different retainment of cellular functions, i.e., metabolic pathways, transport systems, or hormone receptors, may be used to establish new continuous lines more closely resembling the characteristics of the cell type of origin. Fusion of cells from primary cultures with cells from continuous lines delineated from the same nephron cell or nephron segment may help to either immortalize the respective primary culture or help to reexpress lost functions within the continuous cell type.

Genetic approaches[184] may deliver another route to establish new, more ''natural'' permanent cell lines. Transfection or microinjection with either genomic DNA or, if available, with different but defined genes (or oncogenes) could be one of the tools to be applied.[185-188]

These strategies should even offer the possibility to establish cell lines expressing most or all of the functions of human renal epithelia. However, all these trials demand careful selection procedures to isolate the fused hybridoma, the mutated or transfected cells.

V. SUMMARY

Increasing ethical, commercial, and scientific needs have initiated worldwide activities to establish reliable, well-characterized, and appropriate *in vitro* alternatives to animal toxicity testing procedures. The methodologies developed in modern cell and tissue culture techniques nowadays allow growth and maintenance of somatic cells *in vitro* under precisely defined and controlled environmental conditions.

In the last two decades, cell and tissue cultures of continuous renal epithelial cell lines have become powerful tools to study basic renal physiological functions, like transepithelial transport and its regulation by metabolism, hormones, or drugs. Therefore, kidney cells in culture may also represent one of the many *in vitro* approaches for studying drug-induced nephrotoxicity.

In the present chapter, we describe the characteristics of continuous renal epithelial cell lines, the retention in tissue culture of kidney-specific characteristics, and the legitimation to use these cell lines in the *in vitro* assessment of xenobiotic-induced nephrotoxicity and renal cell injury.

ACKNOWLEDGMENTS

We wish to thank Mrs. Edna Nemati and Ms. Evelyn Troppmair for the photographic work. Studies in our laboratory were supported in part by the Austrian Science Foundation, Project P7968-MED, as part of a biotechnology program — BRIDGE-T (PL890388) — of the Commission of the European Communities.

REFERENCES

1. **Kriz, W. and Kaissling, B.,** Structural organization of mammalian kidney, in *The Kidney: Physiology and Pathophysiology,* Seldin, D. W. and Giebisch, G., Eds., Raven Press, New York, 1985, 265.
2. **Wirthensohn, G. and Guder, W. G.,** Renal substrate metabolism, *Physiol. Rev.,* 66, 469, 1986.
3. **Jacobson, H. R.,** Functional segmentation of mammalian nephron, *Am. J. Physiol.,* 241, F203, 1981.
4. **Knepper, M. and Burg, M.,** Organization of nephron function, *Am. J. Physiol.,* 244, F579, 1983.
5. **Bulger, R. E. and Dobyan, D. C.,** Recent advances in renal morphology, *Annu. Rev. Physiol.,* 44, 47, 1982.
6. **Pfaller, W., Gstraunthaler, G., and Kotanko, P.,** Compartments and surfaces in renal cells, in *Renal Biochemistry, Cells, Membranes, Molecules,* Kinnc, R. H. K., Ed., Elsevier Science Publishers, Amsterdam, 1985, 1.
7. **Tisher, C. C.,** Anatomy of the kidney, in *The Kidney,* 2nd ed., Brenner, B. M. and Rector, F. C., Eds., W. B. Saunders, Philadelphia, 1981, 3.
8. **Kriz, W. and Bankir, L.,** A standard nomenclature for structures of the kidney, *Am. J. Physiol.,* 254, F1, 1988; *Kidney Int.,* 33, 1988; *Pflügers Arch.,* 411, 113, 1988.
9. **Brezis, M., Rosen, S., Silva, P., and Epstein, F. H.,** Renal ischemia: a new perspective, *Kidney Int.,* 26, 375, 1984.
10. **Pfaller, W.,** Structure function correlation on rat kidney, *Adv. Anat. Embryol. Cell Biol.,* 70, 1, 1982.
11. **Pfaller, W., Gstraunthaler, G., and Willinger, C. C.,** Morphology of renal tubular damage from nephrotoxins, *Toxicol. Lett.,* 53, 39, 1990.

12. **Venkatachalam, M. J., Bernard, D. B., Donohoe, J. F., and Levinsky, N. G.,** Ischemic damage and repair in the rat proximal tubule: differences among S_1, S_2, and S_3 segments, *Kidney Int.*, 14, 31, 1978.
13. **Kinne, R. K. H.,** Selectivity and direction: plasma membranes in renal transport, *Am. J. Physiol.*, 260, F153, 1991.
14. **Ullrich, K. J. and Rumrich, G.,** Contraluminal transport systems in the proximal renal tubule involved in secretion of organic anions, *Am. J. Physiol.*, 254, F453, 1988.
15. **Ullrich, K. J., Rumrich, G., Gemborys, M. W., and Dekant, W.,** Renal transport and nephrotoxicity, in *Nephrotoxicity. Mechanisms, Early Diagnosis, and Therapeutic Management*, Bach, P. H., Gregg, N. J., Wilks, M. F., and Delacruz, L., Eds., Marcel Dekker, New York, 1991, 1.
16. **Kacew, S. and Bergeron, M. G.,** Pathogenic factors in aminoglycoside-induced nephrotoxicity, *Toxicol. Lett.*, 51, 241, 1990.
17. **Tune, B. M. and Fravert, D.,** Mechanism of cephalosporin nephrotoxicity: a comparison of cephaloridine and cephaloglycin, *Kidney Int.*, 18, 591, 1980.
18. **Tune, B. M. and Hsu, C.-Y.,** Mechanisms of beta-lactam antibiotic nephrotoxicity, *Toxicol. Lett.*, 53, 81, 1990.
19. **Ullrich, K. J. and Greger, R.,** Approaches to the study of tubule transport functions, in *The Kidney: Physiology and Pathophysiology*, Seldin, D. W. and Giebisch, G., Eds., Raven Press, New York, 1985, 427.
20. **Acosta, D., Sorensen, E. M. B., Anuforo, D. C., Mitchell, D. B., Ramos, K., Santone, K. S., and Smith, M. A.,** An *in vitro* approach to the study of target organ toxicity of drugs and chemicals, *In Vitro Cell. Dev. Biol.*, 21, 495, 1985.
21. **Boogaard, P. J., Nagelkerke, J. F., and Mulder, G. J.,** Renal proximal tubular cells in suspension or in primary culture as *in vitro* models to study nephrotoxicity, *Chem.-Biol. Interactions*, 76, 251, 1990.
22. **Gstraunthaler, G., Steinmassl, D., and Pfaller, W.,** Renal cell cultures: a tool for studying tubular function and nephrotoxicity, *Toxicol. Lett.*, 53, 1, 1990.
23. **Williams, P. D.,** The application of renal cells in culture in studying drug-induced nephrotoxicity, *In Vitro Cell. Dev. Biol.*, 25, 800, 1989.
24. **Wilson, P. D.,** Use of cultured renal tubular cells in the study of cell injury, *Mineral Electrol. Metab.*, 12, 71, 1986.
25. **Gstraunthaler, G. J. A.,** Epithelial cells in tissue culture, *Renal Physiol. Biochem.*, 11, 1, 1988.
26. **Green, N., Algren, A., Hoyer, J., Triche, T., and Burg, M.,** Differentiated lines of cells from rabbit renal medullary thick ascending limbs grown on amnion, *Am. J. Physiol.*, 249, C97, 1985.
27. **Hall, H. G., Farson, D. A., and Bissell, M. J.,** Lumen formation by epithelial cell lines in response to collagen overlay: a morphogenetic model in culture, *Proc. Natl. Acad. Sci. U.S.A.*, 79, 4672, 1982.
28. **Karst, W. and Merker, H.-J.,** The differentiation behaviour of MDCK cells grown on matrix components and in collagen gels, *Cell Differ.*, 22, 211, 1988.
29. **McAteer, J. A., Evan, A. P., and Gardner, K. D.,** Morphogenetic clonal growth of kidney epithelial cell line MDCK, *Anat. Rec.*, 217, 229, 1987.
30. **Minuth, W. W. and Rudolph, U.,** A compatible support system for cell culture in biomedical research, *Cytotechnology*, 4, 181, 1990.
31. **Yaoita, E.,** Behavior of rat mesangial cells cultured within extracellular matrix, *Lab. Invest.*, 61, 410, 1989.
32. **Zuk, A., Matlin, K. S., and Hay, E. D.,** Type I collagen gel induces Madin-Darby canine kidney cells to become fusiform in shape and lose apical-basal polarity, *J. Cell Biol.*, 108, 903, 1989.
33. **Handler, J. S., Preston, A. S., and Steele, R. E.,** Factors affecting differentiation of epithelial transport and responsiveness to hormones, *Fed. Proc.*, 43, 2221, 1984.
34. **Kersting, U., Joha, H., Steigner, W., Gassner, B., Gstraunthaler, G., Pfaller, W., and Oberleithner, H.,** Fusion of cultured dog kidney (MDCK) cells. I. Technique, fate of plasma membranes and cell nuclei, *J. Membrane Biol.*, 111, 37, 1989.
35. **Wohlwend, A., Montesano, R., Vassalli, J.-D., and Orci, L.,** LLC-PK1 cysts: a model for the study of epithelial polarity, *J. Cell. Physiol.*, 125, 533, 1985.
36. **Audus, K. L., Bartel, R. L., Hidalgo, I. J., and Borchardt, R. T.,** The use of cultured epithelial and endothelial cells for drug transport and metabolism studies, *Pharmaceut. Res.*, 7, 435, 1990.
37. **Cho, M. J., Thompson, D. P., Cramer, C. T., Vidmar, T. J., and Scieszka, J. F.,** The Madin Darby canine kidney (MDCK) epithelial cell monolayer as a model cellular transport barrier, *Pharmaceut. Res.*, 6, 71, 1989.
38. **Handler, J. S., Green, N., and Steele, R. E.,** Cultures as epithelial models: porous-bottom culture dishes for studying transport and differentiation, *Meth. Enzymol.*, 171, 736, 1989.
39. **Ip, T. K., Galletti, P. M., and Aebischer, P.,** Effects of attachment substrates on the growth and differentiation of LLC-PK_1 cells, *In Vitro Cell. Dev. Biol.*, 26, 162, 1990.

40. **Leiderman, L. J., Tucker, J. A., and Dennis, V. W.,** Growth and differentiation of opossum kidney cells on microscopically transparent microporous membranes, *Tissue Cell,* 21, 355, 1989.
41. **Biber, J., Malmström, K., Reshkin, S., and Murer, H.,** Phosphate transport in established renal epithelial cell lines, *Meth. Enzymol.,* 191, 494, 1990.
42. **Ruedl, C., Gstraunthaler, G., and Moser, M.,** Differential inhibitory action of fungal toxin orellanine on alkaline phosphatase isoenzymes, *Biochim. Biophys. Acta,* 991, 280, 1989.
43. **Fouda, A.-K., Fauth, C., and Roch-Ramel, F.,** Transport of organic cations by kidney epithelial cell line LLC-PK_1, *J. Pharmacol. Exp. Ther.,* 252, 286, 1990.
44. **Handler, J. S.,** Overview of epithelial polarity, *Annu. Rev. Physiol.,* 51, 729, 1989.
45. **Rodriguez-Boulan, E. and Nelson, W. J.,** Morphogenesis of the polarized epithelial cell phenotype, *Science,* 245, 718, 1989.
46. **Simons, K. and Fuller, S. D.,** Cell surface polarity in epithelia, *Annu. Rev. Cell Biol.,* 1, 243, 1985.
47. **Cereijido, M., Ehrenfeld, J., Fernandez-Castelo, S., and Meza, I.,** Fluxes, junctions, and blisters in cultured monolayers of epithelioid cells (MDCK), *Ann. NY Acad. Sci.,* 372, 422, 1981.
48. **Lever, J. E.,** Variant (MDCK) kidney epithelial cells altered in response to inducers of dome formation and differentiation, *J. Cell. Physiol.,* 122, 45, 1985.
49. **Taub, M.,** Retinoic acid modulates dome formation by MDCK cells in defined medium, *J. Cell. Physiol.,* 141, 24, 1989.
50. **Handler, J. S.,** Use of cultured epithelia to study transport and its regulation, *J. Exp. Biol.,* 106, 55, 1983.
51. **Simmons, N. L.,** Ion transport in "tight" epithelial monolayers of MDCK cells, *J. Membrane Biol.,* 59, 105, 1981.
52. **Simmons, N. L.,** Tissue culture of established renal cell lines, *Methods Enzymol.,* 191, 426, 1990.
53. **Pfaller, W., Gstraunthaler, G., Kersting, U., and Oberleithner, H.,** Carbonic anhydrase activity in MDCK cells: evidence for intercalated cell properties, *Renal Physiol. Biochem.,* 12, 328, 1989.
54. **Hidalgo, I. J., Raub, T. J., and Borchardt, R. T.,** Characterization of human colon carcinoma cell line (Caco-2) as a model system for intestinal epithelial permeability, *Gastroenterology,* 96, 736, 1989.
55. **Dharmsathaphorn, K. and Madara, J. L.,** Established intestinal cell lines as model systems for electrolyte transport studies, *Methods Enzymol.,* 192, 354, 1990.
56. **Schaeffer, W. I.,** In the interest of clear communication, *In Vitro Cell. Dev. Biol.,* 25, 389, 1989.
57. **Schaeffer, W. I.,** Terminology associated with cell, tissue and organ culture, molecular biology and molecular genetics, *In Vitro Cell. Dev. Biol.,* 26, 97, 1990.
58. **Gaush, C. R., Hard, W. L., and Smith, T. F.,** Characterization of an established line of canine kidney cells (MDCK), *Proc. Soc. Exp. Biol. Med.,* 122, 931, 1966.
59. **Madin, S. H. and Darby, N. B., Jr.,** Established kidney cell lines of normal adult bovine and ovine origin, *Proc. Soc. Exp. Biol. Med.,* 98, 574, 1958.
60. **Hull, R. N., Cherry, W. R., and Weaver, G. W.,** The origin and characteristics of a pig kidney cell strain, LLC-PK_1, *In Vitro,* 12, 670, 1976.
61. **Keith, D. H., Teplitz, R. L., and Riggs, A. D.,** Metaphase synchronization and chromosome preparation from the OK opossum cell line having a potentially isolatable X chromosome, *In Vitro,* 20, 833, 1984.
62. **Koyama, H., Goodpasture, C., Miller, M. M., Teplitz, R. L., and Riggs, A. D.,** Establishment and characterization of a cell line from American opossum *(Didelphys virginiana), In Vitro,* 14, 239, 1978.
63. **Gstraunthaler, G. and Handler, J. S.,** Isolation, growth and characterization of a gluconeogenic strain of renal cells, *Am. J. Physiol.,* 252, C232, 1987.
64. **Gstraunthaler, G., Pfaller, W., and Kotanko, P.,** Biochemical characterization of renal epithelial cell cultures (LLC-PK_1 and MDCK), *Am. J. Physiol.,* 248, F536, 1985.
65. **Gstraunthaler, G., Gersdorf, E., Fischer, W. M., Joannidis, M., and Pfaller, W.,** Morphological and biochemical changes of LLC-PK_1 cells during adaptation to glucose-free culture conditions, *Renal Physiol. Biochem.,* 13, 137, 1990.
66. **Fauth, C., Rossier, B., and Roch-Ramel, F.,** Transport of tetraethylammonium by a kidney epithelial cell line (LLC-PK_1), *Am. J. Physiol.,* 254, F351, 1988.
67. **Pfaller, W., Gstraunthaler, G., and Loidl, P.,** Morphology of differentiation and maturation of LLC-PK_1 epithelia, *J. Cell. Physiol.,* 142, 247, 1990.
68. **Rabito, C. A.,** Occluding junctions in a renal cell line (LLC-PK_1) with characteristics of proximal tubular cells, *Am. J. Physiol.,* 250, F734, 1986.
69. **Rabito, C. A.,** Reassembly of the occluding junctions in a renal cell line with characteristics of proximal tubular cells, *Am. J. Physiol.,* 251, F978, 1986.
70. **Morel, F. and Doucet, A.,** Hormonal control of kidney functions at the cell level, *Physiol. Rev.,* 66, 377, 1986.
71. **Malmström, K. and Murer, H.,** Parathyroid hormone inhibits phosphate transport in OK cells but not in LLC-PK_1 and JTC-12.P3 cells, *Am. J. Physiol.,* 251, C23, 1986.

72. **Ausiello, D. A., Skorecki, K. L., Verkman, A. S., and Bonventre, J. V.,** Vasopressin signaling in kidney cells, *Kidney Int.*, 31, 521, 1987.
73. **Burnatowska-Hledin, M. A. and Spielman, W. S.,** Vasopressin increases cytosolic free calcium in LLC-PK_1 cells through a V_1-receptor, *Am. J. Physiol.*, 253, F328, 1987.
74. **Tang, M. J. and Weinberg, J. M.,** Vasopressin-induced increases of cytosolic calcium in LLC-PK_1 cells, *Am. J. Physiol.*, 251, F1090, 1986.
75. **Goldring, S. R., Dayer, J. M., Ausiello, D. A., and Krane, S. M.,** A cell strain cultured from porcine kidney increases cyclic AMP content upon exposure to calcitonin or vasopressin, *Biochem. Biophys. Res. Comm.*, 83, 434, 1978.
76. **Wohlwend, A., Malmström, K., Henke, H., Murer, H., Vassalli, J. D., and Fischer, J. A.,** Calcitonin and calcitonin gene-related peptide interact with same receptor in cultured LLC-PK_1 kidney cells, *Biochem. Biophys. Res. Comm.*, 131, 537, 1985.
77. **Garg, L. C., Wozniak, M., and Phillips, M. I.,** Stimulation of phosphoinositide hydrolysis by oxytocin in renal epithelial cells, *J. Pharmacol. Exp. Ther.*, 252, 552, 1990.
78. **Stassen, F. L., Heckman, G., Schmidt, D., Papadopoulos, M. T., Nambi, P., Sarau, H., Aiyar, N., Gellai, M., and Kinter, L.,** Oxytocin induces a transient increase in cytosolic free Ca^{2+} in renal tubular epithelial cells: evidence for oxytocin receptors on LLC-PK_1 cells, *Mol. Pharmacol.*, 33, 218, 1988.
79. **Gstraunthaler, G. and Pfaller, W.,** Modulation of the ammoniagenic response of LLC-PK_1 cultured epithelia. role of transamination, *Mineral Electrol. Metab.*, 15, 371, 1989.
80. **Gstraunthaler, G., Landauer, F., and Pfaller, W.,** Ammoniagenesis in renal epithelial cell culture, *Pflügers Arch.*, 411, R90, 1988.
81. **Sahai, A., Cole, L. A., and Tannen, R. L.,** Pathways and regulation of ammoniagenesis by LLC-PK_1 cells in culture, *J. Lab. Clin. Med.*, 114, 285, 1989.
82. **Sahai, A., Cole, L. A., Clarke, D. L., and Tannen, R. L.,** Rocking promotes differentiated properties in LLC-PK_1 cells by improved oxygenation, *Am. J. Physiol.*, 256, C1064, 1989.
83. **Malmström, K., Stange, G., and Murer, H.,** Identification of proximal tubule functions in the established kidney cell line, OK, *Biochim. Biophys. Acta*, 902, 269, 1987.
84. **Biber, J.,** Cellular aspects of proximal tubular phosphate reabsorption, *Kidney Int.*, 36, 360, 1989.
85. **Helmle-Kolb, C., Montrose, M. H., and Murer, H.,** Parathyroid hormone regulation of Na^+/H^+ exchange in opossum kidney cells: polarity and mechanisms, *Pflügers Arch.*, 416, 615, 1990.
86. **Helmle-Kolb, C., Montrose, M. H., Stange, G., and Murer, H.,** Regulation of Na^+/H^+ exchange in opossum kidney cells by parathyroid hormone, cyclic AMP and phorbol esters, *Pflügers Arch.*, 415, 461, 1990.
87. **Reshkin, S. J., Forgo, J., and Murer, H.,** Functional assymetry of phosphate transport and its regulation in opossum kidney cells: phosphate transport, *Pflügers Arch.*, 416, 554, 1990.
88. **Reshkin, S. J., Forgo, J., and Murer, H.,** Functional assymetry in phosphate transport and its regulation in opossum kidney cells: parathyroid hormone inhibition, *Pflügers Arch.*, 416, 624, 1990.
89. **Rabkin, R., Dahl, D. C., Mahoney, C. A., and Tsao, T.,** Protein catabolism in cultured kidney cells, *Kidney Int.*, 36, S11, 1989.
90. **Yagil, C., Frank, B. H., and Rabkin, R.,** Internalization and catabolism of insulin by an established renal cell line, *Am. J. Physiol.*, 254, C822, 1988.
91. **Yagil, C., Ehmann, U. K., Frank, B. H., and Rabkin, R.,** Insulin binding, internalization, and degradation by a cultured kidney cell line, *Am. J. Physiol.*, 254, E601, 1988.
92. **Takaoka, T., Katsuta, H., Endo, M., Sato, K., and Okumura, H.,** Establishment of a cell strain, JTC-12, from cynomolgus monkey kidney tissue, *Jpn. J. Exp. Med*, 32, 351, 1962.
93. **Takuwa, Y. and Ogata, E.,** Differentiated properties characteristic of renal proximal epithelium in a cell line derived from a normal monkey kidney (JTC-12), *In Vitro Cell. Dev. Biol.*, 21, 445, 1985.
94. **Ishizuka, I., Tadano, K., Nagata, N., Nimura, Y., and Nagain, Y.,** Hormone-specific responses and biosynthesis of sulfolipids in cell lines derived from mammalian kidney, *Biochim. Biophys. Acta*, 541, 467, 1978.
95. **Matsumoto, T., Kawanobe, Y., and Ogata, E.,** Regulation of 24,25-dihydroxyvitamin D-3 production by 1,25-dihyroxyvitamin D-3 and synthetic human parathyroid hormone fragment 1-34 in a cloned monkey kidney cell line (JTC-12), *Biochim. Biophys. Acta*, 845, 358, 1985.
96. **Lang, F., Friedrich, F., Paulmichl, M., Schobersberger, W., Jungwirth, A., Ritter, M., Steidl, M., Weiss, H., Wöll, E., Tschernko, E., Paulmichl, R., and Hallbrucker, C.,** Ion channels in Madin-Darby canine kidney cells, *Renal Physiol. Biochem.*, 13, 82, 1990.
97. **McRoberts, J. A., Taub, M., Saier, M. H., Jr.,** The Madin-Darby canine kidney (MDCK) cell line, in *Functionally Differentiated Cell Lines*, Alan R. Liss, New York, 1981, 117.
98. **Ziyadeh, F. N. and Agus, Z. S.,** Role calcium in chloride-secreting epithelia, *Mineral Electrol. Metab.*, 14, 78, 1988.
99. **Meier, K. E. and Insel, P. A.,** Hormone receptors and response in cultured renal epithelial cell lines, in *Tissue Culture of Epithelial Cells*, Taub, M., Ed., Plenum Press, New York, 1985, 145.

100. **Oberleithner, H., Steigner, W., Silbernagl, S., Vogel, U., Gstraunthaler, G., and Pfaller, W.,** Madin-Darby canine kidney cells. III. Aldosterone stimulates an apical H^+/K^+ pump, *Pflügers Arch.*, 416, 540, 1990.
101. **Oberleithner, H., Vogel, U., Kersting, U.,** Madin-Darby canine kidney cells. I. Aldosterone-induced domes and their evaluation as a model system, *Pflügers Arch.*, 416, 526, 1990.
102. **Oberleithner, H., Vogel, U., Kersting, U., and Steigner, W.,** Madin-Darby canine kidney cells. II. Aldosterone stimulates Na^+/H^+ and Cl^-/HCO_3^- exchange, *Pflügers Arch.*, 416, 533, 1990.
103. **Barker, G. and Simmons, N. L.,** Identification of two strains of cultured canine renal epithelial cells (MDCK cells) which display entirely different physiological properties, *Quart. J. Exp. Physiol.*, 66, 61, 1981.
104. **Richardson, J. C. W., Scalera, V., and Simmons, N. L.,** Identification of two strains of MDCK cells which resemble separate nephron tubule segments, *Biochim. Biophys. Acta*, 673, 26, 1981.
105. **von Bonsdorff, C.-H., Fuller, S. D., and Simons, K.,** Apical and basolateral endocytosis in Madin-Darby canine kidney (MDCK) cells grown on nitrocellulose filters, *EMBO J.*, 4, 2781, 1985.
106. **Stevenson, B. R., Anderson, J. M., Goodenough, D. A., and Mooseker, M. S.,** Tight junction structure and ZO-1 content are identical in two strains of Madin-Darby canine kidney cells which differ in transepithelial resistance, *J. Cell Biol.*, 107, 2401, 1988.
107. **Hansson, G. C., Simons, K., and van Meer, G.,** Two strains of the Madin-Darby canine kidney (MDCK) cell line have distinct glycosphingolipid compositions, *EMBO J.*, 5, 483, 1986.
108. **Nichols, G. E., Lovejoy, J. C., Borgman, C. A., Sanders, J. M., and Young, W. W., Jr.,** Isolation and characterization of two types of MDCK epithelial cell clones based on glycosphingolipid pattern, *Biochim. Biophys. Acta*, 887, 1, 1986.
109. **Nichols, G. E., Shiraishi, T., and Young, W. W., Jr.,** Polarity of neutral glycolipids, gangliosides, and sulfated lipids in MDCK epithelial cells, *J. Lipid Res.*, 29, 1205, 1988.
110. **Simons, K. and van Meer, G.,** Lipid sorting in epithelial cells, *Biochemistry*, 27, 6197, 1988.
111. **van Meer, G. and Simons, K.,** Lipid polarity and sorting in epithelial cells, *J. Cell. Biochem.*, 36, 51, 1988.
112. **Valentich, J. D.,** Morphological similarities between the dog kidney cell line MDCK and the mammalian cortical collecting tubule, *Ann. N.Y. Acad. Sci.*, 372, 384, 1981.
113. **Saier, M. H., Boerner, P., Grenier, F. C., McRoberts, J. A., Rindler, M. J., Taub, M., and Ü, H. S.,** Sodium entry pathways in renal epithelial cell lines, *Mineral Electrol. Metab.*, 12, 42, 1986.
114. **Handler, J. S., Perkins, F. M., and Johnson, J. P.,** Hormone effects on transport in cultured epithelia with high electrical resistance, *Am. J. Physiol.*, 240, C103, 1981.
115. **Perkins, F. M. and Handler, J. S.,** Transport properties of toad kidney epithelia in culture, *Am. J. Physiol.*, 241, C154, 1981.
116. **Lang, M. A., Muller, J., Preston, A. S., and Handler, J. S.,** Complete response to vasopressin requires epithelial organization in A6 cells in culture, *Am. J. Physiol.*, 250, C138, 1986.
117. **Preston, A. S., Muller, J., and Handler, J. S.,** Dexamethasone accelerates differentiation of A6 epithelia and increases response to vasopressin, *Am. J. Physiol.*, 255, C661, 1988.
118. **Kreisberg, J. I. and Wilson, P. D.,** Renal cell culture, *J. Electron Microsc. Technol.*, 9, 235, 1988.
119. **Handler, J. S. and Moran, A.,** Regulation of expression of the sodium-coupled hexose transporter in cultured LLC-PK_1 epithelia, *Pflügers Arch.*, 405, S163, 1985.
120. **Mullin, J. M., Weibel, J., Diamond, L., and Kleinzeller, A.,** Sugar transport in the LLC-PK_1 renal epithelial cell line: similarity to mammalian kidney and the influence of cell density, *J. Cell. Physiol.*, 104, 375, 1980.
121. **Rabito, C. A., Kreisberg, J. I., and Wight, D.,** Alkaline phosphatase and gamma-glutamyl transpeptidase as polarization makers during the organization of LLC-PK_1 cells into an epithelial membrane, *J. Biol. Chem.*, 259, 574, 1984.
122. **Sepulveda, F. V., Burton, K. A., and Pearson, J. D.,** The development of gamma-glutamyltransferase in a pig renal-epithelial-cell line *in vitro*, *Biochem. J.*, 208, 509, 1982.
123. **Yoneyama, Y. and Lever, J. E.,** Induction of microvillar hydrolase activities by cell density and exogenous differentiation inducers in an established kidney epithelial cell line (LLC-PK_1), *J. Cell. Physiol.*, 121, 64, 1984.
124. **Biber, J. and Murer, H.,** Na-P_i cotransport in LLC-PK_1 cells: fast adaptive response to P_i deprivation, *Am. J. Physiol.*, 249, C430, 1985.
125. **Scheinman, S. J.,** Effects of confluence on phosphate transport capacity in cultured renal cell lines, *J. Cell. Physiol.*, 135, 122, 1988.
126. **Kleinman, H. K., Luckenbill-Edds, L., Cannon, F. W., and Sephel, G. C.,** Use of extracellular matrix components for cell culture, *Anal. Biochem.*, 166, 1, 1987.
127. **McDonald, J. A.,** Receptors for extracellular matrix components, *Am. J. Physiol.*, 257, L331, 1989.

128. **Reid, L. M. and Rojkind, M.,** New techniques for culturing differentiated cells: reconstituted basement membrane rafts, *Meth. Enzymol.*, 58, 263, 1979.
129. **Yang, J. and Nandi, S.,** Growth of cultured cells using collagen as substrate, *Int. Rev. Cytol.*, 81, 249, 1983.
130. **Steele, R. E., Preston, A. S., Johnson, J. P., and Handler, J. S.,** Pourous-bottom dishes for culture of polarized cells, *Am. J. Physiol.*, 251, C136, 1986.
131. **Cook, J. R., Crute, B. E., Patrone, L. M., Gabriels, J., Lane, M. E., and van Buskirk, R. G.,** Microporosity of the substratum regulates differentiation of MDCK cells *in vitro, In Vitro Cell. Dev. Biol.*, 25, 914, 1989.
132. **Cott, G. R.,** Modulation of bioelectric properties across alveolar type II cells by substratum, *Am. J. Physiol.*, 257, C678, 1989.
133. **Fantini, J., Verrier, B., Marvaldi, J., and Mauchamp, J.,** *In vitro* differentiated HT 29-D4 clonal cell line generates leakproof and electrically active monolayers when cultured in porous-bottom culture dishes, *Biol. Cell,* 65, 163, 1989.
134. **Anders, M. W.,** Metabolism of drugs by the kidney, *Kidney Int.*, 18, 636, 1980.
135. **Elfarra, A. A. and Anders, M. W.,** Renal processing of glutathione conjugates. Role in nephrotoxicity, *Biochem. Pharmacol.*, 33, 3729, 1984.
136. **Monks, T. J., Anders, M. W., Dekant, W., Stevens, J. L., Lau, S. S., and van Bladeren, P. J.,** Glutathione conjugate mediated toxicities, *Toxicol. Appl. Pharmacol.*, 106, 1, 1990.
137. **Mertens, J. J. W. M., Weijnen, J. G. J., van Doorn, W. J., Spenkelink, B., Temmink, J. H. M., and van Bladeren, P. J.,** Differential toxicity as a result of apical and basolateral treatment of LLC-PK_1 with S-(1,2,3,4,4-pentachlorobutandienyl)glutathione and *N*-acetyl-S-(1,2,3,4,4,-pentachlorobutandienyl)-L-cysteine, *Chem.-Biol. Interactions,* 65, 283, 1988.
138. **Mertens, J. J. W. M., Keukens, E. A. J., Appel, M., Spenkelink, B., Temmink, J. H. M., and van Bladeren, P. J.,** Cytotoxicity of S-(1,2,3,4,4-pentachlorobutandienyl)-L-cysteine after apical and basolateral exposure of LLC-PK_1 monolayers. Involvement of an amino acid transport system, *Chem.-Biol. Interactions,* 75, 119, 1990.
139. **Mertens, J. J. W. M., Sterck, J. G. H., Lau, S. S., Monks, T. J., van Bladeren, P. J., and Temmink, J. H. M.,** Cytotoxicity of nephrotoxic glutathione-conjugated halohydroquinones, *Toxicol. Lett.*, 53, 147, 1990.
140. **Schaeffer, V. H. and Stevens, J. L.,** The transport of S-cysteine conjugates in LLC-PK_1 cells and its role in toxicity, *Molec. Pharmacol.*, 31, 506, 1987.
141. **Stevens, J., Hayden, P., and Taylor, G.,** The role of glutathione conjugate metabolism and cysteine conjugate β-lyase in the mechanism of S-cysteine conjugate toxicity in LLC-PK_1 cells, *J. Biol. Chem.*, 261, 3325, 1986.
142. **Golenhofen, N., Heuner, A., Mildenberger, S., Schwegler, J., and Silbernagl, S.,** Mercapturic acid formation in cultured opossum kidney cells, *Toxicol. Lett.*, 53, 261, 1990.
143. **Endicott, J. A. and Ling, V.,** The biochemistry of the P-glycoprotein-mediated multidrug resistance, *Annu. Rev. Biochem.*, 58, 137, 1989.
144. **Pastan, I. and Gottesman, M. M.,** Multidrug resistance, *Annu. Rev. Med.*, 42, 277, 1991.
145. **Horio, M., Chin, K.-V., Currier, S. J., Goldenberg, S., Williams, C., Pastan, I., Gottesman, M. M., and Handler, J. S.,** Transepithelial transport of drugs by the multidrug transporter in cultured Madin-Darby canine kidney cell epithelia, *J. Biol. Chem.*, 264, 14880, 1989.
146. **Horio, M., Pastan, I., Gottesman, M. M., and Handler, J. S.,** Transepithelial transport of vinblastine by kidney-derived cell lines. Application of a new kinetic model to estimate *in situ* K_m of the pump, *Biochim. Biophys. Acta,* 1027, 116, 1990.
147. **Lieberman, D. M., Reithmeier, R. A. F., Ling, V., Charuk, J. H. M., Goldberg, H., and Skorecki, K. L.,** Identification of P-glycoprotein in renal brush border membranes, *Biochem. Biophys. Res. Comm.*, 162, 244, 1989.
148. **Thiebaut, F., Tsuro, T., Hamada, H., Gottesman, M. M., Pastan, I., and Willingham, M. C.,** Cellular localization of the multi-drug-resistance gene product P-glycoprotein in normal human tissue, *Proc. Natl. Acad. Sci. U.S.A.*, 84, 7735, 1987.
149. **Guder, W. G. and Heidland, A.,** Urine analysis, *J. Clin. Chem. Clin Biochem.*, 24, 611, 1986.
150. **Pfaller, W., Joannidis, M., Gstraunthaler, G., and Kotanko, P.,** Quantitative morphologic changes of nephron structures and urinary enzyme activity pattern in sodium-maleate induced renal injury, *Renal Physiol. Biochem.*, 12, 56, 1989.
151. **Price, R. G.,** Urinary enzymes, nephrotoxicity and renal disease, *Toxicology,* 23, 99, 1982.
152. **Bacon, J. A., Linseman, D. A., and Raczniak, T. J.,** *In vitro* cytotoxicity of tetracyclines and aminoglycosides in LLC-PK_1, MDCK and Chang continuous cell lines, *Toxicol. in Vitro,* 4, 384, 1990.

153. **Eng, S. P. and Lo, C. S.,** Neomycin inhibits mastoparan-induced lactate dehydrogenase release, ethidium bromide accumulation, and intracellular fluorescein depletion in MDCK cells, *Cell Biol. Toxicol.,* 6, 95, 1990.
154. **Hori, R., Yamamoto, K., Saito, H., Kohno, M., and Inui, K.-I.,** Effect of aminoglycoside antibiotics on cellular functions of kidney epithelial cell line (LLC-PK_1): a model system for aminoglycoside nephrotoxicity, *J. Pharmacol. Exp. Ther.,* 230, 742, 1984.
155. **Lever, J. E. and Sari, C. E.,** Effect of tunicamycin on polarized membrane functions of an established kidney epithelial cell line, *Biochim. Biophys. Acta,* 762, 265, 1983.
156. **Cereijido, M., Meza, I., and Martinez-Palomo, A.,** Occluding junctions in cultured epithelial monolayers, *Am. J. Physiol.,* 240, C96, 1981.
157. **Cereijido, M., Ponce, A., and Gonzalez-Mariscal, L.,** Tight junctions and apical/basolateral polarity, *J. Membrane Biol.,* 110, 1, 1989.
158. **Madara, J. L.,** Loosening tight junctions. Lessons from the intestine, *J. Clin. Invest.,* 83, 1089, 1989.
159. **Powell, D. W.,** Barrier function of epithelia, *Am. J. Physiol.,* 241, G275, 1981.
160. **Shaw, A. J., Clothier, R. H., and Balls, M.,** Loss of transepithelial impermeability of a confluent monolayer of Madin-Darby canine kidney (MDCK) cells as a determinant of ocular irritancy potential, *ATLA,* 18, 145, 1990.
161. **Boulpap, E. L. and Seely, J. F.,** Electrophysiology of proximal and distal tubules in the autoperfused dog kidney, *Am. J. Physiol.,* 221, 1084, 1971.
162. **Cereijido, M., Robbins, E. S., Dolan, W. J., Rotunno, C. A., and Sabatini, D. D.,** Polarized monolayers formed by epithelial cells on a permeable and translucent support, *J. Cell Biol.,* 77, 853, 1978.
163. **Rabito, C. A., Tchao, R., Valentich, J., and Leighton, J.,** Distribution and characteristics of the occluding junctions in a monolayer of a cell line (MDCK) derived from canine kidney, *J. Membrane Biol.,* 43, 351, 1978.
164. **Shashby, D. M., Winter, M., and Shashby, S. A.,** Oxidants and conductance of cultured epithelial cell monolayer: inositol phospholipid hydrolysis, *Am. J. Physiol.,* 255, C781, 1988.
165. **Mullin, J. M. and McGinn, M. T.,** Effects of diaclyglycerols on LLC-PK_1 renal epithelia: similarity to phorbol ester tumor promoters, *J. Cell. Physiol.,* 134, 357, 1988.
166. **Sack, K., Marre, R., and Schulz, E.,** Renale Nebenwirkungen von Beta-Laktam-Antibiotika, *Krankenhauspharmazie,* 6, 415, 1985.
167. **Saito, H., Inui, K.-I., and Hori, R.,** Mechanisms of gentamicin transport in kidney epithelial cell line (LLC-PK_1), *J. Pharmacol. Exp. Ther.,* 238, 1071, 1986.
168. **Schwertz, D. W., Kreisberg, J. I., and Venkatachalam, M. A.,** Gentamicin-induced alterations in pig kidney epithelial (LLC-PK_1) cells in culture, *J. Pharmacol. Exp. Ther.,* 236, 254, 1986.
169. **Duffy, P. A. and McNae, F. R.,** *In vitro* toxicity of antibiotics to LLC-PK_1 rabbit kidney cells, *Toxicol. In Vitro.,* 4, 375, 1990.
170. **Linseman, D. A., Raczniak, T. J., Aaron, C. S., and Bacon, J. A.,** Comparative cytotoxicity rankings of four aminoglycoside antibiotics in the Chang, SIRC and LLC-PK_1 cell lines, *ATLA,* 18, 283, 1990.
171. **Williams, P. D., Buening, M. K., Gries, C. L., Hanasono, G. K., Lask, D. A., Tamura, R. N., and Heim, R. A.,** Comparative toxicity of oral cephalosporin antibiotics in the rabbit and in a rabbit kidney cell line (LLC-PK_1), *Toxicol. In Vitro,* 4, 207, 1990.
172. **Montine, T. J. and Borch, R.F.,** Quiescent LLC-PK_1 cells as a model for *cis*-diamminedichloroplatinum(II) nephrotoxicity and modulation by thiol rescue agents, *Cancer Res.,* 48, 6017, 1988.
173. **Mingard, F., Hausel, P., and Dietzi, J.,** Cadmium uptake by proximal tubular cells (LLC-PK_1) *in vitro,* in *Nephrotoxicity, Mechanisms, Early Diagnosis, and Therapeutic Management,* Bach, P. H., Gregg, N. J., Wilks, M. F., and Delacruz, L., Eds., Marcel Dekker, New York, 1991, 367.
174. **Prozialeck, W. C. and Niewenhuis, R. J.,** Cadmium (Cd^{2+}) disrupts intercellular junctions and actin filaments in LLC-PK_1 cells, *Toxicol. Appl. Pharmacol.,* 107, 81, 1991.
175. **Templeton, D. M.,** Cadmium uptake by cells of renal origin, *J. Biol. Chem.,* 265, 21764, 1990.
176. **Paulmichl, M., Gstraunthaler, G., and Lang, F.,** Electrical properties of Madin-Darby canine kidney cells: effects of extracellular potassium and bicarbonate, *Pflügers Arch.,* 405, 102, 1985.
177. **Jungwirth, A., Paulmichl, M., and Lang, F.,** Cadmium enhances potassium conductance in cultured renal epitheloid (MDCK) cells, *Kidney Int.,* 37, 1477, 1990.
178. **Jungwirth, A., Paulmichl, M., and Lang, F.,** Cobalt activates potassium conductance in the plasma membrane of cultured renal epitheloid (MDCK) cells, *Biochim. Biophys. Acta,* 1054, 143, 1990.
179. **Jungwirth, A., Ritter, M., Paulmichl, M., and Lang, F.,** Activation of cell membrane potassium conductance by mercury in cultured renal epitheloid (MDCK) cells, *J. Cell. Physiol.,* 146, 25, 1991.
180. **Goligorski, M. S. and Hruska, K. A.,** Trancytosis in cultured proximal tubular cells, *J. Membrane Biol.,* 93, 237, 1986.

181. **Heyman, M., Crain-Denoyelle, A.-M., Nath, S. K., and Desjeux, J.-F.,** Quantification of protein transcytosis in the human colon carcinoma cell line CaCo-2, *J. Cell. Physiol.*, 143, 391, 1990.
182. **Pfaller, W., Gstraunthaler, G., Prast, H., Rupp, L., Ruedl, C., Michelitsch, S., and Moser, M.,** Effects of the fungal toxin orellanine on renal epithelium, in *Nephrotoxicity. Mechanisms, Early Diagnosis, and Therapeutic Management,* Bach, P. H., Gregg, N. J., Wilks, M. F., Delacruz, L., Eds., Marcel Dekker, New York, 1991, 63.
183. **Oberleithner, H., Schwab, A., Westphale, H.-J., Schuricht, B., Püschel, B., and Koepsell, H.,** Giant MDCK cells: a novel expression system, *Methods Enzymol.*, 191, 437, 1990.
184. **Pouyssegur, J., Franchi, A., L'Allemain, G., Magnaldo, I., Paris, S., and Sardet, C.,** Genetic approach to structure, function, and regulation of the Na^+/H^+ antiporter, *Kidney Int.*, 32, S144, 1987.
185. **Gargus, J. J.,** Mutant isolation and gene transfer as tools in study of transport proteins, *Am. J. Physiol.*, 252, C457, 1987.
186. **Haugen, A., Ryberg, D., Hansteen, I. L., and Amstad, P.,** Neoplastic transformation of a human kidney epithelial cell line transfected with v-Ha-ras oncogene, *Int. J. Cancer,* 45, 572, 1990.
187. **Pastan, I., Gottesman, M. M., Ueda, K., Lovelace, E., Rutherford, A. V., and Willingham, M. C.,** A retrovirus carrying an *MDR1* cDNA confers multidrug resistance and polarized expression of P-glycoprotein in MDCK cells, *Proc. Natl. Acad. Sci. U.S.A.*, 85, 4486, 1988.
188. **Vandewalle, A., Lelongt, B., Geniteau-Legendre, M., Baudoin, B., Antoine, M., Estrade, S., Chatelet, P., Cassingena, R., and Ronco, P.,** Maintenance of proximal and distal cell functions in SV40-transformed tubular cell lines derived from rabbit kidney cortex, *J. Cell. Physiol.*, 141, 203, 1989.

Chapter 9

NEPHROTOXICITY STUDIES WITH FRESHLY ISOLATED CELLS FROM RAT KIDNEY

Lawrence H. Lash

TABLE OF CONTENTS

I. INTRODUCTION

During the last two decades, suspensions of isolated cells from various mammalian tissues have become useful in *in vitro* model systems for the study of cellular function and metabolism and of mechanisms of chemical and pathological cell injury. The advantages of using such systems include convenience, flexibility in terms of alterations in incubation conditions (e.g., temperature, pH, osmolarity, ionic composition, metabolic state), the ability to have paired control samples from the same animal, direct accessibility of administered chemicals to sites of action, and simplicity in that distributional and other extracellular factors are not additional variables. Although it can be claimed that the above-mentioned differences render the model of isolated cells in suspension unphysiological, numerous comparisons of these and similar *in vitro* systems with whole animal and perfused organ studies have demonstrated qualitative and quantitative similarities in functional and biochemical responses. As discussed below, application of several key criteria to isolated cell preparations is necessary and can be performed to validate the integrity of these systems. A wide range of experimental approaches are possible and several toxicologically relevant processes, including measurement of drug metabolism, cellular energetics, membrane transport processes, and effects on specific cellular functions, can be studied with these *in vitro* systems.

Development of *in vitro* models to study renal function, metabolism, and toxicology is complicated by the anatomical and biochemical heterogeneity of the kidneys.[1,2] Cell populations from each region of the nephron differ from one another with respect to membrane structure and hence membrane permeability characteristics, cellular energetics properties, activities of many drug metabolism and other enzymes, presence of transport systems for amino acids, sugars, peptides, and inorganic ions, and cell size and overall morphology. An important consequence of these cell type-specific physiological and biochemical properties is that each cell population exhibits a characteristic susceptibility to various chemical toxicants when exposed to them either *in vivo* or *in vitro*.

Differences in a variety of physicochemical properties among the nephron cell populations can be employed as a means of cell separation. For example, surface markers that are specific to a given renal cell population can be used as immunological markers,[3,4] and surface charge density can be used to purify cell populations by electrophoresis.[5] By far the most common and convenient property to use as a separation factor, however, is that of cell density. Although density-gradient centrifugation in Ficoll[6] or Percoll[7-9] has been used to separate proximal tubular (PT) and distal tubular (DT) fragments, only Ficoll has been employed to enrich PT cells from a suspension of single cortical cells.[10]

In a recent book of methodology of *in vitro* systems for toxicologic investigations, we reviewed procedures for the isolation and use in toxicity experiments of isolated cortical cells from rat kidney.[11] The present chapter concerns an extension of these procedures to the separation and purification of two populations of cells from suspensions of renal cortical cells to enable studies of mechanisms of cell type-specific patterns of chemical and pathological injury.[12]

II. EXPERIMENTAL PROCEDURES

A. ISOLATION OF RENAL CORTICAL CELLS

The collagenase perfusion procedure for the isolation of rat kidney cortical cells is based on the method of Jones et al.[13] and Ormstad et al.,[14] and was reviewed recently.[11] In this chapter, I will review only the key points of this method before describing procedures to fractionate these cells to obtain highly enriched populations of PT and DT cells.

Kidneys are first perfused at 8 ml/min in a retrograde manner through the aorta via a 19-gauge steel cannula with a calcium-free, EGTA-containing Hanks' buffer, pH 7.4, containing (in m*M*): NaCl (137), KCl (5.4), $MgSO_4 \cdot 7H_2O$ (0.8), KH_2PO_4 (0.4), Na_2HPO_4 (0.4), $NaHCO_3$ (25), HEPES (25), EGTA (0.5), and 2% (w/v) bovine serum albumin. All perfusions are performed at 37°C under an atmosphere of 95% O_2/5% CO_2. After approximately 10 min of recirculating perfusion, kidneys are then transferred to a beaker containing Hanks' buffer as above, but without EGTA or bovine serum albumin, and with 4 m*M* $CaCl_2$ and 0.15% (w/v) collagenase (type I from Sigma Chemical Co.) added, and are perfused at 5 ml/min. After an appropriate length of time that produces digestion of the kidneys (generally 15 to 20 min), cells are released into Krebs-Henseleit buffer, pH 7.4, containing (in m*M*): NaCl (118), KCl (4.8), $MgSO_4 \cdot 7H_2O$ (1.2), KH_2PO_4 (0.96), $NaHCO_3$ (25), HEPES (25), $CaCl_2$ (2.5), and 2% (w/v) bovine serum albumin. Cells are filtered through polypropylene mesh (210 μm pore size) and are resuspended in fresh Krebs-Henseleit buffer as above. Yield of cortical cells from 2 kidneys from rats weighing 200 to 300 g are generally 40 to 80×10^6 cells. Filtration of the cells and perfusion with collagenase at no more than 5 ml/min assures that mostly single cells in suspension, rather than tubular fragments or multicellular aggregates, are obtained.[11-14] All subsequent purification procedures after resuspension of cortical cells are performed at 4°C.

B. FRACTIONATION OF RENAL CORTICAL CELLS BY PERCOLL DENSITY-GRADIENT CENTRIFUGATION

1. Separation Conditions

To separate different cell populations from suspensions of renal cortical cells, density-gradient centrifugation with Percoll was chosen because of the apparent inertness of Percoll and the simplicity of the method.[15] In purifying populations of freshly isolated cells from rat kidney, two considerations are crucial to methods development: first, because of the relatively low amounts of material obtained from two adult rat kidneys, any procedure must not have too many steps so that low yields are obtained; second, the fragility of the isolated cells necessitates that separation and purification procedures are not too lengthy so that low viabilities are obtained.

Optimal separation conditions were determined by varying Percoll concentration, centrifugation speed and time, and cell concentration layered on the Percoll.[12] Density marker beads (Sigma Chemical Co.) can be used for calibration of the gradients. Isosmotic Percoll (90%, v/v) is prepared by combining 9 parts stock Percoll with 1 part buffer concentrate (10X Krebs-Henseleit-bicarbonate, pH 7.4, containing 250 m*M* HEPES but 0 calcium and 1.2 m*M* magnesium). A Percoll concentration of 45% (v/v) and centrifugation for 30 min at $20{,}000 \times g$ in an SS34 rotor in a Sorvall RC2B centrifuge gives the best range of densities and gradient shape, the most consistent gradients, and ultimately, the best separation of cell populations. The density-gradient is continuous and concave, ranging between 1.016 g/ml and 1.120 g/ml, and has an inflection point at 1.057 g/ml. Cortical cells (5 ml, 5 to 8×10^6 cells/ml) are layered on 35 ml of the Percoll suspension in 50-ml polycarbonate centrifuge tubes.

2. Assessment of Cell Type Identity and Purity

For analytical purposes, 20 2-ml fractions are collected from the gradient with an automatic pipettor to measure cell recovery and marker enzyme distributions. Alkaline phosphatase (AP; EC 3.1.3.1) and γ-glutamyltransferase (GGT; EC 2.3.2.2) activities are measured as markers of the PT region of the nephron, and hexokinase (HK; EC 2.7.1.1) activity is measured as a marker for the DT region of the nephron.[12] Based on the activity distributions of the marker enzymes, fractions corresponding to PT and DT cells were pooled

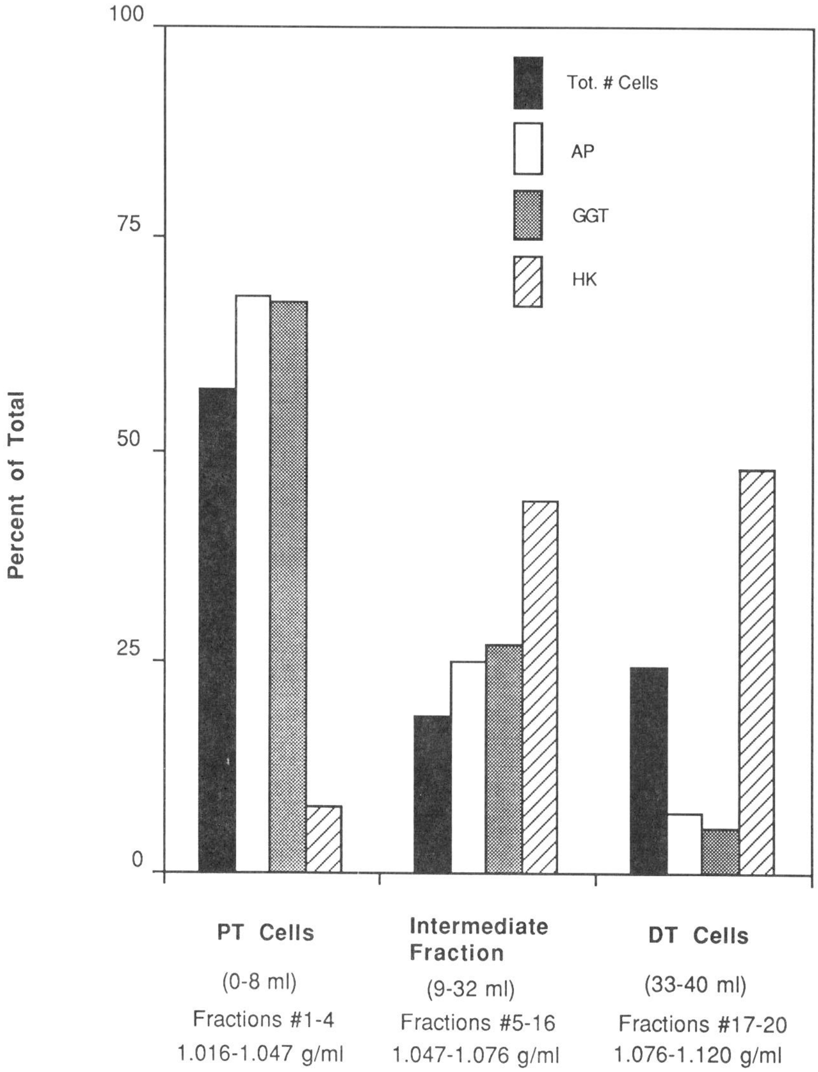

FIGURE 1. Separation of renal proximal tubular and distal tubular cells from suspensions of cortical cells by Percoll density-gradient centrifugation. Isolated renal cortical cells (5 ml, 5 to 8 × 10^6 cells per ml) were layered on 35 ml of 45% (v/v) Percoll solution and were centrifuged at 20,000 × g for 30 min. Fractions (2 ml) were collected and then assayed for cell number and the indicated marker enzymes. Summary results, which are derived from 5 to 11 cell preparations, are shown as the percent of total amount or activity recovered in each pooled fraction.

separately and could then be employed in various studies examining cell type-specific mechanisms of toxicity. As shown in Figure 1, fractions #1 to 4 of the gradient (density = 1.016 to 1.047 g/ml) contain 57.1% of the total cells and 68%, 67%, and 8% of the total AP, GGT, and HK activity, respectively, consistent with identification of these cells as being PT in origin. In contrast, fractions #17 to 20 of the gradient (density = 1.076 to 1.120 g/ml) contain 24.3% of the cells and 7%, 5%, and 48% of the total AP, GGT, and HK activity, respectively, consistent with identification of these cells as being DT in origin.

For preparative purposes, fractions identified as PT and DT cells are separately pooled, are washed with calcium-free, low-magnesium Krebs-Henseleit buffer, and are resuspended in normal Krebs-Henseleit-bicarbonate buffer, pH 7.4, supplemented with 25 m*M* HEPES, 5 m*M* glucose, 5 m*M* glutamine, and 2% (w/v) bovine serum albumin at concentrations of 2 to 4 $\times$ 10^6 cells per ml. The final yield of PT and DT cells from one rat is typically 20 to 40 $\times$ 10^6 cells and 5 to 15 $\times$ 10^6 cells, respectively. The entire procedure, including buffer preparation, surgery, and the various centrifugation steps, takes approximately 3.5 h.

Purity of the two cell populations can be estimated by using the marker enzyme specific activities. Because PT cells comprise approximately 85% of all cellular material in the cortex,[16] the purity of the PT cell preparation is estimated by the formula 100% − (percentage of cells in cortex not of PT origin) $\times$ (specific activity of PT cell marker in DT fraction/specific activity of PT cell marker in PT fraction). Purity of the DT fraction can be estimated similarly. By this method, the PT and DT cell preparations are estimated to have purities of 97% and 88%, respectively.[12] Although this procedure does not yield PT cells derived specifically from either the pars recta or the pars convoluta, it does produce a highly enriched population of PT cells that are substantially free from other nephron cell types. Similarly, although there are some PT cells and possibly some cortical collecting duct cells in the DT cell preparation, the procedure yields predominantly isolated cells from the distal convoluted tubule that are highly enriched. Some sacrifice in purity must be made so that the final cell preparation can be useful for biochemical and toxicological investigations.

C. INCUBATION CONDITIONS AND SAMPLING METHODS

The PT and DT cell preparations are ideal for short-term incubations where drug metabolism or acute mechanisms of chemical or pathological injury are being studied. Incubations can be performed for up to 4 h in Erlenmeyer flasks (siliconized glass or polypropylene) at 37°C in a Dubnoff metabolic shaking incubator (60 cycles/min). Normally, 25-ml Erlenmeyer flasks are used, and the total volume of cell suspension does not exceed 3 ml so that oxygen diffusion to all cell surfaces does not become a limiting factor. Flasks are sealed with rubber serum bottle stoppers and the atmosphere can be equilibrated with any desired gas composition. Because bicarbonate is generally included in the medium, 5% CO_2 is a component of all gas mixtures.

As a matter of normal procedure, cells are maintained on ice after isolation for up to 1 h. Before beginning experiments, cells are preincubated for 15 min at 37°C on the shaking water bath. This period serves to stabilize several parameters of cell function (see below), and thus yields better, more consistent cells. Additions to cell suspensions are made from concentrated stock solutions so that cells are minimally diluted.

Metabolite concentrations in total cell suspensions can be measured by mixing aliquots of the cell suspensions with acid and centrifuging. Acid-soluble supernatants are then processed according to the specific assay of interest. In those cases where it is necessary to separate the cells from the extracellular medium, a convenient method involves layering 0.5 ml of cells on 1.0 ml of 20% (v/v) Percoll in normal saline in 1.5-ml microcentrifuge tubes. The tubes are centrifuged in a microcentrifuge for 30 sec at 10,000 $\times$ g, yielding the supernatant (extracellular medium) and the cell pellet, which can be resuspended in fresh buffer or can be treated with a protein denaturant and processed for a particular assay of interest. Examples of situations where this is necessary include distinguishing between intracellular and extracellular concentrations of metabolites, transport assays, or assays where cells need to be resuspended in different media.

III. CELLULAR FUNCTION AND VIABILITY

Numerous methods are available to assess the competence of cellular function under a variety of toxicological or pathological conditions (Table 1). What is generally termed "cell

TABLE 1
Some Methods to Assess Function and Viability in Suspensions of Isolated Cells

Process measured	Cellular process or site targeted	Time course of observed effect
	Terminal, irreversible injury	
Lactate dehydrogenase release	Plasma membrane damage	0.5–4 h
Trypan blue exclusion	Plasma membrane damage	0.5–4 h
	Functional alterations: reversible or irreversible injury	
Cellular oxygen consumption	Mitochondrial dysfunction	5–120 min
Transmembrane ion distribution (e.g., Ca^{2+}, Na^{+}, K^{+})	Membrane damage, energy depletion, specific inhibition	5–60 min
Membrane potential	Membrane damage, energy depletion	5–60 min
Active transport	Membrane damage, energy depletion, specific inhibition	15–60 min
Protein synthesis	Energy depletion	15–120 min
	Metabolic alterations: reversible injury	
GSH status	Oxidative injury, energy depletion	5–60 min
Adenine nucleotide status	Energy depletion	5–60 min
Intermediary metabolites	Energy depletion, enzyme inhibition	5–60 min

viability'' is defined broadly as the ability of the plasma membrane to separate intracellular and extracellular compartments by maintaining a permeability barrier. Two convenient ways to assess this ability are the lactate dehydrogenase (LDH; EC 1.1.1.27) leakage assay and the trypan blue exclusion test.[11] Both tests quantitate the ability of the plasma membrane to retain its impermeability to normally impermeable substances. The LDH release assay involves measurement of NADH oxidation spectrophotometrically after addition of pyruvate and cells, in the absence and then presence, of a detergent such as Triton X-100 (usually at 0.1%, v/v). The ratio of the slopes in the two cases is equivalent to the fraction of cells that release LDH. Immediately after isolation, PT and DT cells generally exhibit 5 to 15% LDH release and maintain less than 25% LDH release for up to 4 h incubation at 37°C. Trypan blue exclusion involves measurement of the fraction of cells that exclude the vital dye. Immediately after isolation, 85 to 95% of the PT and DT cells exclude trypan blue and this fraction of exclusion is generally above 80% for up to 4 h of incubation at 37°C. These two assays are indicators of irreversible membrane damage and are thus indicators of terminal cell injury. In acute cytotoxicity experiments, LDH release or trypan blue uptake are usually observed at later stages of the incubations, between 0.5 and 4 h, and normally give similar results. The convenience of the LDH release and trypan blue exclusion assays as indicators of irreversible cytotoxicity enables the investigator to use these methods to rapidly and easily screen potentially toxic chemicals and to compare the toxic potencies of various chemicals.

Once it is established that an agent or pathological condition produces cytotoxicity, other assessments of cellular function are needed to provide mechanistic information. These methods are also important tools to assess the functional integrity of control cells and thus the appropriateness of suspensions of isolated renal cells as an *in vitro* model system. Selected examples of these methods are divided into functional alterations and metabolic alterations (Table 1). Functional alterations involve measurements of integrated cellular processes. The examples shown are multistep processes that are generally energy-dependent and are highly regulated. Alterations in these processes occur at early to intermediate times and, depending on the duration and severity of the effect, can be signs of either reversible or irreversible injury.

In some cases, functional alterations can be physiological responses of the cells to maintain metabolic homeostasis. As such, these responses would be considered adaptive. An example is the ability of alterations in cellular energy demand to alter rates of cellular oxygen consumption.[17] Because of the high activity of the plasma membrane (Na^+ + K^+)-stimulated ATPase in renal PT and DT cells, cellular energy demand is rapidly altered by addition of either nystatin to stimulate the ATPase or ouabain to inhibit it.[12] By acting as a monocation ionophore, nystatin uncouples the ATPase and increases cellular ATP demand. In a cell with functionally intact mitochondria, nystatin administration is rapidly followed by increased rates of cellular oxygen consumption. Conversely, by inhibiting one of the principal ATP-consuming processes in the cell, ouabain decreases cellular ATP demand. This alteration is followed by a marked decrease in cellular oxygen consumption. Oxygen consumption is readily measured polarographically in sealed, thermostatically controlled chambers with a Clark-type oxygen electrode.

Measurements of concentrations and distributions of key metabolites can be made to provide assessments of early, usually reversible, effects on cells (Table 1). Parameters such as GSH status and adenine nucleotide status are sensitive indicators of cellular redox and energetic homeostasis, respectively. Key intermediary metabolites can be measured to determine fluxes through given metabolic pathways, such as glycolysis or the citric acid cycle, and changes in patterns of metabolites can be used to identify specific target sites of nephrotoxic chemicals.

IV. COMMENTS AND SUMMARY

With the establishment of methods to assess the functional integrity of the isolated PT and DT cell preparations, these cells can be used as models to study chemical toxicity. We have employed these cells to address two separate but related issues, namely, that of elucidation of biochemical mechanisms of chemical or pathological injury and that of the heterogeneous susceptibility of different nephron cell types to chemical or pathological injury.[12,18-20] Because many parameters of the incubation conditions (e.g., temperature, pH, buffer composition, substrate supply, etc.) are easily known and controlled, effects on metabolism and function can be measured, relative time courses assessed, and important processes identified.

Our approach to studying chemical-induced cytotoxicity in the renal PT and DT cells is to expose cells to specific nephrotoxic chemicals (e.g., cephalosporin antibiotics) in order to study their mechanism of action and to use chemicals representing classes of generalized cytotoxicants as probes to study susceptibility of the two cell populations to chemical injury. These classes of cytotoxic chemicals have included oxidants (*tert*-butyl hydroperoxide, hydrogen peroxide, menadione), alkylating agents that act on either soft nucleophiles (methyl vinyl ketone, allyl alcohol) or hard nucleophiles (*N*-dimethylnitrosamine), and inhibitors of cellular energy metabolism, the so-called "chemical hypoxia" model (iodoacetate + KCN). Additionally, the ability to regulate cellular substrate supply and incubation atmosphere (i.e., oxygen vs. nitrogen) allows modeling of renal hypoxia and ischemia in these *in vitro* systems.

In summary, this brief chapter has reviewed procedures to prepare freshly isolated cells from rat kidney cortex and has described procedures to fractionate these cells into two highly enriched populations derived from the PT and DT regions of the nephron. The versatility of these cell preparations for the study of chemical and pathological injury is illustrated and strategies for characterizing mechanisms of cytotoxicity are discussed. Major advantages of using this methodology for toxicological investigations include the relative ease of preparation, the specification of incubation conditions, the use of paired control and test samples in a single preparation, and the ability to dissect biochemical mechanisms of action by studying time courses of effects on metabolic and functional processes in cells.

ACKNOWLEDGMENT

Research from the author's laboratory was supported by Grant DK-40725 from the National Institute of Diabetes, Digestive and Kidney Diseases.

REFERENCES

1. **Walker, L. A. and Valtin, H.,** Biological importance of nephron heterogeneity, *Annu. Rev. Physiol.,* 44, 203, 1982.
2. **Guder, W. G. and Ross, B. D.,** Enzyme distribution along the nephron, *Kidney Int.,* 26, 101, 1984.
3. **Stanton, R. C., Mendrick, D. L., Rennke, H. G., and Seifter, J. L.,** Use of monoclonal antibodies to culture rat proximal tubule cells, *Am. J. Physiol.,* 251, C780, 1986.
4. **Allen, M. L., Nakao, A., Sonenburg, W. K., Burnatowska-Hledin, M., Spielman, W. S., and Smith, W. L.,** Immunodissection of cortical and medullary thick ascending limb cells from rabbit kidney, *Am. J. Physiol.,* 255, F704, 1988.
5. **Kreisberg, J. I., Sachs, G., Pretlow, T. G., II, and McGuire, R. A.,** Separation of proximal tubule cells from suspensions of rat kidney cells by free-flow electrophoresis, *J. Cell. Physiol.,* 93, 169, 1977.
6. **Scholer, D. W. and Edelman, I. S.,** Isolation of rat kidney cortical tubules enriched in proximal and distal segments, *Am. J. Physiol.,* 237, F350, 1979.
7. **Vinay, P., Gougoux, A., and Lemieux, G.,** Isolation of a pure suspension of rat proximal tubules, *Am. J. Physiol.,* 241, F403, 1981.
8. **Cojocel, C., Maita, K., Pasino, D. A., Kuo, C.-H., and Hook, J. B.,** Metabolic heterogeneity of the proximal and distal kidney tubules, *Life Sci.,* 33, 855, 1982.
9. **Gesek, F. A., Wolff, D. W., and Strandhoy, J. W.,** Improved separation method for rat proximal and distal renal tubules, *Am. J. Physiol.,* 253, F358, 1987.
10. **Kreisberg, J. I., Pitts, A. M., and Pretlow, T. G., II,** Separation of proximal tubule cells from suspensions of rat kidney cells in density gradients of Ficoll in tissue culture medium, *Am. J. Pathol.,* 86, 591, 1977.
11. **Lash, L. H.,** Isolated kidney cells in the study of chemical toxicity, in *In Vitro Toxicology: Model Systems and Methods,* McQueen, C. A., Ed., Telford Press, Caldwell, NJ, 1989, 231.
12. **Lash, L. H. and Tokarz, J. J.,** Isolation of two distinct populations of cells from rat kidney cortex and their use in the study of chemical-induced toxicity, *Anal. Biochem.,* 182, 271, 1989.
13. **Jones, D. P., Sundby, G.-B., Ormstad, K., and Orrenius, S.,** Use of isolated kidney cells for study of drug metabolism, *Biochem. Pharmacol.,* 28, 929, 1979.
14. **Ormstad, K., Orrenius, S., and Jones, D. P.,** Preparation and characteristics of isolated kidney cells, *Methods Enzymol.,* 77, 137, 1981.
15. **Pertoft, H. and Laurent, T. C.,** Sedimentation of cells in colloidal silica (Percoll), in *Cell Separation: Methods and Selected Applications,* Vol. 1, Pretlow, T. G., II and Pretlow, T. G., Eds., Academic Press, New York, 1982, 115.
16. **Schlondorff, D.,** Isolation and use of specific nephron segments and their cells in biochemical studies, *Kidney Int.,* 30, 201, 1986.
17. **Soltoff, S. P.,** ATP and the regulation of renal cell function, *Annu. Rev. Physiol.,* 48, 9, 1986.
18. **Lash, L. H.,** Susceptibility to toxic injury in different nephron cell populations, *Toxicol. Lett.,* 53, 97, 1990.
19. **Lash, L. H. and Tokarz, J. J.,** Oxidative stress in isolated rat renal proximal and distal tubular cells, *Am. J. Physiol.,* 259, F338, 1990.
20. **Lash, L. H. and Woods, E. B.,** Cytotoxicity of alkylating agents in isolated rat kidney proximal tubular and distal tubular cells, *Arch. Biochem. Biophys.,* 286, 46, 1991.

Chapter 10

PRIMARY PROXIMAL TUBULE CULTURES FOR SCREENING NEPHROTOXICANTS

Sue M. Ford and Patricia D. Williams

TABLE OF CONTENTS

I. INTRODUCTION

The renal proximal tubule is the target for the toxicity of numerous therapeutic agents, particularly antibiotics[1,2] and anticancer drugs.[3,4] Determining the nephrotoxic potential of compounds at the earliest possible stage in the drug development process would reduce the cost and the number of animals used in preclinical toxicology studies. Primary renal cultures can be utilized to compare a new drug or chemical entity for nephrotoxic potential relative to agents with known liabilities *in vivo*. This type of evaluation permits the selection from a series of chemical analogs of those agents possessing reduced nephrotoxicity. Such preliminary screening can greatly enhance the probability of success of new agents in *in vivo* nephrotoxicity studies. As a result of these concerns, there has been considerable interest in the development of *in vitro* systems to screen for nephrotoxicity prior to the initiation of animal studies.

A. SENSITIVITY OF THE PROXIMAL TUBULE TO TOXICANTS

The proximal tubule is a highly differentiated epithelium, with biochemical and physiological features that influence the toxicity of several compounds. For example, transport mechanisms on the plasma membrane accumulate xenobiotics to higher concentrations in the proximal tubules than in other cells of the body. Transporters for organic anions are present on the basolateral side of the cell, and the uptake of cephaloridine by this route has been linked to its nephrotoxicity. Accumulation by endocytosis on the apical side of the cell appears to contribute to the tubular damage following gentamicin exposure.[5] Most of the salt and water filtered at the glomerulus is reabsorbed by the end of the proximal tubule, so that xenobiotics remaining in the lumen are concentrated. Consequently, tubular cells are exposed to higher extracellular levels of drugs than are other cells. The proximal tubule is also the location of renal cytochrome P450-dependent enzymes which may produce toxic reactive intermediates in these cells.[6] Another factor contributing to the sensitivity of the proximal tubule to toxicity is the dependency on a high rate of intermediary metabolism, since interruption of critical energy-producing steps may contribute to the deleterious effects of certain agents.[7,8] These and other features which contribute to the susceptibility of the proximal tubule to xenobiotics have been reviewed in several papers.[9,10]

B. ADVANTAGES OF CELL CULTURE FOR NEPHROTOXICITY SCREENING

To accurately predict the nephrotoxicity of potential therapeutic agents *in vitro*, it would be desirable to use a model that retains the specialized functions contributing to the sensitivity of the kidneys to toxicants. Several *in vitro* systems have been invaluable in exploring the toxic mechanisms of known nephrotoxicants,[11] but are limited in their potential for screening. Compared to these conventional techniques, the major advantages of cell culture are the ability to prepare many homogenous treatment units, the extended viability span which permits longer exposure periods, the potential for development of rapid automated toxicity assays, and the ability to grow cells on filters in order to mimic the *in vivo* exposure route.

Cell lines, i.e., cultures that have been serially propagated, have provided a starting point in developing nephrotoxicity screens, but there are several problems with the currently available renal cell lines. Most useful cell lines are those that have been cultured for a prolonged period, in some cases over 30 years. During that time many cumulative genetic changes may have occurred to alter the expression of toxicologically important features. The pig kidney cell line LLC-PK_1 possesses an epithelioid morphology along with several transport systems present in the proximal tubule, but differs from that segment in its adenylate cyclase response to hormones (see below). Additionally, although the cells possess the capacity to transport the prototype organic cation, tetraethylammonium (TEA) bromide,[12,13] transport of the organic anion *p*-aminohippurate (PAH) by LLC-PK_1 cells has not been reported. The rabbit kidney cell line LLC-RK_1 has been studied less than LLC-PK_1; one problem with this line is that its monolayers do not form domes, which are characteristic of cultured salt- and water-transporting epithelia. This suggests that despite the epithelial morphology of the cells,[14] the functional properties of LLC-RK_1 might deviate significantly from those of the proximal tubule.

C. ADVANTAGES OF PRIMARY PROXIMAL TUBULE CULTURES FOR NEPHROTOXICITY SCREENING

Primary proximal tubule cultures are currently undergoing extensive study for use in the screening of nephrotoxicants. Primary cultures are initiated from tissue taken directly from an animal and should have a considerable resemblance to proximal tubular cells *in vivo*. The use of primary cultures also facilitates the study of species variability in toxic responses. Proximal tubules have been successfully cultured from the kidneys of several species, including rats,[15-27] rabbits,[16,28-32] humans,[19,33-36] mice,[37,38] dogs,[39,40] and fish.[41] A further advantage of primary cultures is that the starting tubular material is available, so one can study the success of the purification as well as changes in the cells caused by culturing.[42] The rabbit primary proximal tubule model of Chung and co-workers[29] is particularly attractive because of the ease of isolation of tubules, the large amount of material available from one rabbit, and the widespread use of rabbits in nephrotoxicity testing for therapeutic agents.

II. PRIMARY CULTURE OF RABBIT PROXIMAL TUBULES

A. PREPARATION AND REAGENTS

The sieves used to isolate the tubules are prepared prior to obtaining the kidneys. Squares of nylon nitrix screening material (Tetko, Inc., Lancaster, NY) with meshes of 253 μm (cat. #3-253/46) and 85 μm (cat. #3-85/44) are stretched on plastic embroidery hoops (size 5). The hoops are immersed in 70% ethanol, as is an appropriately sized piece of stiff plastic mesh. The hoops and plastic mesh may be obtained at a hobby or fabric store.

During the isolation procedure, paramagnetic iron oxide particles are used to remove glomeruli from the tubule preparation. Sufficient iron oxide for several experiments can be prepared at one time. NaOH (1.3 g) and 10 g KNO_3 are dissolved in 50-ml O_2-saturated water. $FeSO_4$ (4.5 g) is also dissolved in 50-ml O_2-saturated water. The two solutions are combined in an Erlenmeyer flask, covered with a watch glass, and boiled for 20 min. The solution is cooled to room temperature and a large magnetic stirring bar is added. After the particles have settled, the clear liquid is decanted carefully in order to retain the particles on the stirring bar; the particles are then washed 5 to 10 times with 100 to 200 ml of water. The FeO is resuspended in 500 ml of 0.9% NaCl and 80 ml aliquots are dispensed into 100-ml glass bottles; these are autoclaved for 20 min with a liquid cycle. On the day of the experiment, 40 ml of FeO suspension is diluted 1:1 with basal culture medium (SFFD, see below), and 2 ml of collagenase solution (10 mg/ml SFFD) and 2 ml of soybean trypsin inhibitor solution (1 mg/ml PBS) are added.

The phosphate buffered saline (PBS) routinely used is Dulbecco's PBSA, which lacks calcium and magnesium salts. It can be used when rinsing the kidneys or instruments, but should not be substituted for SFFD in final perfusions or rinses of the tubules because the outgrowth of cells is adversely affected. The water used for the preparation of reagents and media is tissue-culture grade (pyrogen free), and all reagents used during the procedure should be sterile and cold.

B. PROCEDURE FOR RABBIT PRIMARY PROXIMAL TUBULE CULTURES

The tubules are isolated from young adult male New Zealand rabbits weighing 2.0 to 3.0 kg; we and others[43] have observed that outgrowth of cells from the tubules is reduced when older or larger animals are used. Small rabbits may be killed by cervical dislocation in order to avoid the use of drugs;[29] however, we have been using barbiturate overdose (30 to 45 mg/kg by ear vein injection) successfully for several years without any apparent adverse effects on the resulting cultures. Euthanasia by CO_2 is slow for larger animals such as rabbits, so that ischemic damage to the tissue is a concern.

The abdominal cavity of the animal is opened and the kidneys are extirpated along with the renal artery, renal vein, and about an inch of the ureter. Surgical sterility is not required while the renal capsule is intact, but swabbing the abdomen with 70% ethanol before cutting the skin will reduce the amount of fur in the incision. The kidneys are placed in covered sterile beakers with cold medium and kept on ice. Subsequent procedures are carried out in a sterile cabinet using aseptic techniques. It is possible to isolate and cultivate the cells without antibiotics, and some investigators choose not to include them because of the known sensitivity of the proximal tubule to such agents.[30,33] Others use antibiotics during the isolation[17,40,44] or culturing[15,18,19,24,31,35,36] of the tubules; a combination of penicillin and streptomycin is used most often, but gentamicin has also been employed.[16,21,25] A single kidney provides sufficient material for most laboratories to use; the other kidney may be held in reserve in case of a mishap or employed for another purpose.

The kidney is suspended by the ureter with a forceps and rinsed profusely with cold and sterile PBS. It is then transferred to a sterile petri dish where residual fat and fur may be removed. After further rinsing, the kidney is transferred to a clean dish and an 18- to 20-gauge needle (blunted by filing with emory paper) is inserted into the artery and secured tightly with thread or suture (000 or 4-0). A moist gauze pad in the dish will prevent the kidney from moving during the cannulation. The ends of the vein and ureter are clipped, a syringe is attached to the needle, and the kidney is perfused with 30 to 40 ml PBS followed by 30 to 40 ml SFFD until the organ is uniformly blanched. Blood that remains outside of the tissue and underneath the capsule may be ignored. The kidney is perfused with 30 to 40 ml of the FeO/collagenase solution until the surface is uniformly gray.

The blood vessels, ureter, and capsule are then removed and the kidney is rinsed and placed in a clean dish. The cortex is dissected with a scissors or sliced with a razor after saggital bisection of the organ. Care must be taken to avoid including nonperfused cortical areas or the underlying medulla, which can be recognized by the absence of black iron oxide particles. The tissue pieces are minced coarsely and placed in a 15-ml Dounce homogenizer. A few milliliters of SFFD are added and the tubules are separated by four to five strokes with the loose pestle of the homogenizer.

After the cortical homogenate is prepared, the plastic mesh is removed from the ethanol and placed across the rim of a large sterile beaker (1000 ml). The embroidery hoops are stacked on the plastic with the larger mesh (253 μ) screen on top. The hoops and mesh are rinsed thoroughly with PBS and SFFD to remove the ethanol. The homogenate is poured onto the top screen and the tubules slowly rinsed with PBS (250 ml), then SFFD (500 ml), taking care not to overflow the hoops. The debris on the top screen and the filtrate in the beaker are discarded. The bottom (85 μ-mesh) screen retains the proximal tubules and glomeruli; this material is collected with a spatula and suspended in SFFD (35 ml) in a sterile 50-ml screw-cap centrifuge tube. A magnetic stir bar (2″) is added to which the FeO-laden glomeruli will be attracted. After 3 to 4 min, the solution with the tubules is gently decanted into another centrifuge tube containing a clean stir bar; this procedure is repeated 2 to 3 times until most of the glomeruli (which are conspicuous as black specks on the white bar) are removed.

The tubules are poured into a weighed 50-ml centrifuge tube and 1 ml each of the collagenase and soybean trypsin inhibitor solutions are added. The suspension is gently mixed and allowed to stand 2 to 3 min at room temperature, after which it is spun for 5 min at low speed in a table top centrifuge. The supernatant is aspirated, fresh SFFD is added, and the mixture centrifuged again. After removing the supernatant and reweighing the tube, the tubules are suspended in complete culture medium (see below) at a density of 2 mg/ml and inoculated into the culture plates, flasks, or filter inserts. Due to the large and variable sizes of the tubule fragments, it is difficult to obtain a uniform distribution into small multiwell (48- to 96-well) cluster dishes, so larger plates (e.g., $\geq$ 35-mm) and flasks are used. Rabbit tubules adhere immediately to tissue culture-treated plastic; consequently flasks should be placed horizontally immediately after inoculation and promptly swirled to ensure an even distribution of tubules over the culture surface. The cultures are maintained at 37°C with 5% CO_2 in a humidified tissue culture incubator. The medium should be changed after 24 h and every 2 to 4 days thereafter.

Outgrowth from the periphery of the tubules occurs within 24 to 48 hours (Figure 1a). As the cells move out, the tubular structure will degenerate (Figure 1b to d) and the cultures will enter a period of rapid cell proliferation. Proximal tubule cultures grown on plastic form a confluent monolayer in 7 to 9 days; those grown on filters take several days longer. Microscopic evidence of confluency can be corroborated by a plateau in cell number and reduction in ^{3}H-thymidine incorporation. The practical working lifespan of primary cultures is about a week beyond confluency,[27] but longer[45] and shorter[16,21] times have been reported. After confluency, the cells will adhere avidly to each other, making it more difficult to prepare single cell suspensions, yet the cells will detach easily from plastic dishes when the medium is changed. The resultant large holes in the monolayer are especially hard to avoid in cells grown in 35-mm dishes, thus limiting the usefulness of such cultures.

C. STRATEGIES FOR ISOLATING AND CULTURING PROXIMAL TUBULES AND CELLS

Rabbit tubules usually separate easily from each other by gentle dispersion with a Dounce homogenizer, but collagenase may be used to facilitate this process. For the kidneys of other species, collagenase perfusion is required to dissociate the tubules and may be used either alone or in combination with other proteases such as trypsin or hyaluronidase.[16-19,24,26,35,36,39,40] A second purpose for the use of collagenase is to damage the basement membrane and allow the migration of cells from the full length of the tubules. Thus, treating the isolated tubules with collagenase for 2 to 3 min is essential for the outgrowth of the cells.[29,36] The type (grade) and batch of collagenase influences the success of the cultures; this is possibly related to contamination by other proteases. Both Boehringer-Mannheim and Worthington allow investigators to test batches of collagenase in order to select an optimal lot.

We have used the iron oxide perfusion and sieving procedure with rabbit and human kidneys;[9] however, the tubules of other species may not be amenable to this isolation procedure. A commonly used alternative for purifying proximal tubules is separation by density. Hatzinger and Stevens[23] used a simple settling out procedure for rat tubules. Others have employed density gradient centrifugation with Percoll,[16,28,32,39,40] with most authors adapting the method of Vinay and co-workers.[46] Some investigators have cultured cortical explants of tissue that is difficult to perfuse or homogenize (e.g., human biopsy material),[33] relying on the use of serum-free medium to select epithelial cells.[47] At the other extreme of purification, microdissection gives precise control over the segment of the nephron obtained,[31,43] but places practical constraints on the amount of tissue available. Although subculturing can increase the number of cells from microdissected tubules,[43] a loss of brush border has been reported when primary cells are passaged.[16]

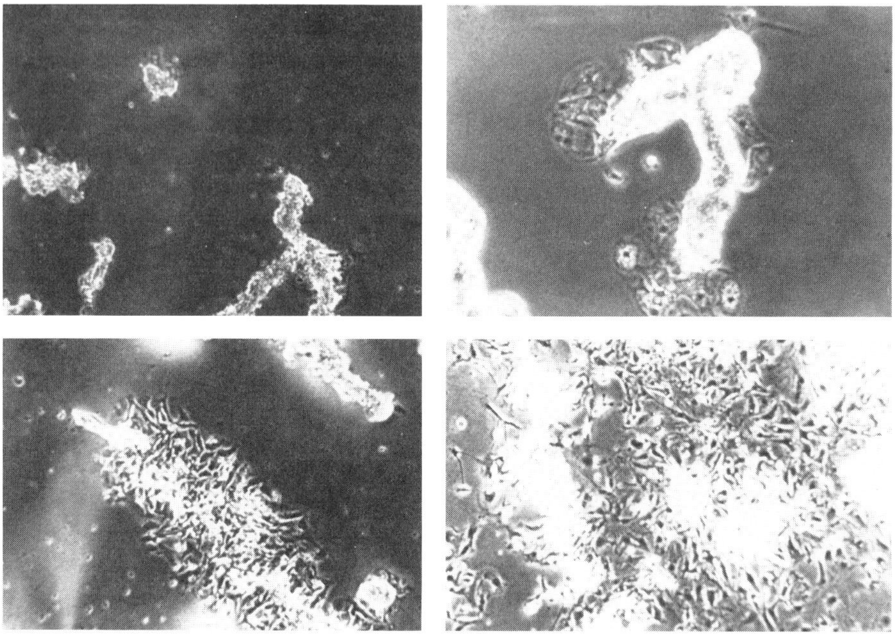

FIGURE 1. Outgrowth of rabbit primary proximal tubules in culture. (a) Day 1 (magnification × 100), (b) day 2 (× 200), (c) day 3 (× 200), and (d) day 4 (× 200).

Isolated cells have been used as the starting material for primary proximal tubule cultures.[15,20,24,25,41,48-50] An advantage is that dispersions of individual cells would be more suitable than tubules or explants to use for smaller treatment units such as 96-well plates. However, the liberation of cells from tubules requires harsher conditions than for dissociation of tubules from each other, generally involving longer treatment with digestive enzymes. Thus, increasing the yield of single cells by this method must be balanced against the cellular damage caused by anoxia or prolonged exposure to the proteases. The survival of cells during a lengthy collagenase treatment can be improved by oxygenating the suspension.[27] For either separated cells or tubules, the material isolated may be purified by gradient density centrifugation[48] or with the use of cell-specific antibodies.[27,38]

The yield of culturable material from a kidney varies with the species and method of isolation. Using collagenase treatment of renal cortical slices followed by density gradient purification, States and co-workers[40] reported that 15 g of slices taken from 2 to 6 dogs provided material for 60 to 80 T-25 flasks. Stanton[27] harvested 10^6 isolated cells from the kidneys of 3 rats and inoculated 200 wells in 24-well plates. In contrast, 3 g of flounder kidneys provided enough material for only eight 35-mm dishes.[41] The procedure of Chung and co-workers[29] described above is fairly rapid (3 to 4 h) and produces a good yield of proximal tubules (750 to 1000 mg per kidney from a single rabbit kidney) with a purity of approximately 90 to 95%. At a density of 2 mg/ml, there is enough material to inoculate 180 to 250 filter inserts (30-mm) or 35-mm dishes. We have found this plating density to be optimal. If the tubules are diluted substantially to seed more plates, the monolayers do not reach confluency. Alternatively, if the density is increased in an attempt to reduce the time to confluency, fewer tubules attach. A similar dependency of culture success on plating density has been reported by others.[18,27]

Rabbit tubules prepared as described above adhere immediately to tissue culture plastic so that neither an attachment period nor special coating of the substrata are necessary; in fact, we have observed that the tubules do not adhere to plates coated with collagen, polylysine, or Matrigel. The proximal tubules of other species or other preparations (e.g., isolated cells) may be more demanding in their requirements. It may be necessary to use special dishes such as Falcon Primaria[35] or to coat the growth surface with collagen,[15,26,28,31,33,40,41] poly-L-lysine,[16,24] fibronectin,[27] or extracellular matrix.[36]

The use of permeable substrata such as membrane filters or floating collagen gels has advantages in nephrotoxicity studies. Several authors have concluded that cells grown on these surfaces display a better retention of differentiated morphology and transport function than the same cells cultured on plastic.[30,51] Growing the cells on filters would also permit access to the basolateral side of the cell, where the transport systems for many nephrotoxicants are located. By increasing both the differentiated state of the cells and the penetration of toxicants to the site of active transport, the sensitivity and specificity of the toxicity assay would be increased for cells grown on permeable supports. Furthermore, such substrata allow measurement of transepithelial resistance and transport functions as indices of cell status and as potential markers of toxicity. Several vendors (Millipore, Costar, Falcon, Anotec) sell prefabricated plate inserts consisting of filters attached to plastic supports which lift the membrane from the bottom of the dish. Plate inserts are manufactured with different types of filters, including transparent membranes and those that are precoated with various matrices. Additionally, 96-well plates are available with a permeable growth substratum comprising the bottom of each well (Poretics Corp., Livermore, CA).

D. GROWTH MEDIA FOR PRIMARY PROXIMAL TUBULE CULTURES

The basal serum-free growth medium for many renal culture models is SFFD, a 50:50 mixture of Dulbecco's Modified Eagles Medium (DMEM) and Ham's Nutrient Mix F12, with 15 m*M* HEPES.[29] SFFD is a good medium for the culturing of many primary cultures and cell lines and is now available in powder or liquid form from several suppliers of tissue culture media. Other basal media have been used, including Waymouth's MB752/1,[15,36] M199,[17,35] Williams' E,[18] DMEM,[20,21,24,25] αMEM,[40] and Hanks' buffered saline solution (HBSS).[50]

Although one investigator has successfully cultured cells in serum-free medium without hormones or growth factors,[26] most cells require such additives for optimal growth. The complete medium, designated RK-1, used for rabbit primary proximal tubule cultures consists of SFFD with added hormones.[29] The final concentrations of these are bovine insulin (5 μg/ml), human or bovine transferrin (5 μg/ml), hydrocortisone (5×10^{-8} *M*), and sodium selenite (10^{-12} *M*). Insulin is prepared as a stock solution of 5 mg/ml in 0.01 *N* HCl, sterilized by filtration with a 0.22 μ-membrane, dispensed in 2- to 4-ml aliquots, and kept refrigerated. Transferrin is dissolved at 5 mg/ml in water, filter-sterilized, and frozen in 2- to 3-ml aliquots. This reagent should not be subjected to more than four freeze-thaw cycles. Hydrocortisone (10^{-3} *M*) is prepared in 100% ethanol, dispensed in 2- to 3-ml aliquots, and refrigerated for no longer than 3 to 4 mo. A stock solution of selenite (10^{-9} *M*) is prepared in SFFD and may be stored indefinitely at 0°C. Aside from insulin, transferrin, hydrocortisone, and selenium, other frequently used additives for proximal tubule cultures include T_3,[27,33,36,39] PGE_1,[27,36,39] and additional amino acids.[16,21,40]

The development of serum-free, hormonally defined media has been a major advancement for the cultivation of mammalian cells.[52] Serum-free media allow the investigator greater control of experimental variables and eliminate the possible toxic effects of serum. For primary kidney epithelial cells, serum-free media also prevent the fibroblast overgrowth that occurs in the presence of serum, as illustrated dramatically in the photomicrographs of Chung and co-workers.[29] Despite the success of defined media, fetal bovine serum remains a valuable reagent and is used by many workers, generally at 3 to 5%[27,36,38-40] or

10%[15-21,24,50] of the volume. In some cases serum-containing medium is used only in the first few days to facilitate the outgrowth of cells, after which it is replaced by hormonally defined medium.[36,38,39]

Medium composition is an important concern for toxicology studies. Hormones and other factors are added to the basal medium to enhance growth of the cells; yet more attention is needed to determine nutrients and additives that will maintain differentiated kidney transport and metabolic functions. Protective compounds such as glutathione or vitamin E and constituents that could interact with the test compounds should also be considered when planning experiments.

III. CORRESPONDENCE OF PRIMARY CULTURES WITH THE PROXIMAL TUBULE *IN VIVO*

A. RETENTION OF EPITHELIAL MORPHOLOGY

Cultured cells which are to be used as models for differentiated tissue should retain the specific characteristics of the tissue from which they were derived. In the past, primary cultures had the tendency to acquire the appearance of fibroblasts ("fibroblast overgrowth"). This was attributed to selection of fibroblasts by the culture conditions or to changes in the epithelial cells such that they more closely resembled the less differentiated fibroblasts. The preferential growth of epithelial cells can be fostered by the use of selective media.[47] For example, substitution of D-valine for L-valine has been used by several groups to inhibit fibroblast growth in primary kidney cultures,[20,21,25] since fibroblasts are unable to utilize the D-isomer. Recent advances in cell culture technology, including the development of serum-free media, have diminished the fibroblast problem; however, it is desirable for investigators to confirm that their cultures are epithelioid in nature.

Several structural criteria can be used to distinguish epithelial cells from fibroblasts. At the light microscope level, fibroblasts are kite-shaped and spindly when subconfluent and form dense mats of narrow fiber-like cells at confluency. In contrast, epithelial cells are polygonal or rounded when subconfluent and have a distinct cobblestone appearance when confluent. Most primary proximal tubule cultures recently reported clearly have an epithelioid appearance under the light microscope.

Ultrastructurally as well, the proximal tubule cultures resemble tubular epithelia. Most authors report a tall, rounded appearance ("cuboidal") of the cells[27,30,31,35,39,53] which contrasts with the thin, flat shape to be expected of fibroblasts. Tight junctions close to the apical side of the cell are further evidence for their epithelial nature.[16,27,28,30,39,41,50] Electrophysiological studies[28,41] reveal that monolayers of these cells grown on filters possess a low transepithelial resistance, which is characteristic of the "leaky" type of tight junctions found in the proximal tubule. Proximal tubule epithelia *in vivo* have a dense covering of microvilli (brush border) on the apical surface which varies in density and height among the regions of the proximal tubule (S1, S2, S3) and among species. Apical microvilli are present on cultured proximal tubule cells from many species,[16,18,27,28,31,37,40,41] but are sparse and shorter compared to the cells *in vivo*. This may be partially due to stretching of the apical side of the cells when they are grown on a flat surface, so that the trapezoidal shape of cells grown in cylindrical tubules[53] is lost. Alternatively, States and co-workers[40] have reported that the density of microvilli for cells grown in αMEM is greater when compared to the same cells grown in DMEM. Proximal tubule epithelial cells have a more complex basolateral surface than do fibroblasts, with interdigitation of adjacent cell membranes and infolding of the basal surfaces. The complexity of the basolateral surface of the cells is present in the primary cultures[16,18,28,31,37,41] though greatly reduced in comparison to that observed for the proximal tubule *in vivo*.

B. RETENTION OF BIOCHEMICAL CHARACTERISTICS OF THE PROXIMAL TUBULE

In addition to confirming the epithelial morphology of the primary cultures, it is important to determine whether they possess the biochemical functions of the proximal tubule, rather than those of other segments of the nephron. Typical characteristics studied include the hormone-responsiveness of adenylate cyclase and the distribution of marker enzymes (summarized in Reference 33), both of which have unique patterns in each segment of the nephron. The proximal tubule *in vivo* exhibits an adenylate cyclase response that is distinguishable from that of other nephron segments[54,55] in being stimulated by parathyroid hormone (PTH) but not antidiuretic hormone (ADH; arginine vasopressin, AVP), isoproterenol, or calcitonin. Primary proximal tubule cultures obtained by various isolation procedures and from different species retain the adenylate cyclase stimulation by PTH, with minimal or no response to ADH or calcitonin.[23,28,29,31,32,35,37,39] In one study,[56] proximal tubule cells on the 4th day of culturing had an increased adenylate cyclase response to PTH, which returned to initial levels by the 8th day. In contrast to primary cultures, the LLC-PK_1 cell line shows marked stimulation of adenylate cyclase activity after exposure to AVP.

Cellular pathways of intermediary metabolism may be targets for or modifiers of toxicity, so the profound changes in energy metabolism that cells undergo in culture are important. Compared to other nephron segments *in vivo,* the proximal tubule relies more on oxidative metabolism and less on glycolysis and possesses the enzymes required for gluconeogenesis.[55] When tubules are placed in culture, the rate of glycolysis and the activities of glycolytic enzymes increase concomitantly with a decrease in aerobic metabolism,[32,50,57] starting from the first hour of tubule isolation.[41] Despite these changes in enzyme activity, the unique metabolic properties of the proximal tubule are qualitatively retained in the resulting cultures. The gluconeogenic enzymes phosphoenolpyruvate carboxykinase (PEPCK) and fructose-6-phosphatase are present in cultures from proximal tubules, but not those from distal tubules.[32,39] Although the activities of hexokinase and other glycolytic enzymes are higher in proximal tubule cultures than in the starting material, they are lower in proximal tubule cultures than in those from the distal tubule.[39,50] Interestingly, in spite of the decreased basal oxygen consumption and increased reliance on anaerobic metabolism, cultured rabbit proximal tubules have higher concentrations of ATP than the starting tissue.[32] Proximal tubule cultures retain the activities of marker enzymes such as gammaglutamyl transferase (GGT), alkaline phosphatase (AP), succinic dehydrogenase (SD), and Na^+/K^+-ATPase,[9,15-18,26,29,37,45,46] also at levels less than in fresh tissue (Table 1). The hydroxylation of vitamin D_3 localized to the proximal tubules,[55] has been detected in cultures from this segment.[37] These differences in pathways of metabolism between cultured cells and the cells *in vivo* may produce critical differences in toxic mechanisms or sensitivity to toxic agents and merit further investigation.

The presence of renal drug metabolizing enzymes, also found in the proximal tubule, often influences the toxicity of xenobiotics to the kidneys.[6,9] When tubules are cultured, the activities of these enzymes are also altered. For example, compared to fresh tubules, the cytochrome P450 and P450-dependent oxidative reactions of cultured cells are decreased, whereas phase II conjugation enzymes and glutathione levels are well maintained.[18,45] The importance of differences in the activity of drug metabolizing enzymes is illustrated by the case of cephalothin, a cephalosporin antibiotic that has low intrinsic nephrotoxicity *in vivo.* To cultured cells, however, this compound is more toxic than known nephrotoxic agents.[58-60] The toxicity of cephalothin to cultured kidney cells is alleviated by coincubation with the 9,000 $\times$ g supernatant (S9) prepared from the renal cortex. The role of renal esterases in the detoxification of this compound is confirmed by the observations that (1) deacetylcephalothin is not toxic to cultured cells,[14] (2) inhibitors of esterases increase the toxicity

TABLE 1
Enzyme Activities in Homogenates of Rabbit Primary Proximal Tubule Cultures (RPTC), a Rabbit Kidney Cell Line ($LLC\text{-}RK_1$), and Fresh Rabbit Renal Cortex (μU/mg protein)[a]

	RPTC	$LLC\text{-}RK_1$	Renal cortex
Na^+/K^+-ATPase	43 ± 5[b,c]	47 ± 8	88 ± 22
Succinic dehydrogenase	15 ± 2	16 ± 1	30 ± 8
Alkaline phosphatase	37 ± 6	21 ± 1	130 ± 24
Glucose-6-phosphate dehydrogenase	37 ± 1	94 ± 9[d]	52 ± 4
Acetylesterase	7 ± .4	1 ± .2[d]	1013 ± 209

[a] One unit (U) will catalyze the metabolism of 1.0 μmol of substrate/minute.
[b] Data are expressed as the mean ± SE of 3 to 5 values.
[c] All values for RPTC primary cultures and $LLC\text{-}RK_1$ cells were different ($p < .05$) from renal cortical homogenate and are not indicated individually.
[d] Significantly different ($p < .05$) from RPTC.

of cephalothin,[60] and (3) cultured kidney cells have less than 1% of the esterase activity of fresh renal cortex (Table 1).

C. TRANSPORT BY PRIMARY PROXIMAL TUBULE CULTURES

The proximal tubule is a transporting epithelium, moving solutes in both the secretory and reabsorptive directions. Solutes and water in the glomerular filtrate are reabsorbed isosmotically in the proximal tubule by the Na^+/K^+-ATPase on the basolateral membrane. The short circuit current and transepithelial potential difference demonstrated in proximal tubules grown on permeable supports[41] provide evidence for the movement of sodium by these cells. Most papers describing the culturing of proximal tubules on plastic report the occurrence of domes, which are fluid-filled blisters in the monolayer (Figure 2). Domes are formed when fluid is transported from the apical (brush border) side of the cell to the basolateral side, lifting the monolayer from the underlying surface.[61] The presence of these structures also confirms that the cells are able to transport salt and water.

The apical membrane of the proximal tubule cell is the site of reabsorption of solutes such as glucose, amino acids, phosphate, and acid equivalents. Rabbit proximal tubules grown on filters are able to move protons from the basolateral to the apical side of the cell[9] and can reabsorb phosphate.[31,62,63] Similarly, all primary proximal tubules described so far, regardless of isolation procedure or culture conditions, reabsorb glucose in a manner similar to the tissue *in vivo*. For example, the transport of the glucose analog α-methylglucoside (AMG) by the cultures is dependent on sodium, is inhibited by phloridzin, and occurs only from the apical side.[16,24,27,29,32,35,37,40,41,64,65] As would be expected, such transport cannot be detected in cultured distal tubules.[39]

The basolateral membrane of proximal tubules *in vivo* possesses transport proteins by which drugs and environmental chemicals may be accumulated within the cell. The presence of secretory transport for the organic anion PAH which is inhibited by probenecid has been reported for primary cultures of flounder,[42] rabbit,[66,67] and rat[68] proximal tubules. This transporter is thought to be the system by which several nephrotoxic agents, including the antibiotic cephaloridine, are concentrated by the proximal tubule cells *in vivo*. Carrier-mediated transport of organic cations such as tetraethylammonium (TEA) has also been demonstrated in kidney cell cultures.[12,13] Growing cells on filters may therefore be important in providing proper access of test compounds to cellular sites of drug entry.

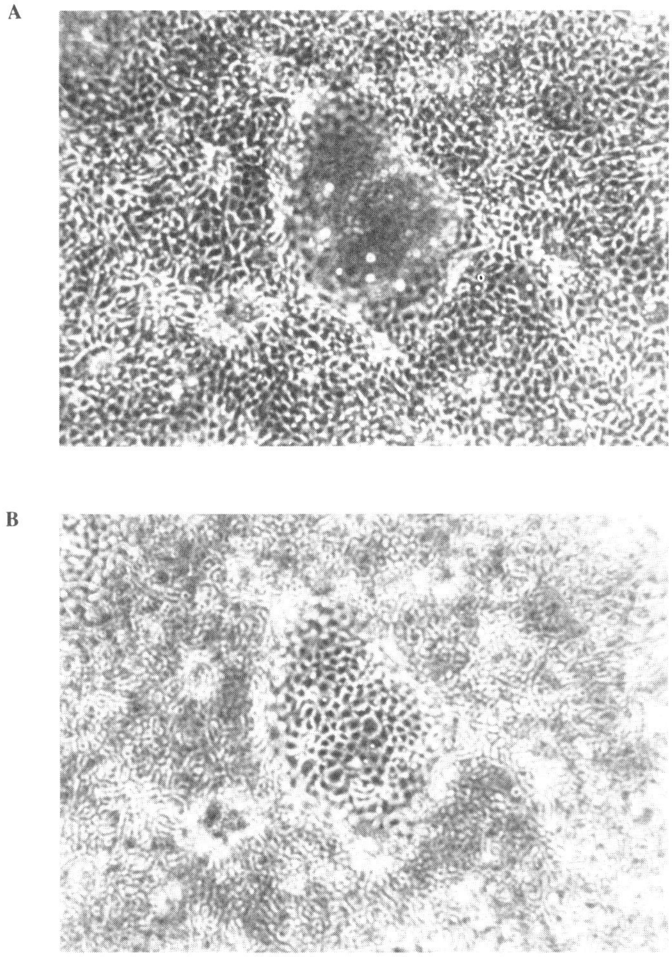

FIGURE 2. Confluent monolayer of rabbit primary proximal tubule cells ($\times$ 200) showing (A) the monolayer in focus, and (B) a dome in focus.

IV. ASSESSMENT OF TOXICITY IN CULTURED PROXIMAL TUBULE CELLS

A. STRUCTURAL DAMAGE

Nephrotoxicants often produce histological damage concomitantly with cellular dysfunction, both *in vivo*[69] and *in vitro*.[70] Borenfreund and Puerner[71] reported a good correlation between morphological changes and functional indices of toxicity for fibroblasts; however, Bacon and co-workers[72] found that morphological examination did not provide an adequate discrimination among test compounds that caused notable differences in LDH release from kidney cells (LLC-PK_1). Although morphometric analysis of toxicity would be unsuitable for screening because of the difficulty in quantifying changes, it is an important adjunct to functional measurements. Some nephrotoxicants produce distinctive structural lesions *in vivo*, and the appearance of these lesions *in vitro* would be an important validation of the model. For example, the myeloid bodies that occur as a result of aminoglycoside exposure *in vivo* have been reproduced in primary kidney cultures,[34,73] as have the inclusion bodies that occur in proximal tubule cells following exposure to lead.[25]

B. CELL VIABILITY

In cultured cells, vitality is most accurately assayed by determining the plating efficiency, a procedure that may take several days. A more convenient estimation of cell viability following exposure to toxic compounds is made by using tests that depend on the integrity of the plasma membrane. Examples include the ability of cells to exclude dyes (nigrosin, trypan blue), the leakage of the intracellular enzyme lactate dehydrogenase (LDH), or the uptake of the dye, neutral red.[71] Such methods should be evaluated carefully, inasmuch as the results may vary among the tests depending on the cell type or the toxic agents employed.[74] The effect of toxicants on cell proliferation has been used as evidence of cytotoxicity in some studies;[34,75,76] however, in renal toxicology we are generally concerned with differentiated, nonproliferating tissue.

C. IMPAIRMENT OF BASIC CELLULAR METABOLISM

Cell death, though an unequivocal endpoint, represents a late event in the development of toxicity. Cell death may be preceded by impairment of one or more vital metabolic processes which could provide an earlier and perhaps more mechanistically relevant parameter of toxicity. For example, syntheses of specific proteins by cultured primary kidney cells were impaired by gallium or arsenic at concentrations that did not cause the release of LDH.[15] The syntheses of macromolecules such as protein and DNA can be quantified by the rate of incorporation of radiolabeled precursors. Protein and DNA syntheses by cultured rat and rabbit proximal tubules are sensitive to the anticancer drug cisplatin.[16,77]

Cellular energy metabolism can also be used to assess sensitivity to test compounds. An assay of mitochondrial function based on the cleavage of a tetrazolium dye by mitochondrial dehydrogenases (MTT test)[78] has been found to correlate well with the neutral red uptake assay in appraising the toxicity of test compounds. ATP concentrations can be conveniently measured in cultured cells and may be a sensitive indicator of toxic damage. For example, the concentrations of ATP are reduced in LLC-PK_1 cells at mercury concentrations lower than those causing ultrastructural damage to mitochondria.[79] Oxygen consumption is a good indicator of toxicity in renal cortical slices[80,81] but may be impractical for cultures because of the large number of cells required to obtain a reliable reading.[32] The capability of treated cells to maintain the transmembrane distribution of sodium and potassium ions has also been used as an endpoint in studies with slices[70] and cultured cells.[82]

D. IMPAIRMENT OF TISSUE-SPECIFIC FUNCTIONS

An approach to the assessment of *in vitro* nephrotoxicity which has also been used in animal studies is to utilize proximal tubule-specific functions. Miyajima and co-workers[69] observed that the accumulation of organic ions by renal cortical slices was a more sensitive indicator of toxicity than was blood urea nitrogen (BUN) concentrations or histological examination of the kidneys. For cultured proximal tubule cells, the rates of organic ion secretion, rates of reabsorption of solutes (glucose, amino acids, phosphate), or the condition of intercellular junctions may be more sensitive and specific criteria of cellular toxicity than viability. The integrity of cellular junctions for monolayers grown on filters can be assessed by determination of transepithelial resistance or by the ability of the cells to impede the movement of labeled inulin across the monolayer.[83] Gstraunthaler and co-workers[84] concluded that electrophysiological measurements on LLC-PK_1 cells grown on filters were more sensitive than morphological analysis or enzyme release as an index of toxicity, and produced a better toxicity ranking of cephalosporin antibiotics.

The number of domes may also be a valuable gauge of cellular toxicity in transporting epithelia such as cultured kidney cells. In addition to depending on the content of Na^+/K^+-ATPase in the basolateral membrane, the formation of domes reflects the provision of ATP for the activity of this enzyme, the strength of intercellular junctions, and the condition of the cytoskeleton.[85] Saito and co-workers[86] reported that the incidence of domes in LLC-PK_1 monolayers was decreased by gentamicin in a dose-dependent manner, and furthermore observed that the ability of aminoglycosides to decrease domes accurately reflected their *in vivo* nephrotoxicity.

Many *in vivo* studies have been done to correlate the urinary excretion of enzymes with exposure to nephrotoxicants. The enzymes most often assayed include the brush border enzymes GGT and AP, and the lysosomal enzyme *n*-acetyl glucosaminidase (NAG). Although the urinary concentration of such enzymes is increased following exposure to certain nephrotoxicants,[87] enzymes have not proved to be dependable indices for assessing nephrotoxicity *in vivo*. However, there may be greater potential for the use of these enzymes under the controlled conditions in cell culture work. Castaing and co-workers[19] found that GGT and AP were released into the culture medium by rat or human kidney cells exposed to 10 μg/ml or greater cisplatin, whereas the effect on NAG was much less. An alternative approach was taken by Hori and co-workers[88] who assayed the enzymes in the monolayer rather than the medium and found that AP, NAG, and Na^+/K^+-ATPase activities were decreased by gentamicin treatment to a greater extent than was viability.

E. MECHANISM-DEPENDENT INDICES OF TOXICITY

The most reliable and sensitive indices of toxicity for cultured cells exposed to a chemical will most likely be measurements representing key events in the pathogenesis of toxicity. Tay and co-workers[77] examined several parameters of cellular function (e.g., mitochondrial and plasma membrane enzymes, protein synthesis) and viability (nigrosin dye exclusion) in rabbit primary proximal tubule cultures exposed to the nephrotoxicant cisplatin and found that the earliest alterations involved inhibition of DNA synthesis. Thus, in examining cisplatin derivatives for potential nephrotoxicity in primary culture, this index may provide the most sensitive measurement. Calcium appears to be a crucial determinant of irreversible cell damage by certain xenobiotics. Trump and co-workers[89] found that the intracellular concentration of calcium was rapidly elevated (within 10 min) after exposure of primary proximal tubule cultures to 10 μ*M* $HgCl_2$. However, for some agents it may be necessary to allow sufficient time (minutes to hours) for a key lesion to be expressed.

The mechanism-specific approach to monitoring toxicity in primary cultures has its disadvantages as well. First, the endpoints established will likely be applicable to a particular chemical series (e.g., cephalosporins, aminoglycosides); so for each new series of compound studied, specific endpoints will need to be established. Second, assumptions regarding the causal relationship between an early endpoint and cell death are often made. Considerable time and effort is required to substantiate such relationships and, in fact, few have been established with certainty in the field of nephrotoxicology. Alternatively, general indicators of cellular function and viability as discussed above may be monitored simultaneously.

V. SCREENING POTENTIAL OF PRIMARY PROXIMAL TUBULE CULTURES

Several studies have been done to evaluate the sensitivity and accuracy of established cells lines in ranking model nephrotoxicants. The pig kidney cell line LLC-PK_1, often used as a model of the proximal tubule, was found to be more sensitive to aminoglycoside or tetracycline toxicity than the dog kidney line MDCK,[72] which has many characteristics of the distal tubule. In contrast, LLC-PK_1 was not any better in predicting aminoglycoside toxicity than either a liver or corneal cell line.[76] Success in using LLC-PK_1 for toxicity testing is dependent on the toxicity endpoint used. LDH leakage[76] viable cell count,[88] ATP

TABLE 2
Toxicity of Cephalosporin Antibiotics to Cultured Kidney Cells[a]

Culture[b]	LLC-RK$_1$		RPC		HPC	
Dose (mg/ml)	5.0	7.5	5.0	7.5	1.0	3.0
Cefazolin	64	42	44	36	52	31
Cephaloridine	39	26	41	29	46	9
Cephalothin	3	0	28	18	6	ND[c]

[a] Data are expressed as the % viable control (%VC) = (no. viable cells in treated group ÷ no. viable cells in control) × 100.
[b] The culture models are LLC-RK$_1$ (rabbit kidney cell line), RPC (rabbit primary proximal tubule cultures), and HPC (human primary renal cortex cultures).
[c] ND: not determined.

concentration,[88] AMG uptake,[90] and inhibition of cell proliferation[34,76] were not satisfactory predictors of aminoglycoside toxicity. In contrast, the number of floating cells, the incidence of domes, and the activity or release of other cellular enzymes were sensitive and accurate indicators of the nephrotoxic potential of aminoglycosides.[88,90] LLC-RK$_1$, a rabbit kidney cell line, has also been used to study antibiotic nephrotoxicity. When the culture medium is supplemented with kidney S9 during the test, these cells rank the toxicity of eight cephalosporins in agreement with their *in vivo* potency.[14,91,92]

Despite the numerous *in vitro* cytotoxicity studies with undifferentiated cells or with kidney cell lines, few studies have examined the screening potential of primary cultures. Those reported with primary cultures have been concerned with determining the toxic mechanism for a single agent.[77,93,94] The ranking studies available suggest that the favorable state of differentiation of the primaries may provide a more accurate ranking of nephrotoxicants. Although LLC-PK$_1$ and primary human kidney cells ranked the toxicity of aminoglycosides in the same order, human cultures were found to be more sensitive.[95] Rabbit primary proximal tubule cultures had a greater ability than LLC-RK$_1$ cells to discriminate among cephalosporin and carbapenem antibiotics having different nephrotoxic potencies (Table 2). In addition, the nontoxic carbapenem BMY-26225 was extremely toxic to LLC-RK$_1$ but not to primary cultures. Similar to the case of cephalothin, the toxicity of BMY-26225 to LLC-RK$_1$ was prevented by including S9 in the test media. Such results suggest that the metabolic capacity of primary cultures is closer than the cell line to that of the proximal tubule *in vivo,* and that the predictive ability of primary cultures will be greater than that of continuous cell lines.

To be efficient, screening studies should be rapid and involve a minimum of time and materials. The use of isolated cells for initiation of cell culture has had the advantage of being able to use microplates (96-well plates) and microplate readers for rapid visible and fluorescent spectrophotometric assays. Although this level of convenience has not been possible with cultures of tubules, equipment has recently become available to read the larger 6-well plates and filter inserts (Cytofluor, Millipore Corp). Thus, cytotoxicity studies and mechanistic experiments (e.g., intracellular calcium) can now be performed with tubule cultures. Functional parameters such as organic ion secretion, amino acid, glucose or phosphate reabsorption, protein synthesis, energy status, and so forth may be more sensitive and rapid than viability in the evaluation of toxicity and would facilitate direct comparison with similar indices *in vivo.*

General considerations for the routine use of *in vitro* toxicity testing have been delineated in a report from the Johns Hopkins Center for Alternatives to Animal Testing.[96] An aspect of testing that is unique to the kidneys concerns the relevancy of concentrations used. As described above, cells in the nephron may be exposed to high extracellular concentrations of xenobiotics due to the reabsorption of fluid from the tubular lumen. Consequently, serum drug levels do not necessarily reflect the concentrations to which proximal tubule cells are exposed, and the use of higher concentrations to obtain a toxic response may be warranted.[97]

VI. SUMMARY

Proximal tubules cultured from various species retain many of the morphological and functional attributes of the original kidney tissue. There is a reduction in the activity or presence of many characteristics, which is probably due to loss of some modulating factors or hormones rather than a permanent ''dedifferentiation'' or genetic alteration. The ability to discriminate among a range of toxicities has been found to be greater for primary cultures than for established cell lines. Therefore, it is likely that as more is learned about the influence of the culture environment on the expression of differentiated characteristics, improvements in the kidney-specific functions of the cells will be possible. In turn, the utility of proximal tubule cultures in predicting nephrotoxic potential will be enhanced. For the present, proximal tubule cell cultures promise to be an efficient tool in the process of compound selection and evaluation, which can significantly reduce the number of animals used in screening activities.

REFERENCES

1. **Appel, G. B. and Neu, H. C.,** The nephrotoxicity of antimicrobial agents. I, *New Engl. J. Med.*, 296, 663, 1977.
2. **Williams, P. D. and Hottendorf, G. H.,** Critical appraisal of animal models for antibiotic toxicity, in *Modern Analysis of Antibiotics*, Aszalos, A., Ed., Marcel Dekker, New York, 1986, 495.
3. **Goldstein, R. S. and Mayor, G. H.,** Minireview: the nephrotoxicity of cisplatin, *Life Sci.*, 32, 685, 1983.
4. **Madias, N. E. and Harrington, J. T.,** Platinum nephrotoxicity, *Am. J. Med.*, 65, 307, 1978.
5. **Cojocel, C. and Hook, J. B.,** Aminoglycoside nephrotoxicity, *Trends Pharmacol. Sci.*, 4, 174, 1983.
6. **Rush, G. F., Smith, J. H., Newton, J. F., and Hook, J. B.,** Chemically induced nephrotoxicity: role of metabolic activation, *CRC Crit. Rev. Toxicol.*, 13, 99, 1984.
7. **Goldstein, R. S., Pasino, D. A., Hewitt, W. R., and Hook, J. B.,** Biochemical mechanisms of cephaloridine nephrotoxicity: time and concentration dependence of peroxidative injury, *Toxicol. Appl. Pharmacol*, 83, 261, 1986.
8. **Rush, G. and Ponsler, G. D.,** Cephaloridine-induced biochemical changes and cytotoxicity in suspensions of rabbit isolated proximal tubules, *Toxicol. Appl. Pharmacol.*, 109, 314, 1991.
9. **Ford, S. M. and Hook, J. B.,** Biochemical Mechanisms of toxic nephropathies, *Sem. Nephrol.*, 4, 88, 1984.
10. **Hewitt, W. R., Goldstein, R. S., and Hook, J. B.,** Toxic responses of the kidney, in *Casarett and Doull's Toxicology: The Basic Science of Poisons*, 4th ed., Pergamon Press, New York, 1991.
11. **Smith, M. A., Hewitt, W. R., and Hook, J. B.,** *In vitro* methods in renal toxicology, in *In Vitro Methods in Toxicology*, Cambridge University Press, Cambridge, 1987.
12. **Inui, K., Saito, H., and Hori, R.,** H^+-gradient-dependent active transport of tetraethylammonium cation in apical-membrane vesicles isolated from kidney epithelial cell line LLC-PK1, *Biochem. J.*, 227, 199, 1985.
13. **Fauth, C., Rossier, B., and Roch-Ramel, F.,** Transport of tetraethylammonium by a kidney epithelial cell line (LLC-PK1), *Am. J. Physiol.*, 254, F351, 1988.

14. **Williams, P. D., Laska, D. A., Tay, L. K., and Hottendorf, G. H.,** Comparative toxicities of cephalosporin antibiotics in a rabbit kidney cell line (LLC-RK_1). *Antimicrob. Agents Chemother.*, 32, 314, 1988.
15. **Aoki, Y., Lipsky, M. M., and Fowler, B. A.,** Alteration in protein synthesis in primary cultures of rat kidney proximal tubule epithelial cells by exposure to gallium, indium, and arsenite, *Toxicol. Appl. Pharmacol.*, 106, 462, 1990.
16. **Barron, E. T., O'Brien, A., and Ryan, M. P.,** Primary cultures of rat and rabbit renal proximal epithelium as models for nephrotoxicity investigations, *Toxicol. Lett.*, 53, 161, 1990.
17. **Bellemann, P.,** Primary monolayer culture of liver parenchymal cells and kidney cortical tubules as a useful new model for biochemical pharmacology and experimental toxicology. Studies *in vitro* on hepatic membrane transport, induction of liver enzymes, and adaptive changes in renal cortical enzymes, *Arch. Toxicol.*, 44, 63, 1980.
18. **Bruggemann, I. M., Mertens, J. J. W. M., Temmink, J. H. M., Lans, M. C., Vos, R. M. E., and van Bladeren, P. J.,** Use of monolayers of primary rat kidney cortex cells for nephrotoxicity studies, *Toxicol. In Vitro*, 3, 261, 1989.
19. **Castaing, N., Merlet, D., and Cambar, J.,** *Cis*-platin cytotoxicity in human and rat tubular cell cultures, *Toxicol. In Vitro*, 4, 396, 1990.
20. **Cherian, M. G.,** Rat kidney epithelial cell culture for metal toxicity studies, *In Vitro Cell. Develop. Biol.*, 21, 505, 1985.
21. **Cherian, M. G.,** The synthesis of metallothionein and cellular adaptation to metal toxicity in primary rat kidney epithelial cell cultures, *Toxicology*, 17, 225, 1980.
22. **Goligorsky, M. S., Menton, D. M., and Hruska, K. A.,** Parathyroid hormone-induced changes of the brush border topography and cytoskeleton in cultured renal proximal tubular cells, *J. Membr. Biol.*, 92, 151, 1986.
23. **Hatzinger, P. B. and Stevens, J. L.,** Rat kidney proximal tubule cells in defined medium: the roles of cholera toxin, extracellular calcium and serum in cell growth and expression of γ-glutamyltransferase, *In Vitro Cell. Develop. Biol.*, 25, 205, 1989.
24. **Larsson, S., Aperia, A., and Lechene, C.,** Studies on the final differentiation of rat renal proximal tubular cells in culture, *Am. J. Physiol.*, C455, 1986.
25. **McLachlin, J. R., Goyer, R. A., and Cherian, M. G.,** Formation of lead-induced inclusion bodies in primary rat kidney epithelial cell cultures: effect of actinomycin D and cycloheximide, *Toxicol. Appl. Pharmacol.*, 56, 418, 1980.
26. **Rosenberg, M. R. and Michalopoulos, G.,** Kidney proximal tubular cells isolated by collagenase perfusion grow in defined media in the absence of growth factors, *J. Cell. Physiol.*, 131, 107, 1987.
27. **Stanton, R. C., Mendrick, D. L., Rennke, H. G., and Seifter, J. L.,** Use of monoclonal antibodies to culture rat proximal tubule cells, *Am. J. Physiol.*, 251, C780, 1986.
28. **Bello-Reuss, E. and Webber, M. R.,** Electrophysiological studies on primary cultures of proximal tubule cells, *Am. J. Physiol.*, 251, F490, 1986.
29. **Chung, S. D., Alavi, N., Livingston, D., Hiller, S., and Taub, M.,** Characterization of primary rabbit kidney cultures that express proximal tubule functions in a hormonally defined medium, *J. Cell Biol.*, 95, 118, 1982.
30. **Ford, S. M., Williams, P. D., Grassl, S., and Holohan, P. D.,** Transepithelial acidification by cultures of rabbit proximal tubules grown on filters, *Am. J. Physiol.*, 259, C103, 1990.
31. **Suzuki, M., Capparelli, A., Jo, O. D., Kawaguchi, Y., Ogura, Y., Miyahara, T., and Yanagawa, N.,** Phosphate transport in the *in vitro* cultured rabbit proximal convoluted and straight tubules, *Kidney Int.*, 34, 268, 1988.
32. **Tang, M.-J., Suresh, K. R., and Tannen, R. L.,** Carbohydrate metabolism by primary cultures of rabbit proximal tubules, *Am. J. Physiol.*, 256, C532, 1989.
33. **Detrisac, C. J., Sens, M. A., Garvin, A. J., Spicer, S. S., and Sens, D. A.,** Tissue culture of human kidney epithelial cells of proximal tubule origin, *Kidney Int.*, 25, 383, 1984.
34. **Sens, M. A., Hennigar, G. R., and Sens, D. A.,** An *in vitro* model for aminoglycoside nephrotoxicity: human proximal convoluted tubular cell culture, *Lab. Invest.*, 52, 61A, 1985.
35. **States, B., Foreman, J., Lee, J., and Segal, S.,** Characteristics of cultured human renal cortical epithelia, *Biochem. Med. Metab. Biol.*, 36, 151, 1986.
36. **Yang, A. H., Gould-Kostka, J., and Oberley, T. D.,** *In vitro* growth and differentiation of human kidney tubular cells on a basement membrane substrate, *In Vitro Cell. Develop. Biol.*, 23, 34, 1987.
37. **Bell, C. L., Tenenhouse, H. S., and Scriver, C. R.,** Initiation and characterization of primary mouse kidney epithelial cells, *In Vitro Cell. Develop. Biol.*, 24, 683, 1988.
38. **Ellis, D., Sothi, T. D., Curthoys, N. P., Ballou, B., and Avner, E. D.,** Regulation of glucocorticoid receptors and Na-K ATPase activity by hydrocortisone in proximal tubular epithelial cells, *In Vitro Cell. Dev. Biol.*, 24, 811, 1988.

39. **Hruska, K. A., Goligorsky, M., Scoble, J., Tsutsumi, M., Westbrook, S., and Moskowitz, D.,** Effects of parathyroid hormone on cytosolic calcium in renal proximal tubular primary cultures. *Am. J. Physiol.*, 251, F188, 1986.
40. **States, B., Reynolds, R., Lee, J., and Segal, S.,** Cystine uptake by cultured cells originating from dog proximal tubule segments, *In Vitro Cell Dev. Biol.*, 26, 105, 1990.
41. **Dickman, K. G. and Renfro, J. L.,** Primary culture of flounder renal tubule cells: transepithelial transport, *Am. J. Physiol.*, 251, F424, 1986.
42. **Lieberman, I. and Ove, P.,** Enzyme activity levels in mammalian cell cultures, *J. Biol. Chem.*, 233, 634, 1958.
43. **Horster, M.,** Primary culture of mammalian nephron epithelia. Requirements for cell outgrowth and proliferation from defined explanted nephron segments, *Pflügers Arch.*, 382, 209, 1979.
44. **Aleo, M. D., Taub, M. L., Nickerson, P. A., and Kostyniak, P. J.,** Primary cultures of rabbit renal proximal tubule cells. I. Growth and biochemical characteristics, *In Vitro Cell. Develop. Biol.*, 25, 776, 1989.
45. **Aleo, M. D., Taub, M. L., Olson, J. R., and Kostyniak, P. J.,** Primary cultures of rabbit renal proximal tubule cells. II. Selected phase I and phase II metabolic capacities, *Toxicol. In Vitro*, 4, 727, 1990.
46. **Vinay, P., Gougoux, A., and Lemieux, G.,** Isolation of a pure suspension of rat proximal tubules, *Am. J. Physiol.*, 241, F403, 1981.
47. **Ham, R. G.,** Selective media, in *Cell Separation: Methods and Selected Applications*, Vol. 3, Academic Press, NY, 1984, 209.
48. **Kreisberg, J. I., Pitts, A. M., and Pretlow, T. G.,** Separation of proximal tubule cells from suspensions of rat kidney cells in density gradients of Ficoll in tissue culture medium, *Am. J. Pathol.*, 86, 591, 1977.
49. **Lash, L. H. and Tokarz, J. J.,** Isolation of two distinct populations of cells from rat kidney cortex and their use in the study of chemical-induced toxicity, *Anal. Biochem.*, 182, 271, 1989.
50. **Trifillis, A. L., Regec, A. L., and Trump, B. F.,** Isolation, culture and characterization of human renal tubular cells, *J. Urology*, 133, 324, 1985.
51. **Handler, J. S.,** The use of cultured kidney cells to study renal toxicology, in *Nephrotoxicity of Antibiotics and Immunosuppressants*, Tanabe, T., Hook, J. B., and Endou, H., Eds., Elsevier Science Publishers, Amsterdam, 1986, 189.
52. **Taub, M.,** The use of defined media in cell and tissue culture, *Toxicol. In Vitro*, 4, 213, 1990.
53. **Kaissling, B. and Kriz, W.,** Structure-function correlation in transporting epithelia, in *The Kidney: Physiology and Pathophysiology*, Seldin, D. W. and Giebisch, G., Eds., Raven Press, NY, 1985.
54. **Jacobson, H. R.,** Functional segmentation of the mammalian nephron, *Am. J. Physiol.*, 241, F203, 1981.
55. **Kurokawa, K., Torikai, S., Wang, M.-S., Klein, K. L., and Kawashima, H.,** Metabolic heterogeneity of the nephron, *Mineral Electrolyte Metab.*, 7, 225, 1982.
56. **Toutain, H., Courjault, F., Vauclin-Jacques, N., and Morin, J. P.,** Adenylate cyclase responses and biochemical characterization of primary rabbit proximal tubular cell cultures and LLC-PK1 cells, *Renal Fail.*, 12, 177, 1990.
57. **Burlington, H.,** Enzyme patterns in cultured kidney cells, *Am. J. Physiol.*, 197, 68, 1959.
58. **Chang, T.-W. and Weinstein, L.,** Toxic effects of various penicillins and cephalosporin derivatives on human amnion cell cultures, *Proc. Soc. Exp. Biol. Med.*, 124, 980, 1966.
59. **Pain, T. F., Jr., Nickell, J. A., and Jarman, S. D.,** Toxicity of cephalothin for McCoy cell cultures, *Proc. Soc. Exp. Biol. Med.*, 125, 1237, 1967.
60. **Hottendorf, G. H., Laska, D. A., Williams, P. D., and Ford, S. M.,** Role of desacetylation in the detoxification of cephalothin in renal cells in culture, *J. Toxicol. Environ. Health*, 22, 101, 1987.
61. **Cereijido, M., Ehrenfeld, J., Fernandez-Castelo, S., and Meza, I.,** Fluxes, junctions, and blisters in cultured monolayers of epithelioid cells (MDCK), in *Hormonal Regulation of Epithelial Transport of Ions and Water*, Scott, W. N. and Goodman, D. B. P., Eds., New York Academy of Sciences, New York, 1981, 422.
62. **Scheinman, S. J. and Ford, S.,** Transepithelial phosphate transport by cultured renal cells: inhibition with phosphonoformic acid (PFA) at the apical surface, *Kidney Int.*, 33, 348, 1988.
63. **Waqar, M. A., Seto, J., Chung, S. D., Hiller-Grohol, S., and Taub, M.,** Phosphate uptake by primary renal proximal tubule cell cultures grown in hormonally defined medium, *J. Cell. Physiol.*, 124, 411, 1985.
64. **Palmoski, M., Masters, B., Flint, O., Ford, S., and Oleson, F.,** Glucose transport in primary rabbit proximal tubule kidney cells grown on filter cultures, *In Vitro*, 26, 55A, 1990.
65. **Sakhrani, L. M., Badie-Dezfooly, B., Trizna, W., Mikhail, N., Lowe, A. G., Taub, M., and Fine, L. G.,** Transport and metabolism of glucose by renal proximal tubular cells in primary culture, *Am. J. Physiol.*, 246, F757, 1984.

66. **Yang, I. S., Goldinger, J. M., Hong, S. K., and Taub, M.,** Preparation of basolateral membranes that transport p-aminohippurate from primary cultures of rabbit kidney proximal tubule cells, *J. Cell Physiol.*, 135, 481, 1988.
67. **Taub, M. L., Yang, I. S., and Wang, Y.,** Primary rabbit kidney proximal tubule cell cultures maintain differentiated functions when cultured in a hormonally defined, serum-free medium, *In Vitro Cell. Develop. Biol.*, 25, 770, 1989.
68. **Boogaard, P. J., Zoeteweij, J. P., van Berkel, T. J. C., van't Noordende, J. M., Mulder, G. J., and Nagelkerke, J. F.,** Primary culture of proximal tubular cells from normal rat kidney as an *in vitro* model to study mechanisms of nephrotoxicity. Toxicity of nephrotoxicants at low concentrations during prolonged exposure, *Biochem. Pharmacol.*, 39, 1335, 1990.
69. **Miyajima, H., Hewitt, W. R., Cote, M. G., and Plaa, G. L.,** Relationships between histological and functional indices of acute chemically induced nephrotoxicity, *Fund. Appl. Toxicol.*, 3, 543, 1983.
70. **Wolfgang, G. H. I., Gandolfi, A. J., and Brendel, K.,** Evaluation of organic nephrotoxins in rabbit renal cortical slices, *Toxicol. In Vitro,* 3, 341, 1989.
71. **Borenfreund, E. and Puerner, J. A.,** Toxicity determined *in vitro* by morphological alterations and neutral red absorption, *Toxicol. Lett.*, 24, 119, 1985.
72. **Bacon, J. A., Linsemen, D. A., and Raczniak, T. J.,** *In vitro* cytotoxicity of tetracyclines and aminoglycosides in LLC-PK_1, MDCK and Chang continuous cell lines, *Toxicol. In Vitro,* 4, 384, 1990.
73. **Chatterjee, S., Trifillis, A. L., and Regec, A. L.,** Morphological and biochemical effects of gentamicin in cultured human renal tubular cells, in *Renal Heterogeneity and Target Cell Toxicity,* Bach, P. H. and Lock, E. A., Eds., John Wiley & Sons, Chichester, 1985, 549.
74. **Bhuyan, B. K., Loughman, B. E., Fraser, T. J., and Day, K. J.,** Comparison of different methods of determining cell viability after exposure to cytotoxic compounds, *Exper. Cell Res.*, 97, 275, 1976.
75. **Horner, S. A., Fry, J. R., Clothier, R. H., and Balls, M.,** A comparison of two cytotoxicity assays for the detection of metabolism-mediated toxicity *in vitro:* a study with cyclophosphamide, *Xenobiotica,* 15, 681, 1985.
76. **Linseman, D. A., Raczniak, T. J., Aaron, C. S., and Bacon, J. A.,** Comparative cytotoxicity rankings of four aminoglycoside antibiotics in the Chang, SIRC, and LLC-PK1 cell lines, *ATLA* (Altern. Lab. Animals), 18, 283, 1990.
77. **Tay, L. K., Bregman, C. L., Masters, B. A., and Williams, P. D.,** Effects of cis-diamminedichloroplatinum (II) on rabbit kidney *in vivo* and on rabbit renal proximal tubule cells in culture, *Cancer Res.*, 48, 2538, 1988.
78. **Mosmann, T.,** Rapid colorimetric assay for cellular growth and survival: application to proliferation and cytotoxicity assays, *J. Immunol. Methods,* 65, 55, 1983.
79. **Bravo, L. and Ford, S. M.,** Cellular ATP levels and ultrastructural changes in mitochondria in LLC-PK_1 cells after $HgCl_2$ and CH_3HgOH insult, *Toxicologist,* 10, 103, 1990.
80. **Ford, S. M., Laska, D. A., Hottendorf, G. H., and Williams, P. D.,** Assessment of the ability of several in vitro models to predict the nephrotoxicity of β-lactam antibiotics, *Toxicologist,* 8, 187, 1988.
81. **Tyson, C. A., Dabbs, J. E., Cohen, P. M., Green, C. E., and Melnick, R. L.,** Studies of nephrotoxic agents in an improved renal proximal tubule system, *Toxicol. In Vitro,* 4, 403, 1990.
82. **Smith, M. A., Acosta, D. A., and Bruckner, J. V.,** Cephaloridine toxicity in primary cultures of rat renal cortical epithelial cells, *Toxicol. In Vitro,* 1, 23, 1987.
83. **Palmoski, M. J., Masters, B. A., Ford, S. M., and Flint, O. P.,** Growth characteristics and measurement of confluency of rabbit primary proximal tubule kidney cells grown on Millicell-HA filters, *J. Tissue Culture Methods,* 13, 169, 1991.
84. **Gstraunthaler, G., Steinmassl, D., and Pfaller, W.,** Renal cell cultures: a tool for studying tubular function and nephrotoxicity, *Toxicol. Lett.*, 53, 1, 1990.
85. **Handler, J. S., Perkins, F. M., and Johnson, J. P.,** Studies of renal cell function using cell culture techniques, *Am. J. Physiol.*, 238, F1, 1980.
86. **Saito, H., Inui, K.-I., and Hori, R.,** Mechanisms of gentamicin transport in kidney epithelial cell line (LLC-PK_1), *J. Pharmacol. Exp. Therap.*, 238, 1071, 1986.
87. **Smith, J. H. and Hook, J. B.,** Experimental nephrotoxicity *in vivo,* in *Nephrotoxicity. Assessment and Pathogenesis,* Bach, P. H., Bonner, F. W., Bridges, J. W., and Lock, E. A., Eds., John Wiley & Sons, Chichester, 1982, 117.
88. **Hori, R., Yamamoto, K., Saito, H., Kohno, M., and Inui, K.-I.,** Effect of aminoglycoside antibiotics on cellular functions of kidney epithelial cell line (LLC-PK1): a model system for aminoglycoside nephrotoxicity, *J. Pharmacol. Exp. Therap.*, 230, 742, 1984.
89. **Trump, B. F., Berezesky, I. K., Elliget, K. A., Smith, M. A., and Phelps, P. C.,** Nephrotoxicity *in vitro:* role of ion deregulation in signal transduction following injury — studies utilizing digital imaging fluorescence microscopy, *Toxicol. In Vitro,* 4, 409, 1990.

90. **Inui, K.-I., Saito, H., Iwata, T., and Hori, R.,** Aminoglycoside-induced alterations in apical membranes of kidney epithelial cell line ($LLC-PK_1$), *Am. J. Physiol.,* 254, C251, 1988.
91. **Duffy, P. A. and McNae, F. R.,** *In vitro* toxicity of antibiotics to LLC-RK1 rabbit kidney cells, *Toxicol. In Vitro,* 4, 375, 1990.
92. **Williams, P. D., Buening, M. K., Gries, C. L., Hanasono, G. K., Laska, D. A., Tamura, R. N., and Heim, R. A.,** Comparative toxicity of oral cephalosporin antibiotics in the rabbit and in a rabbit kidney cell line (LLC-RK1), *Toxicol. In Vitro,* 4, 207, 1990.
93. **Cherian, M. G.,** Studies on toxicity of metallothionein in rat kidney epithelial cell culture, *Dev. Toxicol. Envir. Sci.,* 9, 193, 1982.
94. **Trifillis, A., Regee, A., Hallcraggs, M., and Trump, B.,** Effects of cyclosporin on cultured human renal tubular cells, *Human Toxicol.,* 3, 454, 1984.
95. **Williams, P. D., Laska, D. A., and Hottendorf, G. H.,** Comparative toxicity of aminoglycoside antibiotics in cell cultures derived from human and pig kidney, in *Vitro Toxicol.,* 1, 23, 1986/7.
96. **Frazier, J. M. and Bradlaw, J. A., Eds.,** Technical Problems Associated with *In Vitro* Toxicity Testing Systems, Tech. Rep. No. 1, Johns Hopkins Center for Alternatives to Animal Testing, Baltimore, MD, 1989.
97. **Bach, P. H.,** Detection of chemically induced renal injury: the cascade of degenerative morphological and functional changes that follow the primary nephrotoxic insult and evaluation of these changes by *in vitro* methods, *Toxicol. Lett.,* 46, 237, 1989.

Chapter 11

THE ISOLATED PERFUSED LUNG PREPARATION

David J. P. Bassett and Robert A. Roth

TABLE OF CONTENTS

I. INTRODUCTION

Isolated perfused lungs from several different species have been extensively used for toxicological studies. Such preparations permit the use of physiological routes of exposure for the study of mechanisms of toxicity under conditions where the architecture remains intact and the potential influences of other organs eliminated. Metabolic processes can be investigated under conditions whereby multienzyme pathways are maintained under normal or altered cellular control mechanisms and under the potential influences of other cell types. The perfused lung also offers certain advantages in toxicokinetic studies designed to establish concentration-uptake and metabolism-response relationships. Exposure conditions can be readily controlled and a mass balance between products and precursors can be made in the absence of metabolic contributions from other tissues. In the elucidation of the potential mechanisms by which toxic substances cause lung injuries, isolated perfused lung studies can be conducted using relatively high doses that might be lethal *in vivo*. The isolated perfused lung preparation is also useful for assessing alterations in biochemical and physiological functions following exposures *in vivo* to toxic agents, provided that any changes in pathology do not interfere with the ability to maintain a viable preparation *in vitro*. Unfortunately, the many cell types within the lung often prevent identification of the cell type involved in the toxic response. It should also be noted that isolated perfused organs are a deteriorating preparation and their usefulness is therefore restricted to a few hours.

Since several descriptions and comprehensive reviews on the use of the isolated perfused lung preparation have already been published,[1-11] the present review is designed to focus mainly on the methods used to perfuse small animal lungs and to highlight some of the main approaches used to evaluate the preparation. A brief listing of some of the ways that the preparation has been used in toxicological experiments is also presented. Although the perfusion of rat lungs will mainly be described, similar methods and approaches with minor modifications can be used when perfusing lungs from other species.

II. IMPLEMENTATION

A. ANIMALS

Although the rat represents the most commonly used species for lung perfusion studies, guinea pigs are often used for the study of pharmacological responses of both airway and vascular smooth muscles. Rabbit lungs, being relatively rich in the nonciliated Clara cells of the terminal airways that contain cytochrome P450, have been used extensively for the study of lung xenobiotic metabolism. Mice have been shown to be more sensitive than rats to the damaging effects of oxidants and are available with specific genetic deficiencies. The age of the animals is also a major consideration in certain types of study.

The acquisition and maintenance of animals free of intercurrent infections is essential in lung studies. A procurement and management program should be employed that routinely monitors for Sendai and rodent corona viruses and for mycoplasmal infections.[12] It is recommended that bronchoalveolar lavage fluid for cell content and blood samples for serological testing be taken from at least two animals from each batch before they enter the facilities. Additional animals should be included in long-term experiments for similar analyses 2 to 3 weeks following the end of each experiment. Animals are best kept isolated from other batches of animals in high-efficiency particulate-filtered air to prevent cross-infection. Since most animal bedding either creates dusts that affect baseline phagocyte numbers and activities or stimulate microsomal enzyme activities, it is recommended that animals be housed in suspended wire caging.

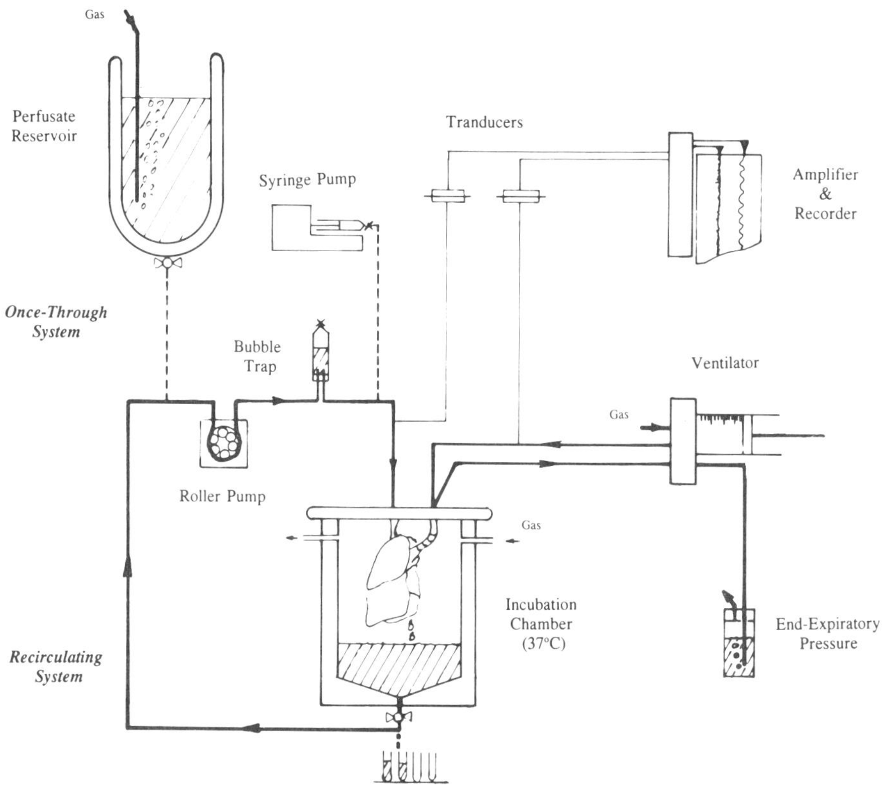

FIGURE 1. Example of a system suitable for perfusing isolated lungs without cannulation of the right atrium, using either recirculation (solid line) or once-through (dashed line) passage of the perfusate.

B. ISOLATION OF THE LUNGS

The species and experimental protocol influence the choice of anesthetic. The most commonly used anesthetic for rats is pentobarbital administered by intraperitoneal injection (50 to 60 mg/kg body wt). In studies to investigate drug metabolism, it might be best not to use an anesthetic that binds too tightly to the microsomal cytochrome P450. Inhalation anesthetics such as halothane (3%) and carbon dioxide (80%) have been used. Following the establishment of an anesthetized state, a cannula (15-gauge blunt needle is suitable for an adult rat) is tied into the trachea. To prevent later collapse of the lungs, the tracheal cannula is connected to a positive pressure respirator through the lid of the incubation chamber (Figure 1). An end-expiratory pressure of 2 to 3 cm H_2O is applied to prevent collapse of the lung, which is controlled by placing the gas outflow line from the respirator under water. Rats are ventilated throughout the isolation procedure at about 60 breaths per min with a tidal volume of 2 ml (approximately 1 ml/100 g body wt).

The lungs are then cleared of blood while remaining within the intact thorax by perfusion with warm isotonic saline via a cannula placed in the portal vein or the inferior vena cava. Blood is released from the circulation by cutting a large abdominal artery. After 1 to 2 min, the thorax is opened by a midline incision and the rib cage carefully fractured close to the posterior lateral thoracic line, ensuring maximal opening of the thorax with as little contact with the lung as possible. A perfusate-filled cannula (18-gauge) is placed into the pulmonary artery following transection of the heart and held in position by a suture placed around both the aorta and pulmonary artery. The left atrium is cut or cannulated to permit free efflux of perfusate. The lungs are then perfused at a relatively low rate of about 5 ml/min to clear any residual blood elements from the vasculature, while being carefully removed from the thoracic cavity, trimmed of nonpulmonary tissue, and then placed within the heated perfusion apparatus (Figure 1). Following the surgical isolation procedure the lungs might have to be hyperinflated in order to remove focal areas of atelectasis. The tidal volume is increased two- to threefold by blocking the expiratory line of the respirator. It is recommended that at any time when hyperinflation is conducted that perfusion be halted in order to prevent the associated increase in vascular resistance that can potentially lead to focal areas of edema formation. The whole procedure from the start of surgery until the lung is positioned in the perfusion apparatus usually takes about 10 min and involves minimal interruption of perfusion and ventilation.

Numerous modifications of this protocol have been used. For example, some investigators have removed the lungs without maintaining continuous ventilation and perfusion.[8] Following cannulation of both trachea and pulmonary artery, lungs are isolated and then carefully inflated while wetted with saline until the surface is smooth. The lung is then deflated and reinflated four to five times until the lung is uniformly inflated and free of any areas of atelectasis. The procedure is conducted prior to the initiation of perfusion. Clearance of blood elements from the vasculature of the lungs is facilitated by intravenous pretreatment with heparin following cannulation of the trachea.[8] However, it should be noted that investigators using continuous ventilation with either abdominal perfusion or direct cannulation of the pulmonary artery have found that no additional improvement in the washout of blood can be achieved by the use of anticoagulants.[1] During the isolation procedure, care should be taken in handling the lung to prevent laceration by the fractured ribs and formation of areas of local increased airway or vasculature pressures. Special care should also be taken to avoid the introduction of air bubbles into the vasculature by ensuring that all cannulae, tubing, and stopcocks are filled with liquid before being introduced into the system.

C. APPARATUS FOR PERFUSING LUNGS

Many different designs of lung perfusion equipment have been described, which in many cases are dependent on the types of experiments to be performed.[1-11] For example, in studies of the uptake and disposition of a circulating drug or xenobiotic, investigators have often utilized a once-through perfusion apparatus that permits measurement of arterial-venous differences in perfusate concentration. Since lung tissue has a high blood flow-rate relative to its mass, many uptake and metabolism studies have employed a recirculating system in order to determine the rate of disappearance of precursors and the subsequent appearance of products in the perfusate. Some of the early lung perfusion experiments used periodic reduction of the air pressure surrounding the lung tissue for ventilation.[4,10] Although this procedure may well provide more even and efficient ventilation of large animal lungs, investigators have more commonly used positive pressure ventilation for perfusion experiments with mice, rats, and guinea pigs.

The apparatus illustrated in Figure 1 represents a relatively simple system for perfusing small animal lungs, which can serve as a base for development of more complicated systems as dictated by the needs of specific investigations. The perfusion apparatus consists of a temperature controlled, water-jacketed (37°C) incubation chamber in which the lungs are suspended by the pulmonary arterial cannula. The lungs are ventilated via the tracheal cannula connected through the lid of the chamber to the inspiratory and expiratory lines of a small animal respirator. The lungs are prevented from collapsing by the application of a 2- to 3-cm H_2O end-expiratory pressure. Some respirators allow adjustment of both inspiratory and expiratory pressures and respiratory rate (Mallard Medical, Irvine, CA), while other positive pressure ventilators force an adjustable fixed volume of gas into the lungs regardless of the required pressure profile (e.g., Model 683, Harvard Apparatus, S. Natick, MA).

Although some investigators have perfused lungs at a constant pressure by pumping perfusate from a reservoir held at a constant level above the lung,[4,5,10] uptake studies require even perfusion of the vasculature that can be best achieved using a constant flow method of perfusion using a peristaltic (e.g., Model 1210, Harvard Apparatus) or a roller pump (e.g., Minipuls 2, Gilson Medical Electronics, Middleton, WI). A simple bubble trap made from an inverted syringe is placed between the perfusate pump and the pulmonary arterial cannula to prevent air emboli from entering the lung circulation and causing edema fluid accumulation. Perfusate is normally allowed to flow freely from the cut pulmonary vein into the incubation chamber from which it is recirculated to the lung by the perfusion pump (Figure 1). A filter (0.45-μm pore size) can be added to the perfusate circuit to remove denatured albumin, fibrin clots, bacteria, and other small particulates. Perfusion and ventilation pressures are monitored using standard equipment based on liquid and air-filled pressure transducers, respectively, amplifiers, and a writing oscillograph (e.g., Grass Instruments, Quincy, MA).

Equipment for once-through perfusion is also illustrated in Figure 1 and includes the use of a temperature controlled reservoir from which perfusate is pumped to the lung pulmonary artery. The compound to be investigated can either be added to the reservoir or administered into the perfusate flow by use of a syringe pump (Figure 1). In this system the incubation chamber is not used as a perfusate reservoir, and effluent samples are collected directly from either the cut pulmonary vein or from a cannula placed in the left atrium. Methods for determining the uptake of agents, based on the bolus addition of the agent of interest with suitable vascular markers, are best done with a cannula placed in the pulmonary vein. It is recommended that such a cannula leave the chamber via a port that is lower than the lung so as to avoid increases in outflow pressure that can potentially result in hydrostatic edema.

Although the perfusion system illustrated in Figure 1 is dependent on the lung for oxygenation of the perfusate, an aeration system can be introduced by recirculating the perfusate over a surface while being exposed to the gas.[1] Alternatively a simple membrane-type oxygenator can be used that involves passing the perfusate through coils of silicone-tubing surrounded by the equilibrating gas in a chamber heated by a water jacket. If a bicarbonate-based buffer system is employed for perfusion, the aeration gas mixture should include 5% CO_2 to maintain perfusate pH. A heating coil can also be introduced in the perfusate line prior to the pulmonary arterial cannula to ensure that the temperature of the perfusate is maintained. Since other modifications in design can be made depending on the application, it is recommended that readers refer to more detailed reviews and papers describing specific applications.[1-11]

The incubation and perfusate reservoirs can easily be constructed using Plexiglas, which permits the easy installation of seals and tube fittings; however, it is not as good as glass for maintaining the temperature of the lung and the perfusate. If glass is used with blood-containing perfusion media, it should be siliconized (Sigmacote, Sigma Chemical Co., St. Louis, MO) to retard clotting and the prevent cell adhesion to the glass. It should be noted that many xenobiotic agents are adsorbed by certain types of tubing, and that in some cases plasticizers leach from the tubing and might affect experimental results. Tubing should be nontoxic (i.e., medical grade). Polyethylene or polypropylene represent the best formulations, although flexible tubing such as vinyl or Tygon is required for the perfusion pump. Except for use in oxygenation, silicone tubing is not recommended, since it is permeable to gases and readily adsorbs proteins. The tubing and the perfusate vessels should be extensively cleaned using dilute detergents or NaOH in combination with a sonicator if available.

D. PERFUSION

Although whole blood has been used to perfuse lungs, it is difficult to obtain and store, has a complex and variable composition, and requires the addition of anticoagulant to prevent clotting. The use of artificial media for lung perfusions is more common. Krebs-Ringer bicarbonate buffer solutions represent a simple solution on which to base more complex media and contains 119 m*M* NaCl, 25 m*M* $NaHCO_3$, 5.9 m*M* KCl, 1.3 m*M* CaCl, 1.8 m*M* Na_2HPO_4, and 1.2 m*M* $MgSO_4$. The osmolality is at the physiological range of about 300 mosm/l and the pH is readily maintained in the range of 7.35 to 7.45 by ventilation of the lung with 5% CO_2 following final adjustment with either dilute HCl or NaOH (0.1 *M*). The buffering capacity can be enhanced if necessary by the addition of such organic buffers as HEPES (*N*-2-hydroxyethylpiperazine-*N'*-2-ethanesulfonic acid, 10 to 20 m*M*).

Prolonged perfusions beyond 20 to 30 min have been found to require the addition of a plasma expander to increase the osmolality of the medium and consequently prevent edema fluid accumulation.[1,8,13] Although Ficoll, dextran, gelatin, and hydroxyethyl starch have been used,[13] most investigators use 3 to 4% bovine serum albumin that might have the added advantage of binding potentially toxic, low molecular weight substances. It should be noted that bovine serum albumin fraction V is contaminated with fatty acids and other serum components that might interfere with the experiment. It is recommended that partially purified preparations be used that are relatively deficient in fatty acids. Albumin may not necessarily be suitable for all types of study since it might bind both precursor and products under study and so influence toxicokinetic determinations. Its ability to scavenge free radical intermediates might also preclude it from use in certain studies.[14]

Since the addition of glucose to the medium has been shown to delay the onset of edema formation,[1,13] it is recommended that it be routinely added to the perfusate. Glucose has been shown to be used by lung tissue for the maintenance of energy supply and for the synthesis of lipids, proteins, and nucleic acids, as well as being required for the production of reducing equivalents (NADPH) needed for fatty acid synthesis and the maintenance of the antioxidant glutathione in its reduced state.[5,15-17] Saturation of lung glucose utilization has been observed with 10 m*M* D-glucose.[18] Some of the lung's intermediary metabolic functions can be supported by other metabolic substrates that include lactate, pyruvate, and palmitate.[19-21]

Uniform perfusion and normal tissue metabolism with a low incidence of edema formation can be obtained by perfusing lungs at approximately a third to a half the physiological rate which for a 250-g rat is about 12 to 18 ml/min. The mean pulmonary artery pressure due to the vasculature resistance of the lung for this flow is about 11 to 17 cm of H_2O. Decreasing the flow-rate for this size rat to below 5 ml/min can potentially lead to uneven perfusate distribution, and raising it to greater than 20 ml/min increases the incidence of edema fluid accumulation. However, inclusion of washed red blood cells to the perfusate has been shown to increase the viability of the isolated perfused lung preparation in experiments that maintain nearly physiological flow-rates for extended periods of time.[4,8] The inclusion of red blood cells has also been shown to slow the deterioration of the pulmonary vasculature[22] and maintain its responsiveness to vasoactive substances.[23] Smooth muscle responses require calcium in the perfusion medium.[23,24]

E. VENTILATION

Isolated rat lungs are usually ventilated with a frequency of 60 to 100 breaths per min and a 1.5 to 2.5 ml tidal volume, which gives an inspiratory pressure of about 6 to 12 cm H_2O. Collapse of the lungs is prevented by the positive end-expiratory pressure of 2 to 3 cm H_2O (Figure 1). Creating an occasional "sigh" by hyperinflating the lungs to 2 to 3 times tidal volume will prevent formation of focal areas of atelectasis. However, as previously mentioned, it is recommended that this should be done in the absence of perfusate flow in order to prevent increases in vascular resistance. The gas mixture used for ventilation usually contains 5% CO_2 for maintenance of the bicarbonate perfusate pH and is humidified before introduction into the apparatus. It should be noted that the gas mixture used for ventilation is also used to maintain the atmosphere within the incubation chamber and in any aeration systems added to the apparatus (Figure 1). Depending on the needs of the experiment, air normally provides the balance of the gas mixture which, with the 5% CO_2, provides a mixture that closely approximates the physiological alveolar gas tensions. Some investigators have used a 95% O_2 and 5% CO_2 mixture to ensure adequate tissue oxygenation. However compared with other tissues, the low oxygen consumption of lung tissue and its short diffusion distances make the use of high oxygen mixtures for lung perfusions unnecessary. High oxygen exposures can increase the possibility of damage to the preparation from increased production of oxygen radicals and lipid peroxides.

III. EVALUATION OF THE PREPARATION

A. CHARACTERISTICS OF THE PREPARATION

Lungs isolated from healthy animals can be perfused for up to 4 to 5 h without rapid accumulation of edema fluid in the alveolar spaces that marks the failure of the preparation. Most rat perfusion experiments are conducted for about 2 h, during which time the preparation has been shown to be stable as indicated by constant ventilation and perfusion pressures and linear metabolic rates. Adenine nucleotide levels are maintained at a relatively high energy state when compared with other perfused organs, giving for rat lung preparations perfused with glucose an ATP/ADP ratio of between 6 and 8 and an energy charge as defined as (ATP + 1/2 ADP)/(ATP + ADP + AMP) of 0.92.[1,15,17] The preparation has also been shown to be under normal metabolic control mechanisms, demonstrated by increased glucose catabolism to lactate on inhibition of mitochondrial metabolism by ventilation with 95% O_2 and 5% CO_2.[15] Mitochondrial carbon dioxide production is enhanced in response to decreased ATP levels brought about by perfusion with the uncoupler of oxidative phosphorylation, 2,4-dinitrophenol.[16] Perfused lung tissue has an active glucose-pentose cycle activity, responsible for the generation of NADPH-reducing equivalents used for maintaining glutathione in its reduced state (GSH) and for the synthesis of fatty acids.[16]

Examination of the preparation by both light and electron microscopy after 15 and 60 min of perfusion has demonstrated normal histology of the alveolar septa with no swelling of the interstitial spaces or alterations in the structure of intracellular organelles.[15,24,25] However, within the first 15 min of perfusion, fluid accumulation has been observed within the perivascular and peribronchial spaces, most likely reflecting the slower rate of drainage associated with these spaces in isolated preparations when compared with the situation *in vivo*.[24-26]

B. INDICATORS OF INJURY

Following exposure of the lung preparation to a potential pneumotoxicant *in vitro,* it may undergo a variety of different responses in altered biochemistry and physiology that will depend on the affected site and mechanism of the toxic action. Measurements of inflow pressure in constant-flow perfusion systems have been used to evaluate the responsiveness of the vascular smooth muscle under different exposure conditions and in the presence of various agonists.[23] Increases in pressure have also been used to indicate changes in vascular resistance resulting from interstitial fluid accumulation associated with alterations in microvascular permeability.[1,15,17] In contrast, changes in peak ventilation pressure during constant volume ventilation, although very useful for measuring bronchoconstriction, are relatively insensitive as an indicator of early airway edema fluid accumulation. Substantial edema fluid accumulation can be detected by increases in lung weight during perfusion or by increases in wet/dry weight ratios measured at the end of the experiment.[24] A decrease in reservoir weight has also been used to assess fluid accumulation in lung preparations. Smaller changes in vascular permeability have been more effectively studied by measurements of the transudation of radiolabeled macromolecules such as albumin or polyethylene glycol from the vasculature into the lung tissue, as well as from the alveolar spaces into the perfusate.[27,28]

The determination of intermediary metabolic rates and steady-state adenine nucleotide levels might represent one of the most sensitive measures of early lung damage, since failure in energy metabolism often precedes the cell damage that subsequently brings about edema fluid accumulation.[1,15,17] Unfortunately it is not practical to use measurements of oxygen utilization to indicate changes in metabolic rates in lung tissue as in other perfused organ systems. However rates of glucose catabolism to carbon dioxide, lactate, and pyruvate can be readily determined during perfusion by use of radiolabeled glucose and standard enzymatic analyses.[5,15-18,29] Failure of the mitochondria to oxidize cytosolic-reducing equivalents is indicated by an increase in the ratio of perfusate lactate to pyruvate ratio, which for perfused rat lungs ventilated with air is in the range of 6 to 10.[15] Since glucose catabolism to carbon dioxide takes place in both mitochondrial and pentose cycle pathways, changes in mitochondrial metabolism can be determined separately by measurements of $^{14}CO_2$ production during perfusion with carbon-14 labeled lactate,[30] pyruvate,[20] and palmitate.[21] The contribution to total carbon dioxide production from glucose by the pentose cycle can be determined by separate perfusions with [U-^{14}C], [1-^{14}C], and [6-^{14}C] D-glucose and then used for estimating the lung turnover of NADPH.[16,17,29]

Following perfusion, bronchoalveolar lavage with isotonic saline can be used to detect the appearance of perfusate macromolecules for indicating permeability changes[31] and for assessing possible changes in the composition and surface properties of the lavaged surfactant. The functional activities of the alveolar inflammatory cells recovered by lavage can also be assessed and include phagocytic activity and ability to generate reactive oxygen intermediates on stimulation with either opsonized zymosan or a phorbol ester.[32] These evaluations might be particularly useful in the study of the early effects of oxidant gas inhalation on a perfused lung preparation where infiltration of inflammatory cells into the lung can be carefully controlled. Measurements of lavage fluid lactate dehydrogenase isoenzyme activities (LDH) might also be useful for detecting damage to specific lung cell types.[31,33] It should be noted that many of the measurements, based on the use of both cellular and noncellular fractions from bronchoalveolar lavage, are more commonly used to evaluate exposures to toxic substances *in vivo,* since they do not necessarily change rapidly enough for detection in the relatively short time used for lung perfusion experiments.

Although the above methods provide useful information into the possible mechanisms by which inhalation and systemic exposures to toxic substances might result in lung injuries, the diversity of cell types within the lung in many cases makes it impossible to identify the specific cellular sites and mechanisms involved. However, the lung conducts a variety of metabolic functions that can often be attributed to specific cell types. For example, the alveolar type II epithelial cells synthesize disaturated phosphatidylcholine and apoproteins as part of their role in the production of the surfactant lining of the alveoli. Interstitial cells, such as fibroblasts, represent a major site of connective tissue protein biosynthesis. It is therefore possible to use measurements of these biosynthetic activities as markers of toxicity to specific cell populations within the lung tissue.

The lung also has some useful metabolic capabilities that have been successfully utilized as markers of early lung capillary damage. An example is the uptake and metabolism of circulating serotonin (5HT) and norepinephrine. These agents are actively taken up by lung endothelial cells by a carrier-mediated process.[19,24,34-36] Following uptake, these biogenic amines are metabolized by monoamine oxidase to more polar products that are less biologically active. The initial removal of these agents from the circulation has been used to indicate changes in endothelial cell function following exposures to toxic substances.[35-39] However, it should be noted that lung clearance of these amines is dependent on specific cell membrane carriers and the endothelial surface area being perfused. The use of amine uptake measurements as a sensitive marker of lung injury in certain types of studies might be limited, since the efficiency of carrier binding to the amines can be influenced by small molecular weight substances and since changes in perfusate distribution can affect the area of endothelium exposed. Enzyme activities associated with the luminal surface of the capillary endothelium and assessed by measurements of perfusate substrate and product levels provide additional methods for evaluating endothelial function following toxic exposures. Such enzymes include angiotensin-converting enzyme (ACE), 5′-nucleosidase,[38,39] and lipoprotein lipase.[40] These activities are also limited by uneven perfusate distribution in the lung vasculature that can in part be accounted for by concomitant measurements of vascular spaces.[37] It should also be noted that these enzyme activities might be released into the perfusate under conditions of endothelial injury. The lung also produces and releases various prostaglandins in response to injury. For example prostacyclin (PGI_2) and thromboxane A_2 are produced in large quantities following endothelial damage and are detected in the perfusate as their respective stable metabolites, 6-keto prostaglandin $F_{1\alpha}$ and thromboxane B_2.[41] Measurements of lung prostanoid release is complicated in a recirculating perfusion system by reuptake by the lung for further metabolism. The ability of the lung to remove certain exogenously added prostanoids from the circulation for metabolism might provide an additional measure of metabolic function as a marker of toxicity.

The activities of lung cytochrome P450 monooxygenases and other xenobiotic metabolizing enzymes have been extensively studied using isolated perfused lung preparations and discussed in detail elsewhere.[1,3,8] Although rabbit and rat lungs differ in their capabilities for xenobiotic metabolism, hydroxylation and demethylation reactions have been identified in both species. The nonciliated bronchiolar Clara cells and the alveolar type II epithelial cells have been identified as major sites of cytochrome P450-linked metabolism, yet other unidentified sites in the lung might contribute to the total metabolism measured using perfused lung preparations. It is interesting that isolated Clara cells and alveolar type II cells demonstrate some differences in their abilities to metabolize certain substrates, which has been attributed to different distribution of cytochrome P450 isoenzymes.[42] Measurement of O-demethylation of *p*-nitroanisole to its product *p*-nitrophenol is an especially useful technique for directly evaluating xenobiotic metabolism in the perfused lung, since the product is colored and can therefore be detected directly in the perfusate using a flow-cell in a spectrophotometer.[43]

The intermediary metabolic functions of the lung involved in energy production, antioxidant processes, and the more cell-specific detoxification and synthetic activities, can also be readily assessed in lungs taken from animals exposed *in vivo* to toxic substances. However, since many toxic responses result in changes in cell population associated with inflammatory and repair responses, interpretation of the results cannot be conducted without concomitant histopathological evaluations. Preparation of lung tissue for both light and electron microscopic examinations requires either intratracheal or intravascular fixation normally conducted with buffered formaldehyde and glutaraldehyde mixtures. For morphometric studies, the degree of lung inflation needs to be carefully controlled and is usually maintained using an inflation pressure of 20 to 25 cm of H_2O. The disadvantage of intratracheal fixation is that the position of inflammatory cells and edema fluid might be altered. Perfusion fixation at a constant lung volume might therefore represent a more suitable approach. Since many lesions in the lung tend to be focal in their distribution, sampling techniques for morphometric studies need to be carefully chosen.[44-46]

IV. APPLICATIONS

Although the various applications of isolated perfused lung preparations to toxicological studies have been more completely reviewed elsewhere,[1,3,7,8] a few examples are listed below. One of the major uses of the isolated perfused lung preparation has been in investigations into the metabolism of various xenobiotic agents. The lung metabolizes a wide range of substances that include methadone, pentobarbital, aldrin, and benzo[a]pyrene. The lung can be exposed via the circulation or by intratracheal administration. It should be noted that some activities present in isolated lung microsomal preparations are sometimes not exhibited by perfused lung preparations, suggesting the presence of permeability barriers. Many xenobiotic agents are lipophilic and are therefore rapidly removed from the pulmonary circulation. Recognizing the fact that the lung takes the whole cardiac output, Wiersma and Roth have demonstrated that lung tissue can be important in the clearance of agents such as benzo[a]pyrene from the blood, even though the liver has a far greater enzyme content.[47,48] Isolated perfused lungs from mice, rats, and rabbits have been used to identify the many pulmonary metabolites of benzo[a]pyrene that are retained within the tissue or released into the perfusate.[9,49] These metabolites include quinones, phenols, dihydrodiols, triols, and tetrols as well as glutathione and glucuronide conjugates. Changes in the pattern of rat lung metabolism of benzo[a]pyrene have also been determined in lungs with altered pathology brought about by exposures *in vivo* to ozone.[49] The initial metabolism of some xenobiotics might be best observed using a single-pass perfusion system, since recirculation of the perfusate and reuptake of the metabolites for further metabolism can complicate interpretation of the data.

A second major use of the isolated perfused lung preparation has been the study of the mechanisms by which specific agents damage the lung. These studies have involved exposures *in vitro* by direct inhalation of such substances as cigarette smoke,[50-52] NO_2,[53] and hyperbaric O_2,[17] and by addition to the circulating perfusate of such compounds as paraquat,[29,54] nitrofurantoin,[54] α-naphthyl-thiourea,[55] and phorbol myristate acetate.[56] For example, in the case of rat and rabbit lung perfusions with the electron acceptors, paraquat and nitrofurantoin, investigators have examined alterations in lung NADPH production and the resulting effects on maintenance of glutathione metabolism.[29,54] A selective paraquat-induced increase in rat lung PGF_2 production has been linked to vasoconstriction and edema formation.[57] Some agents such as the alkaloid monocrotoline require prior hepatic metabolism to a toxic intermediate before they can cause lung damage. In order to demonstrate such a requirement, perfusate collected from livers exposed to monocrotoline were perfused through isolated rat lungs that then exhibited diminished 5HT uptake, consistent with early damage of the endothelium.[58] There has been considerable interest in studying the role of inflammatory cells in lung injury, and lung perfusion studies have been conducted with polymorphonuclear leukocytes in the circulation.[27,41,56,59] This preparation eliminates complication imposed by other blood elements and organs activities that are inherent in studies *in vivo*. For example, Carpenter-Deyo and Roth, in their studies of phorbol myristate acetate damage of the perfused lung, have been able to demonstrate that thromboxane A_2 production is produced from both circulating polymorphonuclear leukocytes and the lung, and that thromboxane A_2 production from both these sources is required for the manifestation of edema.[59]

The isolated perfused lung preparation has also been used to evaluate *in vitro* the effects of exposures *in vivo* to 100% oxygen,[20,37,60] and to pneumotoxic doses of monocrotoline and paraquat,[61] all of which result in impaired uptake of 5HT. Metabolic studies have demonstrated impairment in mitochondrial function within 3 to 6 h of exposure to 100% oxygen that occur prior to any changes in lung histopathology.[20,60] After 3 days of ozone exposure, changes in glucose catabolism and lipid biosynthesis have been observed that are consistent with the increased energy and synthetic needs of a lung undergoing proliferating repair of a damaged epithelium.[62]

In summary, the lung is involved in a wide a range of respiratory and nonrespiratory functions that include the synthesis of the surfactant and mucous-containing airway lining fluids, immune defense mechanisms, and the removal, activation, and detoxification of circulating and inhaled xenobiotic agents. Many of these functions are altered directly or indirectly by exposure to toxic substances and so can be used as markers of injury as well as provide an approach to explore the mechanisms of toxicity. However, because of the cellular complexity of the lung when compared with other tissues, interpretation of the results requires close attention to the physiological condition of the preparation and to any changes in cell population brought about by toxic exposures *in vivo*. Changes in vascular perfusate distribution caused by either vasoconstriction or damage to capillary endothelium can alter the delivery of agents to specific cellular sites within the lung, and the infiltration of inflammatory cells and changes in cell turnover can affect the metabolism and responses to toxic exposures. The isolated perfused lung preparation provides many advantages, but has many limitations and therefore is most effectively used in combination with other *in vitro* and *in vivo* methods.

ACKNOWLEDGMENTS

The authors would like to thank Christine Tucker for her help in preparing the manuscript. David Bassett is currently supported by National Institutes of Health grants HL-34674 and ES-05255. Robert Roth is currently supported by grant ES-02581.

REFERENCES

1. **Fisher, A. B.,** The isolated perfused lung, in *Toxicology of Inhaled Materials*, Witschi, H. P. and Brain, J. D., Eds., *Handbook of Experimental Pharmacology*, Vol. 75, Springer-Verlag, New York, 1985, 149.
2. **Gillis, C. N. and Iwasawa, Y.,** Technique for measurement of norepinephrine and 5-hydroxytryptamine uptake by rabbit lung, *J. Appl. Physiol.*, 33, 404, 1972.
3. **Mehendale, H. M., Angevine, L. S., and Ohmiya, Y.,** The isolated perfused lung — a critical evaluation, *Toxicology*, 21, 1, 1981.
4. **Niemeier, R. W. and Bingham, E.,** An isolated perfused lung preparation for metabolic studies, *Life Sci.*, 11, 807, 1972.
5. **O'Neil, J. J. and Tierney, D. F.,** Rat lung metabolism: glucose utilization by isolated perfused lung and tissue slices, *Am. J. Physiol.*, 226, 867, 1974.
6. **Rhoades, R. A.,** Isolated perfused lung preparation for studying altered gaseous environments, *Environ. Health Perspec.*, 56, 43, 1984.
7. **Roth, J. A.,** Use of the isolated perfused lung in biochemical toxicology, in *Reviews in Biochemical Toxicology*, Vol. 1, Hodgson, E., Bend, J. R., and Philpot, P., Eds., Elsevier/North-Holland, New York, 1979, 287.
8. **Roth, R. A. and Bassett, D. J. P.,** Isolated perfused lung techniques, in *In Vitro Models of Toxicology*, Sipes, G. and McQueen, C. A., Eds., Telford, 1990, 3.
9. **Skelly, M. F. and Shertzer, H. G.,** Benzo(*a*)pyrene metabolism in the isolated perfused mouse lung, *Exper. Lung Res.*, 5, 259, 1983.
10. **Smith, B. R. and Bend, J. R.,** Lung perfusion techniques for xenobiotic metabolism and toxicity studies, *Methods Enzymol.*, 77, 105, 1981.

11. **Tucker, L. D. and Shertzer, H. G.,** Split lung perfusion: a new method to test the effects of chemical agents on pulmonary metabolism, *Toxicol. Appl. Pharmacol.*, 55, 353, 1980.
12. **Hamm, T. E., Jr., Raynor, T. H., and Sherrill, J. M.,** Procurement and management of rodents to minimize disease problems: the CIIT animal management program, in *Complications of Viral and Mycoplasmal Infections in Rodents to Toxicology Research and Testing,* Hamm, T. E., Jr., Ed., Hemisphere, Washington, D. C., 1986, Chapt. 9.
13. **Fisher, A. B., Dodia, C., and Linask, J.,** Perfusate composition and edema formation in isolated rat lungs, *Exper. Lung Res.*, 1, 13, 1980.
14. **Holt, M. E., Ryall, M. E. T., and Campbell, A. K.,** Albumin inhibits human-polymorphonuclear leukocyte luminol-dependent chemiluminescence: evidence for oxygen radical scavenging, *Br. J. Exper. Pathol.*, 65, 231, 1984.
15. **Bassett, D. J. P. and Fisher, A. B.,** Metabolic responses to carbon monoxide by isolated rat lungs, *Am. J. Physiol.*, 230, 658, 1976.
16. **Bassett, D. J. P. and Fisher, A. B.,** Pentose cycle activity of the isolated perfused rat lung, *Am. J. Physiol.*, 231, 1527, 1976.
17. **Bassett, D. J. P and Fisher, A. B.,** Glucose metabolism in rat lung during exposure to hyperbaric oxygen, *J. Appl. Physiol.*, 45, 943, 1979.
18. **Kerr, J. S., Baker, N. J., Bassett, D. J. P., and Fisher, A. B.,** Effect of perfusate glucose concentration on rat lung glycolysis, *Am. J. Physiol.*, 236, E229, 1979.
19. **Fisher, A. B., Steinberg, H., and Dodia, C.,** Reversal of 2-deoxyglucose inhibition of serotonin uptake in isolated guinea pig lung, *J. Appl. Physiol.*, 46, 447, 1979.
20. **Bassett, D. J. P. and Bowen-Kelly, E.,** Pyruvate metabolism of perfused rat lungs after exposure to 100% oxygen, *J. Appl. Physiol.*, 60, 1605, 1986.
21. **Bassett, D. J. P., Hamosh, M., Hamosh, P., and Rabinowitz, J. L.,** Pathway of palmitate metabolism in the isolated rat lung, *Exper. Lung. Res.*, 2, 37, 1981.
22. **Nicolaysen, G.,** Perfusate qualities and spontaneous edema-formation in an isolated perfused lung preparation, *Acta Physiol. Scand.*, 83, 563, 1971.
23. **McMurtry, I. F., Hookway, B. W., and Roos, S. D.,** Red blood cells but not platelets prolong vascular reactivity of isolated rat lungs, *Am. J. Physiol.*, 234, H186, 1978.
24. **Steinberg, H., Bassett, D. J. P., and Fisher, A. B.,** Depression of pulmonary 5-hydroxytryptamine uptake by metabolic inhibitors, *Am. J. Physiol.*, 228, 1298, 1975.
25. **Fisher, A. B. and Pietra, G. G.,** Comparison of serotonin uptake from the alveolar and capillary spaces of isolated rat lung, *Am. Rev. Respir. Dis.*, 123, 74, 1981.
26. **Staub, N. C.,** Pulmonary edema, *Physiol. Rev.*, 54, 678, 1974.
27. **Morganroth, M. L., Till, G. O., Kunkel, R. G., and Ward, P. A.,** Complement and neutrophil-mediated injury of perfused rat lungs, *Lab. Invest.*, 54, 507, 1986.
28. **Lindahl, M., Hede, A. R., and Tagesson, C.,** Lysophosphatidylcholine increases airway and capillary permeability in the isolated rat lung, *Exper. Lung. Res.*, 11, 1, 1986.
29. **Bassett, D. J. P. and Fisher, A. B.,** Alterations of glucose metabolism during perfusion of rat lung with paraquat, *Am. J. Physiol.*, 234, E653, 1978.
30. **Rhoades, R. A., Shaw, M. E., Eskew, M. L., and Wali, S.,** Lactate metabolism in perfused rat lung, *Am. J. Physiol..*, 235, E619, 1978.
31. **Henderson, R. F., Benson, J. M., Hahn, F. F., Hobbs, C. H., Jones, R. K., Mauderly, J. L., McClellan, R. O., and Pickrell, J. A.,** New approaches for the evaluation of pulmonary toxicity: bronchoalveolar lavage fluid analysis, *Fund. Appl. Toxicol.*, 5, 451, 1985.
32. **Esterline, R. L., Bassett, D. J. P., and Trush, M. A.,** Characterization of the oxidant generation by inflammatory cells lavaged from rat lungs following acute exposure to ozone, *Toxicol. Appl. Pharmacol.*, 99, 229, 1989.
33. **Roth, R. A.,** Effect of pneumotoxicants on lactate dehydrogenase activity in bronchopulmonary lavage fluid, *Toxicol. Appl. Pharmacol.*, 57, 69, 1981.
34. **Junod, A. F.,** Uptake, metabolism and efflux of [^{14}C]-5-hydroxytryptamine in isolated perfused rat lungs, *J. Pharmacol. Exper. Therap.*, 183, 341, 1973.
35. **Roth, R. A.,** Biochemistry, physiology and drug metabolism — Implications regarding the role of the lungs in drug disposition, *Clin. Physiol. Biochem.*, 3, 66, 1985.
36. **Roth, R. A. and Wiersma, D. A.,** Role of lung in total body clearance of circulating drugs, in *Handbook of Clinical Pharmacokinetics*, Gibaldi, M. and Prescott, L., Eds., ADIS Health Science Press, New York, 1983, 169.
37. **Block, E. R. and Fisher, A. B.,** Depression of serotonin clearance by rat lungs during oxygen exposure, *J. Appl. Physiol.*, 42, 33, 1977.

38. **Roth, R. A., Wallace, K. B., Alper, R. H., and Bailie, M. D.,** Effect of paraquat treatment of rats on disposition of 5-hydroxytryptamine and angiotensin I by perfused lung, *Biochem. Pharmacol.*, 28, 2349, 1979.
39. **Molteni, A., Ward, W. F., Ts'ao, C. H., Port, C. D., and Solliday, N.,** Monocrotaline-induced pulmonary endothelial dysfunction in rats, *Proc. Soc. Exper. Biol. Med.*, 176, 88, 1984.
40. **Gal, S., Bassett, D. J. P., Hamosh, M., and Hamosh, P.,** Triacylglycerol hydrolysis in the isolated perfused rat lung, *Biochem. Biophys. Acta*, 713, 222, 1982.
41. **Carpenter, L. J. and Roth, R. A.,** Involvement of thromboxane in injury to isolated rat lungs perfused with phorbol myristate acetate in the presence and absence of neutrophils, *Toxicol. Appl. Pharmacol.*, 91, 33, 1987.
42. **Devereaux, T. R.,** Alveolar Type II and Clara cells: isolation and xenobiotic metabolism, *Environ. Health Perspec.*, 56, 95, 1984.
43. **Itakura, N., Fisher, A. B., and Thurman, R. G.,** Cytochrome P-450 linked p-nitroanisole o-demethylation in the perfused lung, *J. Appl. Physiol.*, 43, 238, 1977.
44. **Tyler, W. S., Dungworth, D. L., Plopper, C. G., Hyde, D. M., and Tyler, N. K.,** Structural evaluation of the respiratory system, *Fund. Appl. Toxicol.*, 5, 405, 1985.
45. **Dungworth, D. L., Schwartz, L. W., Tyler, W. S., and Phalen, R. F.,** Morphological methods for evaluation of pulmonary toxicity in animals, *Annu. Rev. Pharmacol. Toxicol.*, 16, 381, 1976.
46. **Weibel, E. R.,** Principles and methods for the morphometric study of the lung and other organs, *Lab. Invest.*, 12, 131, 1963.
47. **Wiersma, D. A. and Roth, R. A.,** Clearance of benzo(a)pyrene by isolated rat liver and lung: alterations in perfusion and metabolic capacity, *J. Pharmacol. Exper. Ther.*, 225, 121, 1983.
48. **Wiersma, D. A. and Roth, R. A.,** The prediction of benzo(a)pyrene clearance by rat liver and lung from enzyme kinetic data, *Molec. Pharmacol.*, 24, 300, 1983.
49. **Bassett, D. J. P., Seed, J., and Bowen-Kelly, E.,** Rat lung benzo(a)pyrene metabolism following three days continuous exposure to 0.6 ppm ozone, *Res. Commun. Pathol. Pharmacol.*, 60, 291, 1988.
50. **Lubawy, W. C. and Isaac, R. S.,** Influence of pretreatment with tobacco smoke condensate or 3-methylcholanthrene on [^{14}C]benzo(a)pyrene metabolism in the isolated perfused rabbit lung, *Toxicol. Lett.*, 7, 153, 1980.
51. **Mannisto, J., Toivonen, H., Hartiala, J., Bakhle, Y. S., and Uotila, P.,** The effect of cigarette smoke on the metabolism of arachidonic acid in isolated hamster lungs, *Prostaglandins*, 22, 195, 1981.
52. **Uotila, P.,** Effect of cigarette smoke on glucuronide conjugation in hamster isolated lungs, *Res. Commun. Chem. Pathol. Pharmacol.*, 38, 173, 1982.
53. **Postlewaite, E. M. and Mustafa, M. G.,** Formation of N-nitrosomorpholine in isolated rat lungs during nitrogen dioxide ventilation, *Carcinogenesis*, 4, 777, 1983.
54. **Dunbar, J. R., DeLucia, A. J., and Bryant, L. R.,** Glutathione status of isolated rabbit lungs. Effects of nitrofurantoin and paraquat perfusion with normoxic and hyperoxic ventilation, *Biochem. Pharmacol.*, 33, 1343, 1984.
55. **Pankhania, J. J. and Bakhle, Y. S.,** Effect of pulmonary oedema induced by alpha-naphthylthiourea on synthesis of cyclo-oxygenase products in rat isolated lungs, *Prostaglandins*, 30, 37, 1985.
56. **Carpenter, L. J., Johnson, K. J., Kunkel, R. G., and Roth, R. A.,** Phorbol myristate acetate produces injury to isolated rat lungs in the presence and absence of perfused neutrophils, *Toxicol. Appl. Pharmacol.*, 91, 22, 1987.
57. **Lindenschmidt, R. C., Patterson, C. E., Forney, R. B., and Rhoades, R. A.,** Selective action of prostaglandin F_2 alpha during paraquat-induced pulmonary edema in the perfused lung, *Toxicol. Appl. Pharmacol.*, 70, 105, 1983.
58. **Lafranconi, W. M. and Huxtable, R. M.,** Hepatic metabolism and pulmonary toxicity of monocrotaline using isolated perfused liver and lung, *Biochem. Pharmacol.*, 33, 2479, 1984.
59. **Carpenter-Deyo, L. and Roth, R. A.,** Cyclooxygenase inhibition in lungs or in neutrophils attenuates neutrophil-dependent edema in rat lungs perfused with phorbol myristate acetate, *J. Pharmacol. Exper. Therap.*, 251, 983, 1989.
60. **Bassett, D. J. P., Bowen-Kelly, E., and Reichenbaugh, S. S.,** Rat lung glucose metabolism after 24 h of exposure to 100% oxygen. *J. Appl. Physiol.*, 66, 989, 1989.
61. **Hilliker, K. S., Bell, T. G., Lorimer, D., and Roth, R. A.,** Pneumotoxicity and thrombocytopenia after a single injection of monocrotaline, *Am. J. Physiol.*, 242, H573, 1982.
62. **Bassett, D. J. P. and Bowen-Kelly, E.,** Rat lung metabolism after 3 days continuous exposure to 0.6 ppm ozone, *Am. J. Physiol.*, 250, E131, 1986.

Chapter 12

THE USE OF MECHANICAL STIMULATION IN *IN VITRO* MODELS

Louis C. Almekinders

TABLE OF CONTENTS

I. INTRODUCTION

The use of cell culture systems has become a cornerstone in toxicology and pharmacology research. While it avoids the use of humans and animals, it also allows a precise control of otherwise virtually uncontrollable variables. Nutrition, temperature, cell density, and especially exposure to xenobiotics can be carefully controlled. In this manner the response to a xenobiotic can be studied at a cellular and subcellular level at a relatively low cost. Once such studies have been completed, however, it remains difficult to extrapolate the results to the *in vivo* situation. Certain variables cannot be simulated in an *in vitro* system and therefore the response *in vivo* may be altered. One profound difference between the *in vitro* and *in vivo* situation is mechanical stimulation. Virtually all living structures undergo constant deformation due to internal and external forces. This motion has been shown to have profound effects on the cellular metabolism and may significantly alter the response of a cell to a chemical stimulus. This chapter will briefly review the effects of mechanical stimulation on cell metabolism and cell injury. This is followed by a description of an *in vitro* system for mechanical stimulation.

II. EFFECTS OF MECHANICAL STIMULATION

All living cells are subjected to mechanical stimulation. This can be caused by external forces such as barometric pressure, as well as internal forces such as muscle contraction, pulsatile flow, and cell-to-cell stimulation due to multiplication. Using *in vivo* systems, profound effects have been observed of both increasing and decreasing this mechanical stress. Virtually all tissues and cell types appear to respond to a change in the mechanical environment.

Ligaments have been studied extensively. Knee ligaments have been shown to increase in strength in response to exercise[1] and weaken as a result of stress deprivation.[2] Immobilization or stress deprivation resulted in change from an anabolic to catabolic state.[3] A significant increase in lysozomal enzyme activity was found following disuse. Increased activity in a different study resulted in an increase in protein synthesis.[4]

Other tissues have been shown to respond in a similar manner. Immobilization of bone results in marked catabolism with resulting osteoporosis.[5] Both strength as well as mineral content is affected in osteoporosis. Muscle exhibits marked atrophy with loss of many oxidative enzymes following disuse.[6] In most tissues these effects can be reversed with increased use and stress. Increased stress has been shown to result in bone production[7] and muscle hypertrophy.[8]

However, there is probably a point where a continued increase in stimulation ceases to be physiologic. Beyond that point an increase in stress will result in cell injury. This has been clearly shown in muscle tissue.[9] The transition from stimulated anabolic state to injury due to excessive stimulation is still poorly defined in many other tissues.

The effects of mechanical stimulation in *in vitro* systems have been studied in various ways. Cellular as well as subcellular responses can be found in many cell types undergoing mechanical stimulation. Stress deprivation is difficult to define in cell culture systems. Most conventional solid-bottomed culture dishes essentially represent a stress-deprived environment. Only when cell growth becomes confluent is there some form of internal cell-to-cell mechanical stimulation.

Stimulation beyond the minimal cell culture forces in solid-bottomed wells has received more attention in the past several years. Several systems have been developed that can be used for this purpose. Early studies show that an increase in *in vitro* mechanical stimulation can stimulate cell duplication. Both accelerated cell cycling and DNA synthesis have been observed[10,11] in normal cells. Much like the *in vivo* system, the mechanical stress induces an anabolic state. At a subcellular level, the synthesis of proteins as well as proteoglycans can be stimulated through mechanical stimulation. Collagens, metalloproteinases, and noncollagenous proteins are produced in response to mechanical stress.[12-14] Not only normal cells but also cells obtained from injured structures such as healing ligaments have been studied.[15] They appear to respond in a similar manner.

Many of the above-mentioned experiments use tensile mechanical stress. In particular, tendon and ligament fibroblast are thought to undergo mainly tensile stresses *in vivo*. Cartilage, however, is mainly subjected to compressive stresses. Studies have shown that even compressive stresses in chondrocytes can induce similar changes in cell duplication and protein synthesis.[16]

In cell cultures, stimulation beyond a certain level is also likely to result in a certain degree of cell injury. Studies are currently underway to determine that level. It seems probable that this level will depend on the cell type being used. For instance, skinned muscle fibers can be easily stretched without any evidence of microscopic injury.

From the above-mentioned studies it becomes clear that a certain level and type of mechanical stress can determine the biological activity of the indidivual cell. Whether function follows form completely as postulated by Watson[17] remains to be decided by future investigation. Already several pathways by which mechanical stimulation is translated into biochemical changes have been identified (mechanotransduction). One of the first to be identified was stretch-activated ion channels. These channels may be coupled with protein synthesis[18] and volume regulatory responses.[19,20] Another possible mechanotransductor is the Na^+/H^+ exchanger. It is possible that cellular attachment to a surface activates the Na^+/H^+ exchanger which may result in cytoplasmatic alkalinization and an increase in DNA synthesis and growth.[21] Finally, second messengers such as cyclic AMP and inositol-(1,4,5) triphosphate have been implicated in translation of mechanical stimuli to biochemical changes.[22,23] Most recent studies have implicated prostaglandin E_2 in this process as well. PGE_2 possibly provides a negative feedback on the cyclic AMP synthesis.[24]

III. *IN VITRO* MODELS

Mechanical stimulation of cells in culture is not an entirely new concept. Roller culture bottles and spinner cultures are forms of mechanical stimulation. Also, individual cell stimulation using micropipettes has been used before.[5] However, recent new technology has made it possible to mechanically stimulate cells in culture in a very controlled manner. Several systems are currently used,[26-28] but most of them involve the use of flexible-bottomed culture dishes. These flexible bottoms can undergo a controlled deformation due to the generation of positive or negative pressure underneath the culture dish. In one of the systems, the Fexercell unit, the culture dishes fit in a baseplate sealed with a gasket which is connected to a microprocessor-controlled pressure module. The entire baseplate with culture dishes is placed in the incubator. A pressure tube connects the baseplate inside the incubator to the control unit outside the incubator. At the start of the stimulation, the microprocessor is programmed with the amount of negative or positive pressure delivered per cycle, frequency, and duration of the stimulation. During each cycle, a preset amount of positive or negative pressure is generated underneath the culture wells. The degree of deformation corresponds with amount of pressure (see Figure 1). Since the flexible culture bottoms are fixed at the edge of the well, the deformation is not evenly distributed over the bottom. With negative pressure, a largely uniaxial gradient is generated. The maximum amount of stretch occurs near the periphery and the least amount near the center. This may be a disadvantage since cells may respond differently depending on the degree of stretch. However, by harvesting

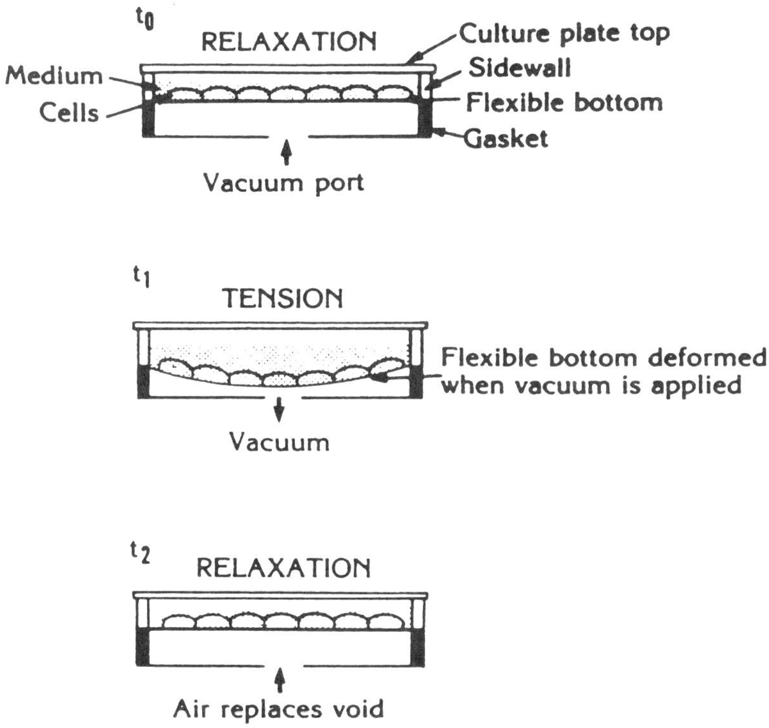

FIGURE 1. One cycle of mechanical stimulation using an *in vitro* system.

the outer cells separately from the inner cells, this problem can be accommodated. Other possibilities include placing a disk in the center of the well to avoid cell growth in this area. With positive pressure, a more uniform, biaxial gradient is produced. Graphs are available that allow the user to determine the maximum amount of stretch with a certain amount of positive or negative pressure. Usually negative pressure is used to stimulate cells in culture which stretches the bottom downwards. Depending on the system that is used, different types of bottoms are used. The Flexercell system and others[28] use a silicone elastomer well bottom which is coated with a special substratum. Most often genetic type I bovine collagen is used, but elastin or fibronectin-coated well bottoms are also used. Other systems use a Pellethane membrane.[26] With the Flexercell unit, pressures in excess of 17 kilopascals can be generated. This corresponds to 27% deformation at the periphery. The wells themselves tolerate maximum deformation up to 200%. Physiologic strains *in vivo* rarely exceed 4% for connective tissue. Cycle frequency of 60 to 70 Hz and over can be used since a positive pressure source is used to force the flexible bottom back in its resting position.

IV. THE USE OF THE FLEXERCELL UNIT

Any type of cell that displays attachment to bottoms of culture wells can be used in the Flexercell system. Initially, cells are cultured from isolates or explants using standard tissue culture techniques. Once enough cells are obtained, they are placed in Flex culture well at a density of approximately 10^5 cells per well. For most experiments, 2 ml of culture medium is used in each well. For cells derived from connective tissue, ascorbic acid (0.5 m*M*) is occasionally added to the medium to stimulate collagen production. The cells are allowed to adhere, grow to confluence, and produce some matrix before actual mechanical stimulation is started. At the start of stimulation the medium is changed.

The stimulation program is entered in the computer prior to the start of the stimulation. The program allows any possible deformation regimen, including high and low frequencies, alternating episodes of rest and stimulation, and varying lengths of stimulation. Subcellular responses such as generation of second messengers (prostaglandins, cAMP) can already be found after several minutes of stimulation. Stimulation for several hours or days may be needed to observe slower processes like cell division. The frequency may depend on the cell type that is being studied. For instance, endothelial cells are often stimulated at frequencies similar to the human heart rate. At the start of the stimulation, the pressure is calibrated using the vacuum gauge on the unit. For long stimulation experiments, the medium may have to be changed before the completion of the experiment. In order to do this, the program is temporarily interrupted. The baseplate is disconnected from the vacuum system and then can be removed from the incubator. Since some forms of stimulation greatly enhance cell metabolism, medium exchange may be needed more frequently than usual.

At the completion of the experiments, cells and supernatants can be harvested in the usual fashion. It is also possible to harvest inner and outer cells separately. Prior to removing the cells from the bottom of the wells, photomicrographs of the cells can give important information regarding their spatial arrangement in response to the stimulation. Fibroblasts will tend to arrange themselves in a circular fashion around the center of the wells.

V. CONCLUSION

The use of mechanical stimulation in *in vitro* models is a result of recently developed technology. Already numerous changes in cellular metabolism have been noted in response to the stimulation. Future studies will determine where physiologic stimulation becomes excessive stimulation resulting in cell injury. Both forms of stimulation can be useful in *in vitro* models. Physiologic stimulation will allow simulation of motion that is experienced by all cells in living tissue. Excessive stimulation can allow study of cells that have undergone an injury but which do not necessarily result in cell death. The combination of mechanical and chemical stimulation of cells *in vitro* can bring *in vitro* testing another step closer to the *in vivo* situation.

REFERENCES

1. **Tipton, C. M., James, S. I., Mergner, W., and Tcheng, T. K.,** Influence of exercise on strength of medial collateral ligaments of dogs, *Am. J. Phys.*, 18, 894, 1970.
2. **Noyes, F. R.,** Functional properties of knee ligaments and alteration induced by immobilization, *Clin. Orthop. Relat. Res.*, 123, 210, 1977.
3. **Gamble, J. G., Edwards, C. C., and Max, S. R.,** Enzymatic adaptation in ligaments during immobilization, *Am. J. Sports Med.*, 12, 221, 1984.
4. **Vailas, A. C., Tipton, C. M., Matthes, R. D., and Gart, M.,** Physical activity and its influence of the repair process of medial collateral ligaments, *Connect. Tissue Res.*, 9, 25, 1981.
5. **Gillespie, J. A.,** The nature of bone changes associated with nerve injuries and disuse, *J. Bone Joint Surg.*, 36B, 464, 1954.
6. **Rifenbireck, D. H., Gamble, J. G., and Max, S. R.,** Response of mitochondrial enzymes to decreased muscular activity, *Am. J. Physiol.*, 225, 1295, 1973.
7. **Goodship, A. E., Lanyon, L. E., and McFie, H.,** Functional adaptation of bone to increased stress, *J. Bone Joint Surg.*, 61A, 539, 1979.

8. **Ianuzzo, C. D., Gollnick, P. D., Armstrong, R. B.,** Compensatory adaptations of skeletal muscle fibre types to a long term overload, *Life Sci.*, 19, 1517, 1976.
9. **Almekinders, L. C. and Gilbert, J. A.,** Healing of experimental muscle strains and the effects of non-steroidal anti-inflammatory medication, *Am. J. Sports Med.*, 14, 303, 1986.
10. **Curtis, A. S. G. and Seehar, G. M.,** The control of cell division by tension or diffusion, *Nature*, 274, 52, 1978.
11. **Brunette, D. M.,** Mechanical stretching increases the number of cells synthesizing DNA in culture, *J. Cell. Sci.*, 69, 35, 1984.
12. **Leung, D. Y. M., Glagoo, S., and Matthew, M. B.,** Cyclic stretching simulates synthesis of matrix components by arterial smooth muscle cells *in vitro, Science*, 191, 475, 1976.
13. **Meikle, M. C., Sellers, A., and Reynolds, J. J.,** Effect of tensile mechanical stress on synthesis of metalloproteinases by rabbit coronal sutures *in vitro, Calcif. Tissue Int.*, 30, 77, 1980.
14. **Hasegawa, S., Sato, S., Saito, S., Suzuki, Y., and Brunette, D. M.,** Mechanical stretching increases the number of cultured bone cells synthesizing DNA and alter their pattern of protein synthesis, *Calcif. Tissue Int.*, 37, 431, 1985.
15. **Sutker, B. D., Lester, G. E., Banes, A. J., and Dahners, L. E.,** Cyclic strain stimulates DNA and collagen synthesis in fibroblasts cultured from rat medial collateral ligaments, *Trans. 36th Annu. ORS*, 15, 130, 1990.
16. **Gray, M. L., Pizzanelli, A. M., Grodzinsky, A. J., and Lee, R. C.,** Mechanical and physicochemical determinants of chondrocyte biosynthetic response, *J. Orthop. Res.*, 6, 777, 1988.
17. **Watson, P. A.,** Function follows form: generations of intracellular signals by cell deformation, *FASEB*, 5, 2013, 1991.
18. **Kent, R. L., Hoober, J. C., and Cooper, G.,** Load responsiveness of protein synthesis in adult mammalian myocardium: role of cardiac deformation linked to sodium influx, *Circ. Res.*, 64, 74, 1989.
19. **Eveloff, J. L. and Warnock, D. G.,** Activation of ion transport systems during cell volume regulation, *Am. J. Physiol.*, 252, F1, 1987.
20. **Morris, L. E.,** Mechanosensitive ion channels, *J. Membr. Biol.*, 112, 93, 1990.
21. **Ingber, D. E., Prusty, D., Fangioni, J. V., Cragoe, E. J., Lechene, C., and Schwartz, M. A.,** Control of intracellular pH and growth by fibronectin in capillary endothelial cells, *J. Cell. Biol.*, 110, 1803, 1990.
22. **Watson, P. A., Haneda, T., and Morgan, H. E.,** Effect of higher aortic pressure on ribosome formation and cAMP concentration in rat heart, *Am. J. Physiol.*, 256, 1257, 1989.
23. **Von Harsdorf, R., Lang, R., Fullerton, M., Smith, A. I., and Woodcock, E. A.,** Right atrial dilation increases inositol- (1,4,5) triphosphate accumulation, *FEBS Lett.*, 233, 201, 1988.
24. **Harrell, A., Dekel, S., and Binderman, I.,** Biochemical effect of mechanical stress on cultured bone cells, *Calcif. Tissue Res.*, Suppl 22, 202, 1977.
25. **Sachs, F.,** Baroreceptor mechanism at a cellular level, *Fed. Proc.*, 46, 12, 1987.
26. **Brighton, C. T., Stafford, B., Gross, S. B., Leatherwood, D. F., Williams, J. L., and Pollack, S. R.,** The proliferative and synthetic response of isolated calvarial bone cells of rats to cyclic biaxial mechanical strain, *J. Bone Joint Surg.*, 73A, 320, 1991.
27. **Banes, A. J., Link, G. W., Gilbert, J. W., Tran Son Tay, R., and Monbureau,** Culturing cells in a mechanically active environment, *Am. Biotech. Lab.*, 8, 12, 1990.
28. **Vandernburgh, H. H. and Karlisch, P.,** Longitudinal growth of skeletal myotubes *in vitro* in a new horizontal mechanical cell stimulator, *In Vitro Cell Develop. Biol.*, 25, 607, 1989.

Chapter 13

HUMAN LEUKOCYTES AS AN *IN VITRO* MODEL FOR STUDYING PCB TOXICITY

Tee-Ping Lee

TABLE OF CONTENTS

I. INTRODUCTION

A. PCBs AND PCB POISONING

Polychlorinated biphenyls (PCBs) once were widely used in industry, where their high stability contributed to both their commercial usefulness and their long-term deleterious environmental and health effects. There have been several reports concerning the toxic effects of PCBs in association with occupational exposure due to dermal contact with these chemicals.[1-12] In addition, there have been two major outbreaks of poisoning, one in Japan in 1968 (Yusho poisoning,[5,13,14]) and the other in Taiwan during 1976 (Yu-Cheng poisoning,[15-17]) Both incidents involved the consumption of rice bran oil contaminated with PCBs.

The most prominent symptoms associated with Yusho or Yu-Cheng patients are dermal and ocular abnormalities such as hyperpigmentation of the skin and mucosal membrane, acne-like eruptions, swelling of the eyelids and meibomian glands, and hypersecretion of cheese-like materials from the eyes. Patients also displayed signs of neuropathy,[5,16-19] abnormal hepatic functions,[5,15,16,20,21] and immunosuppression.[5,6,15,16]

The prevailing symptoms suffered by the majority of orally PCB-poisoned patients, such as hyperpigmentation, abnormal eye discharge, abnormal liver function, and immune suppression, were rare among workers who had had occupational exposure to PCBs due to dermal contact.[7,22,23] PCBs are known to contain different mixtures of homologues and various toxic impurities such as polychlorinated dibenzofurans (PCDFs), polychlorinated quarterphenyls (PCQs), and polychlorinated naphthalene.[1,5,24-29] Some of the impurities (e.g., PCDFs) are more toxic than PCBs[25,29-32] and may be responsible for symptoms associated with oral poisoning.[28]

B. IMMUNOSUPPRESSION ASSOCIATED WITH PCB POISONING

In animal experiments, exposure to PCBs and the related halogenated aromatic hydrocarbons by feeding, injection, or dermal application leads to a wide range of immune suppression. The toxic effects include increased susceptibility to microorganism, virus and endotoxins, atrophy of the cortex of thymus, reduction in the number of germinal centers in the spleen and lymph nodes, decreased immunoglobulin concentration, decreased hypersensitive response, reduced number of circulating leukocytes and lymphocytes, and decreased T cell response to mitogen.[1,25,29,33-46]

Yusho and Yu-Cheng patients also showed signs of immune suppression, such as persistent skin infection, bronchitis-like respiratory symptoms,[5,15] a moderate decrease in immunoglobulin concentration, e.g., IgM and IgA,[5,47] and suppression of delayed hypersensitive response to streptokinase and streptodornase.[48] Laboratory studies have shown that the number of T cells, but not B cells, was decreased. Certain population of T cells (e.g., active T cells and helper T cells) was greatly depressed by PCBs, while other types of T cells (suppressor T cells) were not affected.[47-49] The activities of B cells are regulated by various types of T cells.[50] Suppression of helper T cells might be responsible for the observed decrease in IgM and IgA concentrations.

The percentages of phagocytes (e.g., neutrophil and monocytes) bearing Fc or complement receptors were lower in Yu-Cheng patients.[49,51] These receptors are associated with full expressions of cellular function (e.g., adherence, chemotaxis, phagocytosis).[52,53] Lower percentage of phagocytic cells bearing Fc and/or complement receptors may be responsible for impaired cellular function and, consequently, increased incidence of infection.

In addition to the immune system, the function of the liver and several endocrine glands such as adrenal, thyroid, and pancreatic islets are also affected by halogenated aromatic hydrocarbons (HAHs). These effects lead to the abnormal metabolism of biogenic amines, steroids (e.g., cortisol, androgen, and estrogen), hormones (e.g., thyroxine and insulin), and vitamins[1,2,5,6,16,25,54-56]. Biogenic amines, thyroxine, steroids, and vitamins affect the immune function.[31,54,57-59] Therefore, it is not clear whether the immunosuppressive effects of PCBs are due to the indirect effect of these chemicals on the other organ systems. The study of the effects of PCBs and the related HAHs on leukocyte activity *in vitro* appears to offer an opportunity to solve the controversial issue of direct vs. indirect toxicity and to elucidate the biochemical mechanism involved.

II. PREPARATION OF LEUKOCYTES FROM HUMAN PERIPHERAL BLOOD

Peripheral blood containing heparin, EDTA, or citrate as an anticoagulant is centrifuged at 400 × g for 20 min. The leukocyte-rich fraction is removed, diluted with saline, and layered over Ficoll-Paque (sp gr 1.077) in a centrifuge tube. After centrifugation at 400 × g for 40 min, granulocytes and RBCs are sedimented to the bottom of the tube. Mononuclear cells are in a layer on the upper part of the Ficoll-Paque.[60,61] The mononuclear cell suspension contains both lymphocytes and monocytes.

A. LYMPHOCYTES AND MONOCYTES

Mononuclear cells are removed, suspended in saline, and centrifuged at low speed (100 × g) to remove platelets. In experiments which require the separation of lymphocytes and monocytes, the cells are resuspended in RPMI 1640 containing 10% serum and incubated in a glass bottle previously coated with AB serum for 1 h at 37°C. After 60 min, the cells remaining in the suspension are lymphocytes and the cells attached to the glass surface are mostly monocytes. Lymphocytes are then obtained by decanting the suspension. Fresh medium is added to this bottle and monocytes are removed by scraping the surface with a clean rubber policeman.[62] The composition of the cell population is determined by examination of smears stained by Wright's stain or by using the Quantigen rosette assay (Ortho Diagnostics, Raritan, NJ). The purity of the leukocytes obtained by this method is about 90% for lymphocytes and 75% for monocytes.

B. NEUTROPHILS

The cells (granulocytes and RBCs) at the bottom of the Ficoll-Paque centrifuge tube are suspended in 0.9% ammonium chloride for 5 min to lyse RBCs. After ammonium chloride is removed by centrifugation, the granulocytes are suspended in fresh media. More than 95% of the cells obtained in this fraction are neutrophils.[60,61]

III. ASSESSMENT OF CHEMICAL TOXICITY

PCBs and the related halogenated hydrocarbons are hydrophobic and dissolved in organic solvents (e.g., dimethylsulfoxide, DMSO). The effects of the solvent on cellular and biochemical parameter must be evaluated. In addition, hydrophobic chemicals tend to adhere to the surface of the laboratory wares (e.g., test tubes, pipette tips). Consequently, the actual concentration of the chemical in solution, depending on the composition of the experimental condition (e.g., the presence or the absence of serum), may be far less than the theoretical concentration. Ideally, the actual concentration of the chemical in question should be monitored by spiking with the corresponding radioactive chemical as the internal standard.

To evaluate the toxicity of PCBs on leukocytes, suspension of leukocytes is treated with solution of the tested chemicals and assayed for various cell activities. Inhibition of cell activity may be due to cell mortality, impaired cell functions, or both. Chemical toxicity is studied at the concentrations which impaired only cell functions but not viability. After chemical treatment, cell viability is determined by: (1) the recovery of the number of intact cells, (2) exclusion of trypan blue dye (0.2% in saline), and (3) the absence of cytoplasmic enzyme, lactate dehydrogenase (LDH), in the extracellular media.

IV. EVALUATION OF LYMPHOCYTE FUNCTIONS

A. LYMPHOCYTE MITOGENIC RESPONSE

Lymphocytes can be stimulated by a variety of mitogens, the most common being phytohemagglutinin (PHA), pokeweed mitogen (PWM), and concanavalin A (Con A). These stimulants are nonspecific and can induce transformation of normal lymphocytes. PHA stimulates T lymphocytes. Numerous metabolic changes take place following PHA stimulation: increased membrane phospholipid synthesis, increased glucose, amino acid and calcium transport, increased glycolysis and hexose monophosphate shunt activities, phosphorylation of nuclear proteins, and increased RNA, protein, and DNA synthesis.[63,64] The incorporation of radioactive thymidine into acid precipitable fraction (DNA) has been widely used as an indicator of mitogenic response of lymphocytes.

To evaluate the mitogenic response, suspension of mononuclear cells (1×10^6 cells per ml) is incubated with mitogens such as PHA, PWM, Con A, PMA, or ionophore A23187 for 72 h at 37°C in an atmosphere containing 5% CO_2 in air. ^{3}H-Thymidine (0.1 μCi) is then added and the mixture is incubated for another 24 h. The radioactive thymidine, which is incorporated into DNA fraction, is precipitated with acetic acid (3%). The amount of acetic acid precipitable radioactivity indicates the extent of DNA synthesis. Our preliminary data indicated that Aroclor 1254 at the concentrations of 0.1 and 1.0 μM would inhibit thymidine incorporation by $16 \pm 5\%$ and $85 \pm 3\%$, respectively ($\bar{x} \pm$ SD, n = 6).

B. ROSETTE FORMATION (E-ROSETTES)

Similar to mitogenic response to PHA, rosette formation between human lymphocytes and sheep red blood cells (SRBCs) is characteristic of thymus dependent lymphocytes (T cells). Intact metabolic pathways for glycolysis and protein and nucleic acid metabolism are required for full expression of rosette activity.[65]

Suspension of mononuclear cells or lymphocytes (0.1 ml, 4×10^6 cells per ml) is mixed with equal volume of 1% SRBCs in RPMI 1640 containing fetal calf serum (FCS). The mixture of the cells is then centrifuged at $400 \times g$ for 10 min. E-rosettes are determined after incubation of the pellets of cells at 4°C overnight.[66] Before the determination of the rosettes, the pellets are gently resuspended into medium. A rosette is defined as a lymphocyte which has three or more SRBCs attached to it. Aroclo 1254 at the concentration of 1.0 μM exerted little effect on E-rosette formation.

C. REMOVAL AND REGENERATION OF RECEPTORS FOR ROSETTES

Suspension of lymphocytes (10^6 cells per ml in RPMI 1640) is treated with trypsin (1 mg/ml) in the presence of DNAase (10 μg/ml) for 30 min at room temperature. After incubation, the cells are washed with RPMI by centrifugation. The treated cells form no rosettes with SRBCs. The incubation of the suspension of treated cells in the presence of serum leads to the recovery of rosette forming abilities.[65]

The regeneration of the receptors in trypsin-treated lymphocytes is inhibited by PCBs. Our preliminary data indicated that Aroclor 1254 at the concentration of 0.1 and 1.0 μM would inhibit the regeneration of E-rosettes by $23 \pm 2\%$ and $37 \pm 4\%$ ($\bar{x} \pm$ SD, n = 6), respectively. It has been reported that in PCB-exposed human subjects, there was a marked decrease in the percentage of E-rosette-forming lymphocytes.[49] The decrease in E-rosette-forming lymphocytes may be partially attributed to the diminished ability to synthesize membrane receptors.

D. LYMPHOKINE SECRETION

Lymphokines are nonantibody proteins synthesized and secreted by active lymphocytes that act as intercellular mediators of the immunologic responses.[67-69] While many of the lymphokines are still measured by bioassay, some are detectable by radioimmunoassay (RIA). A RIA procedure of human interleukin-2 (IL-2) is described as follows:

IL-2 is a glycoprotein that serves as a growth factor for activated T cells.[70-72] Abnormalities in the ability of T cells to produce and secrete IL-2 have been detected in several pathologic states including acquired immunodeficiency state, malignancies, and autoimmune disorders.[73-75] PHA-treated lymphocytes secrete IL-2 which peaks at 24 h.[76]

For the measurement of IL-2, lymphocytes (1×10^6 cells in 2 ml of medium) are incubated with PHA for different lengths of time and the supernatant removed by centrifugation. Assays are performed in 5 ml (12×75 mm) glass tubes in a total assay volume of 1.0 ml. For the construction of standard curves, assay mixtures containing 0.1 ml of a solution of rabbit antibody (IgG) against human IL-2 (commercial stock solution diluted 1:1000 in PBS, pH 7.4), 0.1 ml of iodinated IL-2 (3 nCi/tube, equivalent to 10 pg), and unlabeled IL-2 at different concentration diluted in PBS are added to tubes containing 0.5 ml of control culture medium. The final volume per tube is made up to 1 ml with PBS. For the assay of supernatant fluid of lymphocyte cultures, 0.5 ml of supernatant is added to 0.5. ml of an assay mixture that contained rabbit antibody (IgG) to human IL-2 and radioactive IL-2 (3 nCi/tube). Assay mixtures are incubated overnight at 4°C and 0.1 ml of a solution of purified rabbit IgG (1 mg/ml) is added to each tube as carrier. Rabbit IgG is then precipitated with goat antibody to rabbit IgG (0.1 ml of commercial stock, titer 1:16 per tube). The radioactivities in the supernatant and the pellet fractions are counted and analyzed. Under these conditions, in the absence of added unlabeled IL-2, approximately 30 to 40% of the radioactive IL-2 added is associated with the precipitate fraction. The nonspecific binding, measured in the presence of 10,000-fold excess unlabeled IL-2, accounted for less than 4% of the radioactivity added.

All pipettes, tips, and test tubes used for the RIA are coated with BSA by incubation for 1 h at 37°C with a solution containing 20 mg/ml BSA in a coating buffer (50 m*M* sodium bicarbonate, 0.02% sodium azide, pH 9.6), following which they are twice rinsed with distilled water.

V. EVALUATION OF NEUTROPHIL FUNCTIONS

A. CHEMOTAXIS

Human neutrophils, *in vitro*, respond to several kinds of attractant, e.g., bacteria cultural fluid and zymosan activated serum. To prepare the bacterial factor, the bacteria are removed by centrifigation, and the supernatant is filtered through 0.45-μ Millipore filter before use. To prepare zymosan-activated serum, the supension of zymosan in serum (25 mg/ml serum) is incubated at 37°C for 30 min. After the removal of zymosan particles by centrifugation, the activated serum is removed and diluted with medium (1:10 dilution) for use as an attractant. For the assay of neutrophil chemotaxis, a modified Boyden chamber method is used in which the cells are made to migrate upward against gravity.[77,78] Suspension of neutrophils (3×10^6 cells per ml, 0.1 ml aliquot) is deposited on the surface of Millipore filter paper (5 μ) in a circular area of 0.28 cm^2. The deposited cells are sandwiched by the placement of another filter paper. The two filter papers with neutrophils are placed on the blind well chamber (Neuro Probe, Bethesda, MD) with culture medium in the lower compartment. Chemotactic attractant is added to the upper chamber. Thus, the procedure makes the chemotactic movement upward.[77,78]

After incubation at 37°C for 1 to 4 h, the filter papers are separated and dipped in methanol and then placed in phosphate buffer-formalin solution (cell side up). The cells on the filter papers are fixed for a minimum of 10 min to overnight. After fixation, the cells are stained with hematoxylin and then mounted on a microscope slide for observation under a microscope. The field is observed first with low power to select a representative area for counting. High power is then used for actual counting. Five selected counts are made and an average is made from these counts. Under the described conditions, the normal value is about 120 ± 20 cells per high power field (HPF). Aroclor 1254 at the concentration of 10 μM would inhibit chemotaxis by 14 ± 2% ($\overline{X}$ ± SD, n = 6).

B. NEUTROPHIL LYSOSOMAL ENZYME RELEASE

The exposure of neutrophils to zymosan-activated serum or opsonized zymosan particles leads to the release of lysosomal enzymes.[61,79] For the assay of neutrophil B-glucuronidase release, neutrophil suspension (3×10^6 cells per ml) is incubated with cytochalasin B (5 μg/ml) for 5 min at 37°C. Cytochalasin B inhibits phagocytosis of zymosan particles by neutrophils and enhances lysosomal enzyme release.[61,79,80] Autologous serum and zymosan suspension (10 mg/ml) are added to neutrophil suspension. The incubation is continued for another 30 min with constant shaking (120 excusions per min) at 37°C in a Dubnoff metabolic shaker (Precision Scientific Co., Chicago, IL). After incubation, the tubes are centrifuged at 4°C for 2 min at 1000 × g. The cell-free supernatant is removed for the determination of the enzymes released during incubation. Two control tubes are used for the determination of total enzyme activity. The addition of Triton X-100 (1.0%) to the neutrophil suspension releases all the lysosomal and cytoplasmic enzymes into the supernatant. Therefore, total enzyme activity can be measured. The extent of lysosomal enzyme release from neutrophils under different incubating conditions is calculated as follows:

$$\%\text{ of enzyme release} = \frac{\text{enzyme activity in supernatant after incubation}}{\text{total enzyme activity (Triton X-100 treated)}} \times 100$$

The activity of β-glucuronidase is measured by the formation of phenolphthalein from phenolphthalein glucuronide.[81] The activity of LDH is measured by the formation of NADH (absorbance at 340 nM) from lactate and NAD.[82] The absence of LDH in the supernatant and the exclusion of trypan blue indicates that cells are viable and intact.

The exposure of neutrophil suspension to PCBs led to the inhibition of β-glucuronidase release. The degree of inhibition was time and dosage dependent. Optimal inhibition was obtained with 30 min preincubation of neutrophils with PCBs. The results suggested that PCBs caused some reversible metabolic change in neutrophils.[80] Aroclor 1254 at the concentrations of 1.0 and 10.0 μM inhibited β-glucuronidase release by 20 ± 3% and 30 ± 2%, respectively.[80]

C. PHAGOCYTOSIS (OIL RED O)

Oil red O dye is dissolved in diisodecyl phthlate (paraffin oil) and the O.D. at 525 nM is measured. After sonicating the dye containing oil with bacteria endotoxin (*E. coli* lipopolysaccharide endotoxin; Difco Laboratory, Detroit, MI), the mixture is treated with AB serum for 25 min at 37°C. Suspension of neutrophils is incubated with opsonized oil at 37°C for 5 min. The reaction is stopped by centrifugation. The oil droplets which are not ingested by neutrophil are in the supernatant. Pellets of neutrophil containing oil and dye are extracted with DMSO. The O.D. of dye-containing extract is measured at 525 nM. From the O.D. of the original dye-containing oil solution, the amount of oil in the extract (neutrophil ingested) can be calculated.[83] Aroclor 1254 at the concentration of 10 μM inhibited oil ingestion by 25 ± 3%.

D. OXYGEN CONSUMPTION

Oxygen consumption by neutrophil suspension is measured by an oxygraph with a Clark electrode.[84] The Clark electrode measures the oxygen concentration in the solution. The suspension of neutrophils is incubated with PMA. PMA stimulates neutrophil oxygen consumption. Consequently, the concentration of oxygen in the medium is decreased. The decrease of oxygen concentration in the neutrophil suspension reflects the amount of oxygen consumed by neutrophils. Aroclor 1254 at a concentration of up to 10 μM did not affect neutrophil oxygen consumption.

E. PHAGOCYTOSIS AND BACTERIOCIDAL ASSAY *(STAPHYLOCOCCUS)*

The purpose of this procedure is to assess how well the isolated neutrophils phagocytized and killed *Staphylococcus* 502A.[85]

Neutrophils are adjusted to a concentration of 10^7 cells per ml. *Staphylococcus aureus* is adjusted to 10^8 colony-forming units/ml. AB serum is diluted to 20% with Hanks' balance salt solution (HBSS) and is used as an opsonin. The neutrophils, bacteria, and serum are combined to yield the following concentrations, respectively: neutrophils 5×10^6 cells per ml, *Staphylococcus* 10^7 cells per ml, and AB serum 8%. The sample of this mixture is taken at zero time to determine the baseline bacterial concentration. At 30 min and 120 min, samples are taken and the cells are lysed by vortexing at high speed for 30 sec to get the total intracellular and extracellular viable bacteria (TVB). Also, at 30 and 120 min, samples are taken, the extracellular bacteria are killed with lysostaphin which is then inactivated by trypsin, and the cells are lysed to release the intracellular bacteria (IB). Thus at 30 min and at 120 min both TVB and IB are determined by plating, and colonies are counted on tryptic soy agar plates. The number of extracellular bacteria (EB) is determined by subtracting the IB from the total bacteria (TVB − IB = EB).

VI. SUMMARY

There are many aspects of leukocyte activities that can be studied by *in vitro* methods, e.g., antibody production, leukocyte interactions. It is not the intention of the present review to cover all these aspects of cell activities. The available data suggest that PCBs and the related HAHs have a direct effect on human leukocytes. The reported immunosuppression found in experimental animals and human subjects following PCB exposure may be due to the direct effect of PCBs on lymphoid tissues.

There are differences in the susceptibilities to PCBs, between different types of cells and between different aspects of cellular function of a given cell type. The expression of immune function involves the cooperative interaction between several cell types. The study of leukocyte activity *in vitro* provides an opportunity to determine the primary target cells affected and to elucidate the biochemical mechanism involved.

At the present time the exact molecular basis of the immunotoxicity caused by HAHs is not clear. One of the most popular hypothesis derived from the study of 2,3,7,8-TCDD is that the genetically controlled cytoplasmic aromatic hydrocarbon receptor (Ah receptor) mediated the toxicity of HAHs, including PCBs.[25,31,86-88] The presence of high affinity receptors in target tissue appears to be an important determinant of toxicity in specific tissues.[89] Structure-toxicity relationship appears to be related to the affinity of the individual isomers for binding to Ah receptor.[90]

The spectra of toxic effects induced by PCBs are similar to effects produced by 2,3,7,8-TCDD and the related HAHs. PCB molecules with configurations similar to 2,3,7,8-TCDD can bind to the Ah receptor and are the most toxic congeners.[25] The immunotoxic effects of PCBs, 2,3,7,8-TCDD, and the related HAHs compounds may all have been mediated through Ah receptors.[25,31,86] But recently, there is increasing evidence suggesting the involvement of an Ah receptor-independent process as well.[88,91]

PCBs inhibit the activities of Mg-ATPase and Na^+/K^+-ATPase prepared from several tissues.[92] Aroclor 1254 added *in vitro* decreases leukocyte glucose uptake[93] and intracellular ATP concentration.[94]

2,3,7,8-TCDD added *in vitro* to rat thymocytes caused an increase in cytosolic calcium ion concentrations. The activation of a calcium ion-depedent endonuclease lead to DNA fragmentation and cell mortality.[95] 2,3,7,8-TCDD increases the activities of tyrosine kinase[96] and nonphospholipid-dependent protein kinase.[97]

The regulation of ATPase activities, ATP concentration, glucose uptake, calcium ion homeostasis, and protein kinase activities are essential for mammalian cells, not only for the control of cellular metabolism but for mediation of a diverse variety of cellular activities.

In summary, PCBs and the related HAHs affect various types of cell activities as well as different enzymes and biochemical systems. By studying the *in vitro* effects of these chemicals on leukocytes, we may be able to elucidate not only the molecular basis of their toxicities but also the role of different biochemical parameters in the regulation of various cell functions.

REFERENCES

1. **Fishbein, L.,** Toxicity of chlorinated biphenyls, *Annu. Rev. Pharmacol.*, 14, 139, 1974.
2. **Kimbrough, R.,** Human health effects of PCBs and PBBs, *Annu. Rev. Pharmacol. Toxicol.*, 27, 87, 1974.
3. **Nelson, N.,** Polychlorinated biphenyls: environmental impact, *Environ. Res.*, 5, 253, 1972.
4. **Zitco, V. and Choi, P. M. K.,** PCB and other industrial halogenated hydrocarbons in the environment, *Fish. Res. Board Can. Tech. Rep.* 272, 2, 1971.
5. **Higuchi, K.,** *PCB Poisoning and Pollution*, Academic Press, New York, 1976.
6. **Buckley, J. L.,** National Conference on Polychlorinated Biphenyls, Environmental Protection Agency, Washington, D.C., 1976.
7. **Fischbein, A., Wolff, M., Lilis, R., Thornton, J., and Selikoff, I. J.,** Clinical finding among PCB-exposed capacitor manufacturing workers, *Ann. N.Y. Acad. Sci.*, 320, 703, 1979.
8. **Meigs, J., Albom, J., and Kartin, B. L.,** Chloracne from an unusual exposure to Aroclor, *J. Am. Med. Assoc.*, 154, 1417, 1954.
9. **Ouw, K. H., Simpson, G. R., and Siyali, D. S.,** The use and health effects of Aroclor 1242, *Arch. Environ. Health*, 31, 189, 1976.
10. **Schwartz, L.,** Dermatitis from synthetic resins and waxes, *Am. J. Public Health*, 26, 586, 1936.
11. **Schwartz, L.,** An outbreak of halowax acne among electricians, *J. Am. Med. Assoc.*, 122, 158, 1942.
12. **Warshaw, R., Fischbein, A., Thornton, J., Miller, A., and Selikoff, I. J.,** Decrease in vital capacity in PCB-exposed workers in a capacitor manufacturing facility, *Ann. N.Y. Acad. Sci.*, 320, 277, 1979.
13. **Kuratsune, M., Yoshimura T., Matsuzaka, J., and Yamaguchi, A.,** Epidemiologic study on Yusho, *Environ. Health Perspect.*, 1, 119, 1972.
14. **Urabe, H., Koda, H., and Asahi, M.,** Present state of Yusho patients, *Ann. N.Y. Acad. Sci.*, 320, 273, 1979.
15. **Chang, K. J., Chen, J. S., Huang, P. C., and Tung, T. A.,** Study of patients with PCB-poisoning, *J. Formosan Med. Assoc.*, 79, 304, 1980a.
16. **Wong, C. K.,** PCB poisoning. Special issue, *Clin. Med.*, 7, 1, 1981.
17. **Hsu, S., Ma, C., Hsu, S., Wu, S., Hsu, N., and Yeh, C.,** Discovery and epidemiology of PCB poisoning in Taiwan, *Am. J. Ind. Med.*, 5, 71, 1984.
18. **Lee, Y. Y., Wong, P. N., Lu, Y. C., Sun, C. C., Wu, Y. C., Lin, R. Y., Jee, S. H., Ng, K. Y., and Yeh, H. P.,** An outbreak of PCB poisoning, *J. Dermatol.*, 7, 435, 1980.
19. **Chen, R. C., Chang, Y. C., Chang, K. J., Lu, F. J. and Tung, T. C.,** Peripheral neuropathy caused by chronic PCB poisoning, *J. Formosan Med. Assoc.*, 80, 47, 1981.
20. **Hirayama, C.,** Hepatocellular dysfunction in patients with PCB poisoning, *Fukoka Acta Med.*, 70, 238, 1979.

21. **Lu, Y. and Wong, P.,** Dermatological, medical and laboratory findings of patients in Taiwan and their treatments, *Am. J. Ind. Med.*, 5, 81, 1984.
22. **Emmett, E., Maroni, M., Schmith, J., Levin, B., and Jefferys, J.,** Studies of transformer repair workers exposed to PCBs, *Am. J. Ind. Med.*, 13, 415, 1988.
23. **Takamatsu, M., Oki, M., Maeda, K., Inoue, Y., Hirayama, H., and Yoshizuka, K.,** PCBs in blood of workers exposed to PCBs and their health status, *Am. J. Ind. Med.*, 5, 59, 1984.
24. **Bowes, G., Mulvihill, M., Simoneit, B., Burlingame, and Riserbough, R.,** Identification of chlorinated dibenzofurans in American PCBs, *Nature* (London), 256, 305, 1975.
25. **Safe, S.,** PCBs and PBBs: biochemistry, toxicology and mechanism of action, *CRC Crit. Rev. Toxicol.*, 13, 319, 1984.
26. **Masuda, Y. and Yoshimura, H.,** Polychlorinated biphenyls and dibenzofurans in patients with Yusho and their toxicological significance, *Am. J. Ind. Med.*, 5, 31, 1984.
27. **Chen, P., Luo, M., Wong, C., and Chen, C.,** PCBs, PDCFs and PCQs in the toxic rice bran oil and PCBs in the blood of patients with PCB poisoning in Taiwan, *Am. J. Ind. Med.*, 5, 133, 1984.
28. **Kunita, N., Kashimoto, T., Miyata, H., Kukushima, S., Hori, S., and Obana, H.,** Casual agents of Yusho, *Am. J. Ind. Med.*, 5, 45, 1984.
29. **Vos, J. G., Koeman, J. H., Van der Hass, H. I., ten Noever de Brauw, M. C., and de Vos, R. H.,** Identification and toxicological evaluation of chlorinated dibenzofuran and chlorinated naphthalene in PCBs, *Food Cosmet. Toxicol.*, 8, 625, 1970.
30. **Goldstein, J.,** The structure-activity relationship of halogenated biphenyls are enzyme inducers, *Ann. N.Y. Acad. Sci.*, 320, 164, 1979.
31. **Safe, S.,** Comparative toxicology and mechanism of action of polychlorianted dibenzo-p-dioxions and dibenzofurans, *Annu. Rev. Pharmacol. Toxicol.*, 26, 371, 1986.
32. **Holsapple, M., Morris, D., Wood, S., and Snyder, N.,** 2,3,7,8-TCDD induced changes in immunocompetence: possible mechanism, *Annu. Rev. Pharmacol. Toxicol.*, 31, 73, 1991.
33. **Luster, M. I., Blank, J. A., and Dean, H. J.,** Molecular basis of chemically induced immunotoxicology, *Annu. Rev. Pharmacol. Toxicol.*, 27, 23, 1987.
34. **Thomas, P. T. and Faith, R. E.,** Adult and perinatal immunotoxicity induced by halogenated aromatic hydrocarbons, in *Immunotoxicology and Immunopharmacology*, Dean, J. H., Luster, M. I., Munson, A. E., and Amos, H. E., Eds., Raven Press, New York, 1985, 305.
35. **Vos, J. G. and Koeman, J. H.,** Comparative toxicology study with PCBs in chickens, *Toxicol. Appl. Pharmacol.*, 17, 656, 1970.
36. **Allen, J. R.,** Response of the non-human primate to PCB exposure, *Fed. Proc.*, 34, 1675, 1975.
37. **Subba Rao, D. S. and Glick, B.,** Pesticide effects on the immune responses of chicken lymphocytes, *Proc. Soc. Exp. Biol. Med.*, 154, 27, 1977.
38. **Vos, J. G.,** Toxicology of PCBs for mammals and for birds, *Environ. Health Perspects.*, 1, 105, 1972.
39. **Wasserman, M., Wasserman, D., Gershon, A., and Zellermayer, L.,** Effect of organochlorine insecticides on body defense systems, *Ann. N.Y. Acad. Sci.*, 160, 393, 1969.
40. **Vos, J., Faith, R., and Luster, H.,** Immune alterations, in *Halogenated Biphenyls, Terphenyls, Hapthalenes, Dibenzodioxins and Related Products*, Kimbrough, R., Ed., Elsevier/North-Holland Biomedical Press, New York, 1980, 241.
41. **Flick, D. F., O'Dell, R., and Childs, V.,** Studies of the chick edema disease, *Poult. Sci.*, 44, 1460, 1965.
42. **Loose, L., Silkworth, J., Pittman, K., Benitz, K., and Mueller, W.,** Imparied host resistance to endotoxin and malaria in PCB-treated mice, *Infect. Immun.*, 20, 30, 1978.
43. **Thomas, P. T. and Hinsdill, R. D.,** Effects of PCBs on the immune responses of rhesus monkeys and mice, *Toxicol. Appl. Pharmacol.*, 44, 41, 1978.
44. **Koller, L. D. and Thigpen, J. E.,** Reduction of antibodies to pseudorabies virus in PCB exposed rabbits, *Am. J. Vet. Res.*, 34, 1065, 1973.
45. **Friend, M. and Trainer, D.,** PCB: interaction with duck hepatitis virus, *Science*, 170, 1314, 1970.
46. **Vos, J. G. and DeRoij, T.,** Immunosuppressive activity of a PCB preparation on the humoral immune response in guinea pig, *Toxicol. Appl. Pharmacol.*, 21, 549, 1972.
47. **Chang, K. J., Hsieh, K. H., Lee, T. P., Tang, S. Y., and Tung, T. C.,** Immunologic evaluation of patients with PCB-poisoning: determination of lymphocyte subpopulations, *Toxicol. Appl. Pharmacol.*, 61, 58, 1981.
48. **Chang, K. J., Hsieh, K. H., Tang, T. Y., Tung, T. A., and Lee, T. P.,** Immunologic evaluation of patients with PCB-poisoning: evaluation of delayed-type skin hypersensitive response and its relation to clinical studies, *J. Toxicol. Environ. Health*, 9, 217, 1982.
49. **Lee, T. P. and Chang, K. J.,** Health effects of PCBs, in *Immunotoxicology and Immunopharmacology*, Dean, J., Luster, M., Munson, A., and Amos, H., Eds., Raven Press, New York, 1985, 415.
50. **Moretta, L., Webb, S., Grossi, C., Lydyard, P., and Cooper, M.,** Functional analysis of two human T-cell subpopulations, *J. Exp. Med.*, 146, 184, 1977.

51. **Chang, K. J., Hsieh, K. H., Lee, T. P., and Tung, T. A.,** Immunologic evaluation of patients with PCB-poisoning: determination of pathocytic Fc and complement receptors, *Environ. Res.*, 28, 329, 1982.
52. **Klempner, M. and Gallin, J.,** Separation and functional characterization of human neutrophil subpopulations, *Blood*, 51, 659, 1978.
53. **Cline, M., Lehren, R., Territo, M., and Gold, D.,** Monocytes and macrophages, *Ann. Intern. Med.*, 88, 78, 1978.
54. **Rozman, K., Rozman, T., and Greim, H.,** Effects of thyroidectomy and thyroxine on TCDD induced toxicity, *Toxicol. Appl. Pharmacol.*, 72, 372, 1984.
55. **Gallo, M., Hesse, E., Macdonald, G., Umbreit, T.,** Interactive effects of estradiol and 2,3,7,8-TCDD on hepatic cytochrome P-450 and mouse uterus, *Toxicol. Lett.*, 32, 123, 1986.
56. **Loo, J. C., Tryphonas, H., Jordan, N., Brien, R., Karpinski, K. F., and Arnold, D. L.,** Effects of Arochlor 1254 on hydrocortisone levels in adult rhesus monkeys *(Macaca mulatta), Bull. Enrivon. Contam. Toxicol.*, 43, 667, 1989.
57. **Bourne, H. R., Melmom, K. L., Weinstein, Y., and Shearer, G. M.,** Pharmacologic regulation of antibody release *in vitro*, in *cAMP, Cell Growth and the Immune Response*, Braun, W., Lichenstein, L. M., and Parker, C. W., Eds., Springer-Verlag, New York, 1973, 99.
58. **Baxter, J. D. and Forsham, P. H.,** Tissue effects of glucocorticoids, *Am. J. Med.*, 53, 573, 1972.
59. **Panda, B. and Combs, G. F.,** Impaired antibody production in chicks fed diets low in vitamin A, Pantothenic acid or riboflavin, *Proc. Soc. Exp. Biol. Med.*, 113, 530, 1963.
60. **Boyum, A.,** A one stage procedure for isolation of granulocytes and lymphocytes from human blood, *Scan. J. Lab. Invest.*, 21, 51, 1968.
61. **Busse, W. and Lee, T. P.,** Decreased adrenergic responses in lymphocytes and granulocytes in atopic eczema, *J. Allergy Clin. Immunol.*, 58, 586, 1976.
62. **Koller, C., King, G., Hurtubise, P. E., Sagone, A. L., and LuBuglio, A. E.,** Characterization of glass-adherent human mononuclear cells, *J. Immunol.*, 111, 1610, 1973.
63. **Hirschhorn, R.,** The effect of exogenous nucleotides on the response of lymphocytes to PHA PWM and Con A, in *Cyclic AMP, Cell Growth and the Immune Response*, Braun, W., Lichtenstin, M., and Parker, C. W., Eds., Springer-Verlag, New York, 1974, 45.
64. **Campbell, A. K.,** Lymphocyte Activation, in *Intracellular Calcium*, Campbell, A. K., Ed., John Wiley & Sons, New York, 1983, 376.
65. **Bushkin, S. C., Pantic, V. S., and Good, R. A.,** RNA and protein synthesis in spontaneous rosette formation by T-lymphocytes, *J. Immunol.*, 115, 866, 1975.
66. **Dolen, J. G. and Park, B. H.,** An improved micro-method for enumeration of human B-cell rosettes with mouse red blood cells, *Immunol. Commun.*, 7, 677, 1978.
67. **Dumonde, D. and Hamblin, A.,** Lymphokine, in *Immunology in Medicine*, Holborow, E. and Reeves, W., Eds., Grune & Stratton, New York, 1983, 121.
68. **Sorg, C.,** Lymphokines, monokines, cytokines, *Chem. Immunol.*, 49, 82, 1990.
69. **Arai, K., Lee, F., Miyajima, A., Miyatake, S., Arai, N., and Yokota, T.,** Cytokines: coordinators of immune and inflammatory responses, *Annu. Rev. Biochem.*, 59, 783, 1990.
70. **Morgan, D. A., Ruscetti, F. W., and Gallo, R. C.,** Selective *in vitro* growth of T-lymphocytes from normal human bone marrow, *Science*, 193, 1007, 1976.
71. **Cantrell, D. and Smith, K. A.,** The Interleukin-2 T cell system: a new cell growth model, *Science*, 224, 1312, 1984.
72. **Smith, K. A.,** Interleukin-2: inception, impact, and implications, *Science*, 240, 1169, 1988.
73. **Fauci, A. S.,** The acquired immunodeficiency syndrome: an update, *Ann. Int. Med.*, 102, 800, 1985.
74. **Linker-Israeli, M., Bakke, A. C., Kitridou, S., et al.,** Defective production of Interleukin-1 and Interleukin-2 in patients with systemic lupus erythematosus (SLE), *J. Immunol.*, 130, 2651, 1983.
75. **Gehman, L. O. and Robb, R. J.,** An ELISA based assay for quantitation of human Interleukin-2, *J. Immunol. Methods*, 74, 39, 1984.
76. **Lee, T. P., Mookerjee, B. K., and Pauly, J. L.,** A simple radioimmunoassay of human interleukin-2, *J. Immunoassay*, 9, 193, 1988.
77. **Park, B. H., Dolen, J. ,and Synder, B.,** Defective chemotactic migration of PMNs in patients with Pelger-Huet Anomaly, *Proc. Soc. Exp. Biol. Med.*, 155, 51, 1977.
78. **Lee, T. P., Moscati, R., and Park, B.,** Effects of pesticide on human leukocyte function, *Res. Comm. Chem. Pathol. Pharmacol.*, 23, 597, 1979.
79. **Zurier, R., Weissman, G., Hoffstein, S., Kammerman, S., and Tai, H.,** Mechanism of lysosomal enzyme release from human leukocytes, *J. Clin. Invest.*, 53, 297, 1974.
80. **Lee, T. P.,** The inhibition of PMN β-glucuronidase release by Aroclor 1254, *Environ. Res.*, 25, 386, 1981.
81. **Glaser, J. H. and Sly, W.,** β-glucuronidase deficiency in mucopolysaccharidosis, *J. Lab. Clin. Med.*, 82, 969, 1973.

82. **Beutler, E.,** Red cell metabolism. A manual of biochemical methods, 2nd ed., Grune & Stratton, New York, 1975.
83. **Stossel, T., Root, R., and Vaughan, M.,** Phagocytosis in chronic granulomatous disease and the Chediak-Higashi syndrome, *N. Engl. J. Med.*, 286, 120, 1972.
84. **Reiss, M. and Roos, D.,** Differences in oxygen metabolism of phagocytosing monocytes and neutrophils, *J. Clin. Invest.*, 61, 480, 1978.
85. **Tan, J., Watanakunakorn, C., and Phair, J.,** A modified assay of neutrophil function: use of lysostaphin to differentiate defective phagocytosis from impaired intracellular killing, *J. Lab. Clin. Med.*, 78, 316, 1971.
86. **Silkworth, J. and Vecchi, A.,** Role of the Ah receptors in halogenated aromatic hydrocarbon immunotoxicity, in *Immunotoxicology and Immunopharmacology,* Dean, J., Luster, M., Munson, A., and Amos, H., Eds., Raven Press, New York, 1985, 263.
87. **Kerkvliet, N., Baecher-Steppan, L., Smith, B. B., Youngberg, J. A., Henderson, M. C., and Buhler, D. R.,** Role of the Ah locus in suppression of cytotoxic T lymphocyte activity by halogenated aromatic hydrocarbons (PCBs and TCDD): Structure-activity relationships and effects in C57Bl/6 mice congeneic at the Ah locus, *Fund. Appl. Toxicol.*, 14, 532, 1990.
88. **Holsapple, M. P., Morris, D. L., Wood, S. C., and Snyder, N. K.,** 2,3,7,8-Tetrachlorodibenzo-p-dioxin-induced changes in immunocompetence: possible mechanisms, *Annu. Rev. Pharmacol. Toxicol.*, 31, 73, 1991.
89. **Roberts, E. A., Shear, N. H., and Okey, A. B.,** The Ah receptor and dioxin toxicity: from rodent to human tissues, *Chemosphere,* 14, 661, 1985.
90. **Bandiera, S., Safe, S., and Okey, A. B.,** Binding of polychlorinated biphenyls classified as either phenobarbital, 3-methylchlolanthrene, or mixed type inducers to cytosolic Ah receptor, *Chem. Biol. Interact,* 39, 259, 1982.
91. **Holsapple, M., McCay, J., and Barnes, D.,** Immunosuppression without liver induction by subchronic exposure to 2,7-DCDD in adult female mice, *Toxicol. Appl. Pharmacol.*, 83, 445, 1986.
92. **Yap, H., Desaiah, D., and Cutkomp, L.,** Sensitivity of fish ATPase to PCBs, *Nature,* 233, 61, 1971.
93. **Lee, T. P. and Park, B. H.,** Effect of Aroclor 1254 on leukocyte glucose uptake, *J. Toxicol. Environ. Health,* 6, 607, 1980.
94. **Lee, T. P. and Park, B. H.,** Biochemical basis of Aroclor 1254 and pesticide toxicity *in vitro, Res. Comm. Chem. Pathol. Pharmacol.*, 25, 597, 1979.
95. **McConkey, D. J., Hartzell, P., Duddy, S. K., Hakansson, H., and Orrenius, S.,** 2,3,7,8-tetrachlorodibenzo-p-dioxin kills immature thymocytes by calcium-mediated endonuclease activation, *Science,* 242, 256, 1988.
96. **Germolec, D., Clark, G., Blank, J., and Luster, M.,** Protein phosphorylation and tyrosine kinase activity in TCDD exposed B-lymphocytes, *Toxicologist,* 10, (Abstr.), 288, 1990.
97. **Kramer, C., Johnson, K., Dooley, R., and Holsapple, M.,** 2,3,7,8-TCDD enhances antibody production and protein kinase activity in murine B cells, *Biochem. Biophys. Res. Commun.*, 145, 25, 1987.

Chapter 14

IN VITRO METHODS FOR ASSESSING CHEMICAL OR DRUG TOXICITY AND METABOLISM IN PRIMARY HEPATOCYTES

Nicholas J. DelRaso

TABLE OF CONTENTS

I. INTRODUCTION

The Johns Hopkins Center for Alternatives for Animal Testing estimates that approximately 17 to 22 million animals are used annually in U.S. laboratories and that testing of a new chemical will cost approximately 1.5 million dollars. Furthermore, pressures from animal rights groups will result in a need for alternatives to whole animal testing. Because the liver is the major site of chemical and drug biotransformation, it is the tissue of choice for metabolism and toxicity studies. Primary hepatocytes that maintain their *in vivo* characteristics make them ideal candidates for these types of studies. Therefore, it is not surprising to find that many *in vitro* toxicity and metabolism studies over the past 25 years have been conducted using primary hepatocytes. Additional information on the use of primary hepatocytes for toxicity screens can be found in a number of reviews.[18,21,88,93]

Total replacement of whole animal testing is not realistic at this time. However, animal reduction and refinement are achievable. It has recently been reported that animal use has been reduced by the employment of *in vitro* methods.[89] While many different cell types can be isolated and used for toxicity studies, the scope of this chapter will be limited only with primary hepatocytes. It should also be noted that no one cell type will substitute for whole animal studies. More than likely, a battery of assays using multiple cell types will be required to make predictions concerning toxicity with a high degree of confidence. It will also be important to conduct parallel *in vivo* studies with *in vitro* studies so that correlating of toxicity can be done. These studies require careful collaborative planning by both the toxicologist and cell biologist so that *in vitro* systems can be validated against *in vivo* toxicological data.

II. RATIONALE

The rationale for using primary hepatocytes to predict hepatotoxicity is that chemicals or drugs that exert a toxic effect on the isolated cell will exert that same effect on the whole organ. Recent advances in cell culture technology have led to the establishment of primary cultures of hepatocytes that maintain their *in vivo* functions for extended periods of time in culture. Furthermore, isolated cells can easily be fractionated for studies of toxic mechanisms at the subcellular level.

Two important mechanisms in normally functioning hepatocytes are phase I and phase II metabolic reactions. Phase I reactions are oxidation/reduction reactions of metabolism that involve, to a large extent, cytochrome P_{450}s. Frequently, metabolism of chemicals or drugs results in the production of toxic intermediate metabolites. These metabolites are detoxified by phase II conjugation reactions with cellular macromolecules such as glutathione. Therefore, it is important when using primary hepatocytes for chemical or drug toxicity studies that phase I and phase II cellular reactions are maintained. The advantage of using primary hepatocytes to screen chemical or drug hepatotoxicity is a savings in time, cost, and animal use. This is accomplished because *in vitro* screens identify compounds that are worthy of further study and result in better designed *in vivo* studies.

III. PRIMARY HEPATOCYTE ISOLATION AND CULTURE

A. LIVER PERFUSION MEDIA

The perfusion of the liver *in situ* (or of biopsy specimens) for the isolation and enrichment of primary hepatocytes involves a two-step method of blood removal and digestion. Removal of blood is accomplished by perfusing the liver or biopsy sample with a wash-out medium lacking calcium and magnesium and containing heparin. The formulation of this medium is shown in Table 1. This medium is sterilized by vacuum filtration through a 0.22-μm cellulose acetate membrane. The pH of the medium is adjusted as needed to 7.2 using sterile 1 *N* HCl or 1 *N* NaOH. Digestion is accomplished by perfusing the liver or biopsy sample, without interruption of flow, with a medium containing calcium, magnesium, and collagenase (*Clostridium histolyticum*). The formulation of this medium is presented in Table 2. This medium is also filter sterilized and pH adjusted as described above. Collagenase is not added to the digestion medium until the day it is to be used. There are a number of different types of collagenase sold commercially, and the choice of collagenase will depend on what works best for the researcher. Liver biopsy samples are perfused with a digestion medium containing a cruder collagenase preparation.

B. *IN SITU* RAT LIVER PERFUSION

Primary hepatocyte isolation *in situ* from the rat is performed according to the method by Berry and Friend[1] as described by Bonney[2] and Oldam et al.[3] with modifications. Prior to initiating the *in situ* rat liver perfusion, an operating board is placed in a drain pan to catch excess perfusion medium draining from the abdominal cavity. The wash-out and digestion media are placed in a waterbath at 39°C in relative proximity to the operating board. The perfusion tubing is constructed by attaching each end of two 1-ft sections of silicon tubing to the short arm of two 6-inch "L"-shaped Pyrex glass tubes (5 mm diameter), respectively. The other ends of these 1-ft sections of silicon tubing are attached to 2 arms of a Teflon "Y"-shaped connector. A 3-ft section of silicon tubing is then attached to the remaining arm of the "Y"-shaped connector. The Pyrex glass tubes are then inserted through two rubber stoppers, respectively. A second short length of Pyrex glass tubing is also inserted into the two stoppers for pressure equilization during perfusion. The rubber stoppers with inserted Pyrex glass tubing and all attached silicon tubing are autoclavable. The sterile stoppers are placed into the neck of the two perfusion media bottles, respectively. The media bottles are then allowed to incubate at 39°C for 30 min. A section of the 3-ft silicon tubing between the ends is placed into the pump head of a peristaltic pump. The free end of this 3-ft silicon tubing is attached to an aseptically cut (at the finger rests) 1-cm^3 syringe barrel. A sterile 22-ga indwelling catheter is then attached to the other end of the syringe barrel. The peristaltic pump is calibrated to deliver the perfusion media at a flow rate of 25 to 35 ml/min. Air is removed from the perfusion tubing by priming the 1-ft sections of silicon tubing with wash-out and digestion media through the Teflon "Y" connector, respectively, and then continuing through the 3-ft section with wash-out medium. The 1-ft section of

TABLE 1
Preparation of Wash-Out Liver Perfusion Medium for Blood Removal

Reagents	
10X Hanks' balanced salt solution (HBSS) (without magnesium and calcium)	100 ml
Sodium bicarbonate	2.2 g
HEPES	2.83 g
EGTA	0.19 g
Heparin solution (1000 U/ml)	2.0 ml
Distilled water	qs to 1 l

TABLE 2
Preparation of Liver Digestion Perfusion Medium

Reagents	
10X HBSS (complete)	100 ml
Sodium bicarbonate	2.2 g
HEPES	2.83 g
Collagenase (*Clostridium histolyticum*)	0.05–0.1%
Distilled water	qs to 1 l

Note: The amount of collagenase activity per mg will vary depending on the manufacturer. The collagenase (Boehringer Mannheim, IN) used in our laboratory has activity measured in Wunsch Units and is used at 0.26 U/ml.

silicon tubing leading from the digestion medium is clamped off when priming with wash-out medium.

A rat (200 to 300 g) is anesthetized by an intraperitoneal injection (1 ml/kg) with a mixture of ketamine (70 mg/ml) and xylazine (6 mg/ml). After the rat is anesthetized, it is prepared for surgery by shaving the abdominal area and then wiping this area with a disinfectant. The rat is then placed on its back on the operating board and the front and hind legs are secured. All of the following steps should be implemented aseptically. Using a scalpel, a vertical cut is made down the abdomen through the skin and subcutaneous tissue. Using straight scissors and forceps, a horizontal cut is then made through the muscular wall at the midline of the vertical incision at the lower abdomen. Complete opening of the abdominal cavity is accomplished by making a vertical cut through the muscular wall of the abdomen up to the sternum, making sure not to puncture the diaphragm or the liver. Two horizontal cuts are then made through the muscular wall of the lower abdomen below the kidneys, and the two flaps of tissue are held down using Vulsellum forceps. Curved forceps are used to remove connective tissue and fat from around the posterior vena cava between the renal vein and the liver. Two pieces of surgical thread are then pulled under the posterior vena cava, just above the renal vein, with a curved forcep and the threads loosely tied around the vein. With the 22-ga indwelling catheter primed with wash-out medium, the posterior vena cava is canulated one quarter inch below the threads and continuing within the vein beyond the threads. The threads are then tightened around the vein and catheter to prevent back pressure leakage of the perfusion medium. The chest cavity is quickly opened using scissors, and the posterior vena cava anterior to the diaphragm is clamped with a curved

TABLE 3
Preparation of Primary Hepatocyte Cell Wash Medium

Reagents	
10X HBSS	100 ml
Sodium bicarbonate	2.2 g
HEPES	2.83 g
Bovine serum albumin (BSA; fraction V)	1.0 g
Distilled water	qs to 1 l

hemostat. Immediately, the peristaltic pump is activated to force the wash-out medium containing heparin through the liver. The pressure within the liver is allowed to increase for 10 to 15 sec, and then the hepatic portal vein is cut to allow drainage of the perfusion media. It is necessary to massage the lobes of the liver with sterile moist cotton swabs to complete the removal of the blood. Periodically during the perfusion, sterile saline is gently syringed over the liver to keep it moist. After 10 to 12 min of perfusion with the wash-out medium, the tubing leading from the wash-out medium bottle is clamped off and the clamp on the tubing leading from the digestion medium bottle is removed. This step is performed without turning off the peristaltic pump. After 10 to 12 min of perfusion with the digestion medium, remove the liver with straight forceps and scissors and place into a sterile 100-mm petri dish containing ca. 20 ml of cell-wash medium (Table 3). Single cells are expelled from the liver by making incisions in each lobe of the liver with sterile scissors and then gently shaking the liver from side to side in the dish. Further release of cells is achieved by combing the lobes of the liver with a sterile 50-mm dog comb. After combing the lobes of the liver, the remainder of the liver is transferred to a second 100-mm petri dish containing ca. 20 ml of cell-wash medium, and the combing is repeated. The hepatocyte cell suspension from both petri dishes is pooled and transferred to a sterile 100-ml beaker. Stromal tissue is removed from the cell suspension by successive gentle vacuum filtrations through 250- and 62-μm pore size monofilament nylon mesh (Small Parts, Inc., Miami, FL) housed in sterile funnels on sterile 125-ml flasks, respectively. The filtered cell suspension is then transferred to sterile 50-ml centrifuge tubes and washed two times by centrifugation in cell-wash medium at 50 × g for 3 min.

C. PRIMATE LIVER BIOPSY DIGESTION

The perfusion of primate, or other species including human, liver biopsy specimens requires the use of an aseptic recirculating system. The perfusion apparatus is similar to that used to perfuse rat liver *in situ*, except that a second set of "L"-shaped Pyrex tubes are inserted through the rubber stoppers and into the perfusion media bottles. A second set of silicon perfusion tubing (two 1-ft and one 3-ft sections) with a teflon "Y" connector is made and the 1-ft sections are attached to the new "L"-shaped Pyrex tubes of the stoppers. The open end of the 3-ft section of silicon tubing is placed in a sterile reservoir. The middle section of this tubing is then inserted into the pump head of a second peristaltic pump. The purpose of this second perfusion tubing setup is to return the perfusion medium, draining from the liver biopsy specimen, back to their respective bottles. A sterile reservoir is placed directly below a sterile wire mesh that is placed on a ring stand. The biopsied liver specimens that are to be perfused are placed on the sterile wire mesh. The liver perfusion drain-off in the reservoir from the first 5 min of perfusion with each of the perfusion solutions is discarded.

For maximal yield of primary hepatocytes from biopsied material, specimens should be ca. 3.0 g with single cut surfaces. Exposed vessels on the cut surfaces of the biopsied liver specimens are perfused via a 22-ga indwelling catheter attached to the silicon perfusion tubing as described above. These liver specimens are perfused at a flow rate of 6 to 10 ml/min, with random movement of the catheter between 3 to 4 exposed vessels per specimen. The perfusion media are returned to their respective bottles at a flow rate comparable to that of the forward flow rate so that the recirculating closed system is in equilibrium with respect to flow. The wash-out and digestion media used to perfuse biopsied liver specimens are the same as that used to perfuse livers *in situ,* except that a cruder collagenase preparation with higher activity (317 U/ml; Sigma, St. Louis, MO) is used in the digestion medium. The biopsied specimens are perfused with the wash-out medium for ca. 30 min and with the digestion medium for 60 min. The digested liver specimens are then transferred to a sterile 100-mm petri dish, and the hepatocytes are released by gentle combing with a sterile 50-mm dog comb. Viable parenchymal hepatocytes are enriched as described below.

D. PRIMARY HEPATOCYTE ENRICHMENT

After washing the isolated hepatocyte suspension by centrifugation, the parenchymal hepatocytes are enriched by a low-speed iso-density Percoll (Pharmacia, Piscataway, NJ) centrifugation procedure described by Kreamer et al.[4] Stock isoosmotic Percoll (SIP) is made by adding 1 vol of 10X Hank's balanced salt solution (HBSS) to 9 vol of Percoll (d = 1.12 g/l). For experimental purposes, 21.6 ml of Percoll and 2.4 ml of 10X HBSS are added to sterile 50-ml conical centrifuge tubes. The pH of the SIP solution is adjusted to 7.2 by the addition of 0.1 ml of 1 *N* HCl to each centrifuge tube. The SIP tubes can be stored at 4°C for 2 mo. Parenchymal hepatocytes are enriched by first gently layering 26-ml aliquots of cell suspension onto 24-ml SIP solutions (d = 1.06 g/l). The centrifuge tubes are then inverted five times to ensure a homogeneous cell suspension. These tubes are then centrifuged at 50 × g for 10 min at 4°C. Viable parenchymal hepatocytes will pellet at the bottom of the centrifuge tubes. Nonparenchymal cells and nonviable cells will form a flocculent layer at the top of the centrifuge tubes. The supernate from this centrifugation step is carefully and aseptically aspirated off and the enriched hepatocytes are washed two times by centrifugation in cell-wash medium at 50 × g for 3 min. After the final wash, the hepatocytes are resuspended in supplemented Williams E (or Leibovitz's L-15) culture medium (pH 7.2; Table 4). If the hepatocytes are to be cultured in plates, they should be resuspended in Williams E culture medium (Table 4) supplemented with dexamethasone (200 ng/ml).

E. HEPATOCYTE CELL CULTURE

There are two types of experimental culture systems that can be employed for chemical or drug cytotoxic and metabolic studies using primary hepatocytes. The two types of culture systems are suspension and attachment cultures. Although suspension culture studies are rapid and relatively easy to utilize, there are limitations to be considered. The viability of primary hepatocytes in suspension decreases precipitously over time. Suspension cultures are suitable for chemical or drug toxicity and/or metabolism studies only for a 4- to 5-h exposure period.[5] Because primary hepatocytes in suspension maintain their cytochrome P_{450} levels for only a short period of time, they can be utilized for rapid evaluation of chemical or drug metabolism. However these cells lack the cell-to-cell association inherent in the intact organ. Furthermore, the membranes of these cells are impaired as a result of the isolation procedure, and enzymes and cofactors are leaked. Under appropriate culture conditions, attached primary hepatocyte cultures remain viable over longer culture times, retain a number of differentiated liver functions, and recover from injury sustained during isolation.[6] These characteristics make attached primary hepatocyte cultures ideally suited for acute and chronic toxicity and/or metabolism studies. However, it should be noted that cytochrome P_{450} will diminish with time in culture. Some cell culture techniques have resulted in the maintenance of cytochrome P_{450} levels for long periods of time in culture that are comparable

TABLE 4
Composition of Primary Hepatocyte Culture Medium

Reagents	
Williams E (or Leibovitz's L-15) powdered medium	1 l pkg
Fetal calf serum	5%
Insulin/transferrin/sodium selenite solution	5.0 ml
HEPES	2.83 g
Sodium bicarbonate	2.2 g
5-Aminolevulinic acid	17.0 mg
Gentamicin solution (10 mg/ml)	5.0 ml

to *in vivo* levels.[7–10] The procedures for utilizing the two types of primary hepatocyte culture are described below.

1. Suspension Cultures

Washed hepatocytes from the Percoll centrifugation are resuspended in Williams E medium (pH 7.2; Table 4) at a cell density of 5×10^5 cells/ml. Suspension cultures for experimental use are established by placing 4.0 ml of the resuspended cell suspension into 25-ml siliconized glass Erlenmeyer flasks. These cells can then be exposed to desired test agents. After initial exposure, suspension culture flasks are placed on a clinical rotator at 90 rpm and incubated for up to 5 h at 37°C in an incubator with 95% air and 5% CO_2.

2. Attachment Cultures

Prior to seeding isolated hepatocytes on tissue culture plates, the plates are coated with a biomatrix material so that differentiated cell functions can be maintained over an extended period of time in culture. Primary hepatocytes can also attach to other biomatrix coated material such as nylon mesh. The need for an extracellular matrix to maintain normally functioning hepatocytes has been previously demonstrated.[11] Once the distribution of the extracellular components in rat liver had been demonstrated,[12] the various components such as laminin, collagen type I, collagen type IV, and fibronectin were used to coat tissue culture surfaces. Although attachment efficiency and longevity of primary hepatocytes on these various substrates are indistinguishable, specific components of the extracellular matrix have been shown to modulate differentiated function and replication of hepatocytes in culture.[13–15] Therefore, for acute toxicity studies (<2 week) any of these biomatrix components may be suitable whereas chronic (>2 week) studies may require multiple extracellular components.[16,17] The procedure described below for coating tissue culture plates or nylon mesh with collagen type I is the one used in our laboratory for acute cytotoxicity screening.

a. Collagen-Coated Plates and Mesh

Collagen type I (or type IV) solution (4 mg/ml in 0.02 *N* acetic acid) can be prepared in the laboratory or purchased commercially. Using a micropipetter with sterile tip, 50-μl aliquots of collagen solution are pipetted into 60-mm tissue culture plates. The collagen solution is evenly spread over the plates using a sterile "L"-shaped glass rod. These plates are then placed into an ammonia vapor chamber, a desiccator jar containing gauze or cotton saturated with ammonium hydroxide. After 5 min, the plates are removed from the ammonia vapor jar to a laminar flow hood and 5.0 ml of sterile distilled water is added to each plate. The plates are allowed to stand at room temperature for 1 h and then the water is aseptically aspirated off. The steps of addition and aspiration of water are repeated two more times to rid the collagen gel of the cytotoxic ammonia. The last addition of water is allowed to remain in the plates overnight at 4°C. On the following day, the final plate rinse is aseptically aspirated and 4.0 ml of sterile culture medium containing fetal calf serum (FCS; 2 to 5%) is added. These plates can be stored at 4°C until needed. It is important that these collagen gels not be allowed to dry, or decreased hepatocyte viability and function may result. The procedure for collagen-coating nylon mesh is similar to that described above for plates. Sterile nylon mesh (20- to 62-μm pore size) is first placed into sterile 100-mm tissue culture plates, and collagen solution is evenly dispersed over the mesh as described above. The amount of collagen solution added to the mesh will depend on the size of the mesh being coated. The lids of the 100-mm plates are then returned to the plates, and the plates are placed in the ammonia vapor chamber for 5 min. The steps following the ammonia vapor exposure to set the collagen gels are the same as that described above for tissue culture plates.

b. Rat Hepatocytes, Plates

The washed isolated hepatocytes described above are resuspended at a cell density of 1 $\times$ 10^6/ml in Williams E (or Leibovitz's-15) culture medium (Table 4) supplemented with dexamethasone (200 ng/ml). The addition of dexamethasone is required to enhance hepatocyte attachment. Two-ml aliquots of the hepatocyte suspension are added to collagen gel-coated culture plates and the cells are allowed to attach for 3 to 4 h at 37°C in a 95% air/5% CO_2 incubator. After the hepatocytes have attached, the attachment culture medium is aseptically removed and 2.0 ml of fresh culture medium (without dexamethasone) is added back to the plates. The plates are then returned to the incubator for 24 h to allow hepatocytes damaged during the isolation procedure to recover. Following the recovery period, the culture medium is removed and fresh medium is added back. These plates can then be exposed to soluble or solubilized liquid or solid compounds for cytotoxicity and/or metabolism assessment.

c. Primate Hepatocytes, Plates

Primary primate hepatocytes are resuspended in attachment medium and seeded into collagen gel-coated plates as described above for rat hepatocytes. A problem that arises when establishing plate cultures of primary primate hepatocytes is the eventual fibroblastic overgrowth of the cultures. Therefore, Williams E culture medium lacking serum is added back to the cultures after hepatocyte attachment. This medium is supplemented with a commercially available serum-free media supplement solution (StimuCYTE, Upstate Biotechnology, Lake Placid, NY) at 2 to 5%. Alternately, specially formulated cell culture medium containing D-valine can be used, supplemented with 2 to 5% FCS. These two types of culture conditions allow parenchymal hepatocytes to survive while inhibiting fibroblastic growth. Primary primate hepatocyte cultures are incubated and exposed to soluble compounds as described above for rat hepatocytes.

d. Micro Roller Bottle, Mesh

Recent development of an airtight micro roller bottle (Figure 1; patent pending) in our laboratory, and the fact that primary hepatocytes attach to collagen-coated nylon mesh, has led to the establishment of an *in vitro* system for screening volatile compounds for cytotoxicity. The newly developed micro roller bottle is a modified Pyrex glass 20-ml gas chromatography (GC) sample vial with two open ends. The micro roller bottle is 40 mm in length with a circumference of 95 mm and can receive a 35 $\times$ 85-mm strip of collagen gel-coated nylon mesh. The micro roller bottle is made airtight by the insertion of Mininert valves (Pierce, Rockford, IL) into the open ends of the bottle. Before hepatocytes can be

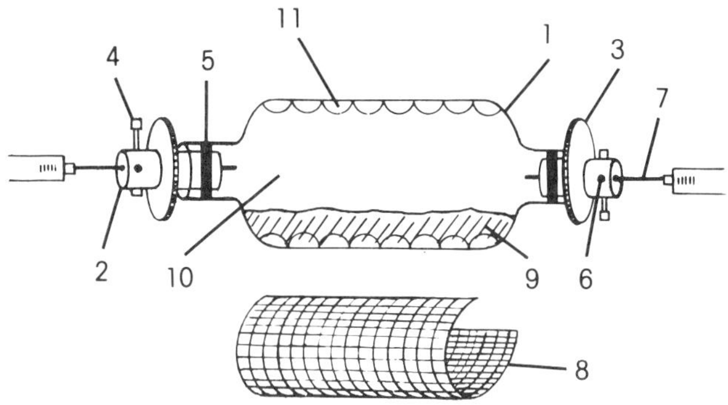

FIGURE 1. Schematic representation of micro roller bottle sytem for *in vitro* exposure to volatile compounds. (1) Pyrex glass roller bottle; (2) Mininert valve; (3) Mininert valve thumb wheel; (4) Mininert valve open/close button; (5) Mininert valve "O"-ring seal; (6) Mininert valve silicon injection septum; (7) side port needle; (8) 20- to 62-micron pore size nylon mesh; (9) hepatocyte culture medium; (10) roller bottle head space; and (11) cells.

exposed to volatile compounds in this micro roller bottle, they must be attached to the collagen gel-coated nylon mesh strip. The collagen gel-coated meshes are formed in 100-mm culture plates as described above. The Williams E culture medium containing FCS covering these stored mesh strips (4°C) is removed before the hepatocytes are added to them. Primary hepatocytes are first concentrated to a cell density of 5×10^5/0.1 ml in Williams E culture medium (Table 4) supplemented with dexamethasone so that 2×10^6 hepatocytes (0.4 ml) can be distributed over the mesh in a volume of medium that would minimize cell runoff from the mesh. While the hepatocytes are attaching to the mesh, the micro roller bottles are set up to receive the mesh by placing a Mininert valve into one end of the bottle. Just prior to adding the mesh to the micro roller bottles, 1.0 ml of Williams E culture medium (lacking dexamethasone) is added. Using forceps, a corner of the mesh in the culture plate is grasped and the mesh is rolled into a narrow tube. The narrow tube of mesh is then inserted into the roller bottle and the mesh is unrolled. Because there is medium in the roller bottle, the free end of the mesh is pulled to the glass surface and held in place. The forceps can then be released, and by gently rolling the roller bottle the mesh will unroll itself. Before placing the other Mininert valve into the roller bottles, 1.0 ml of Williams E culture medium is added bringing the total volume of culture medium in the roller bottles to 2.0 ml. The micro roller bottles are exposed to volatile compounds injected into the roller bottles with a 60-cm^3 syringe and side port needle. Volatile compounds of different concentrations are withdrawn from previously formulated standard bags using the 60-cm^3 syringe with side port needle and inserted through the Mininert valves of the micro roller bottles, respectively. Before flushing the micro roller bottle chamber with the volatile test compound, a second side port needle is inserted through the Mininert valve at the opposite end of the roller bottle to prevent excessive pressure build up during injection. After flushing the micro roller bottle chamber with test agent, the two side port needles are removed and both Mininert valves are closed. Control roller bottles are flushed with an incubator atmosphere of 95% air/5% CO_2. An atmosphere sample is then taken from all the micro roller bottles, except controls, and analyzed by GC to determine the concentration of test agent in the roller bottles. A second sample is taken at the termination of exposure to ensure that the test agent is present at a concentration of at least 95% of that measured at dosing. When the micro roller bottle is placed on a modified roller apparatus in an incubator at 37°C, hepatocytes are rotated so that they are exposed to both the medium and the experimental atmosphere. Medium samples for cellular lactate dehydrogenase (LDH) and aspartate aminotransferase (AST) leakages (assays discussed below), after various times of exposures, can be taken through the Mininert

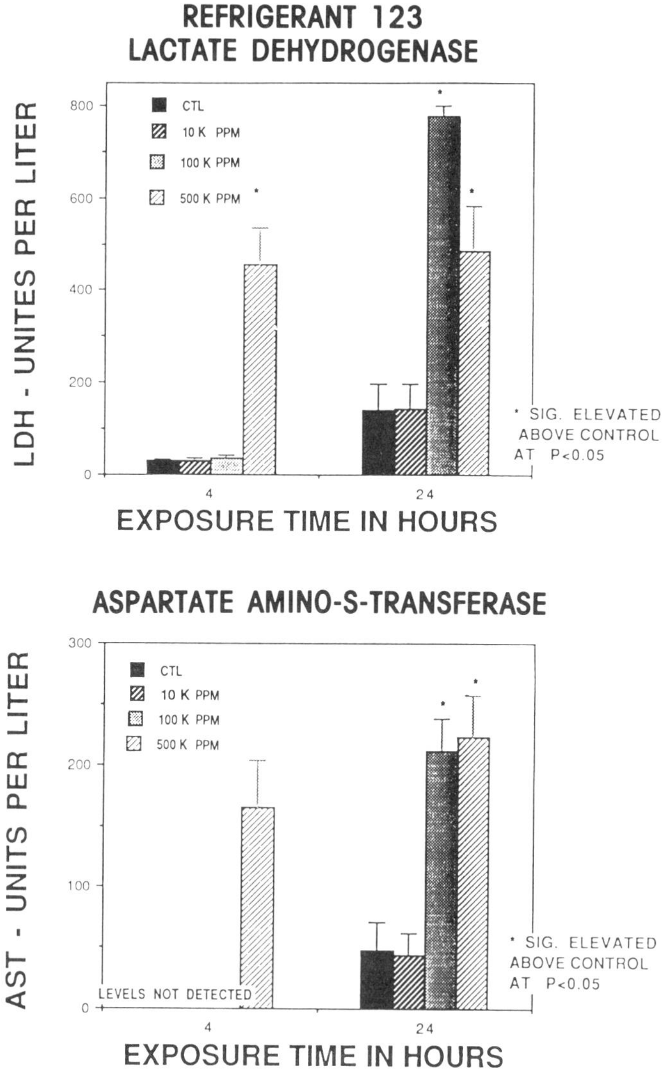

FIGURE 2. Leakage of LDH and AST from hepatocytes exposed to various concentrations of the volatile hydrochlorofluorocarbon refrigerant 2,2-dichloro-1,1,1-trifluoroethane (HCFC-123) for 4 and 24 h using a novel *in vitro* system.

valve, using a side port needle, without violating the experimental exposure conditions (Figure 2).

IV. CYTOTOXICITY ASSAYS

In order to assess chemical or drug cytotoxicity, alterations in cellular function and structure that lead to irreversible cell damage must be detected. Considering the vast number of biochemical pathways that exist in cells, there are a variety of biochemical indicators available that can be chosen to acquire information at the cellular, subcellular, and molecular levels. Deciding on which assay to perform and by which method can be difficult. A number of factors such as species specificity, sensitivity, reproducibility, and reliability must be taken into consideration when choosing an assay or method. A number of reviews have been written on the use of biochemical indicators for *in vitro* mechanistic and cytotoxic screening studies.[19–23] Because of the wide choice of biochemical indicators that can be used for cytotoxicity measures, only those used in our laboratory to assess hepatotoxicity will be discussed. The methods described below are not intended to provide an all-inclusive list of biochemical indicators for hepatocyte toxicity, but only those that we have found convenient and applicable to our experimental design.

A. CELL SAMPLE PREPARATION

Treated or untreated hepatocytes in 60-mm culture plates to be used in biochemical assay determinations are collected in 150 μl of cold 50-m*M* Tris-HCl/154-m*M* KCl buffer (pH 7.2). After the addition of this buffer to the plates, the cells (1.5 to 2.0 mg cell protein) are scraped using a rubber policeman and transferred to 1.5 ml conical microcentrifuge tubes on ice. After each plate has been harvested, the samples are sonicated 5 times for 5 sec at 50% maximum output. The samples are kept on ice until needed. Hepatocyte cell suspensions can also be used for biochemical determinations. Suspension cultures are centrifuged in 1.5-ml conical centrifuge tubes at 50 × g for 3 min and the supernate is discarded. The cell pellet is then resuspended in 150 μl of cold Tris-HCl/KCl buffer and sonicated as described above. A 5-μl sample of each cell sonicate is removed and placed into a 16 × 100-mm test tube containing 995 μl of phosphate-buffered saline (pH 7.2). The protein concentration in these tubes is then determined by the method described by Bradford[24] using a Coomasie brilliant blue G-250-based reagent. This reagent can be obtained commercially. The protein concentration of the samples is important because most of the cytotoxicity assays described below are normalized to cell protein.

B. CELL MEMBRANE INTEGRITY

Although the definition of cell death is still a matter of debate, it can be viewed functionally as the point when severe and irreversible injury leads to a biologically inactive cell. The integrity of the plasma membrane is directly related to a cell's ability to function normally and maintain its viability. A number of indicators such as trypan blue dye, fluorescein diacetate, or ethidium bromide can be used to assess irreversible membrane damage. The most commonly used indicator, especially for suspension cultures of cells, is trypan blue dye exclusion and will be described below. Because it has been generally accepted that the leakage of the cytosolic enzyme LDH correlates very well with viability, and is more precise than dye exclusion, it is very useful as an indicator of plasma membrane damage (Table 5). Furthermore, the high content of AST in the mitochondria[25] makes possible its use as an indicator of mitochondrial membrane integrity. These two enzymes (LDH and AST) should be monitored at the same time because certain chemicals or drugs may affect one or the other or both types of membranes (Figure 3). The automated procedures for both LDH and AST will be discussed below. It should be noted that it is possible to have enzyme leakage results that do not accurately reflect damage to the plasma membrane due to chemical- or drug-induced enzyme inhibition.[26]

1. Trypan Blue Dye Exclusion

A stock solution of trypan blue (0.4%) is prepared by weighing out 0.4 g into a 150-ml beaker containing 100 ml of 15 m*M*-4-(2-hydroxyethyl)-1-piperazineethanesulfonic acid (HEPES) buffered HBSS (pH 7.2). After stirring the solution for 5 min, the beaker is placed into a laminar flow hood and vacuum filter sterilized through a 0.2-μm pore filter. Because trypan blue is a suspected carcinogen, the contaminated filter should be disposed of by incineration. A working solution of trypan blue (0.08%) is made by aseptically adding 20 ml of the stock trypan blue solution to 80 ml of sterile HEPES-buffered HBSS. The pH of this solution is adjusted to 7.2 as necessary with sterile 1 *N* HCl or 1 *N* NaOH.

TABLE 5
Viability and LDH Leakage of Primary Hepatocytes Exposed to Increasing Concentrations of 2,3,4-TMP for 4 h in Suspension Cultures

TMP dose (m*M*)	Percent viability[a]	Percent LDH in cells
7.9	100[b](±2)	97 (±1)
12.0	99[c](±4)	92[c](±2)
15.7	86 (±5)	87 (±2)
19.1	63[c](±17)	51[c](±2)
31.5	0	0

[a] Viability was determined by trypan blue dye exclusion (0.08%).
[b] values represent the aveage mean (and one SEM) from four experiments incorporating replicate flasks.
[c] Values reflect three experiments (modified from DelRaso et al.[87]).

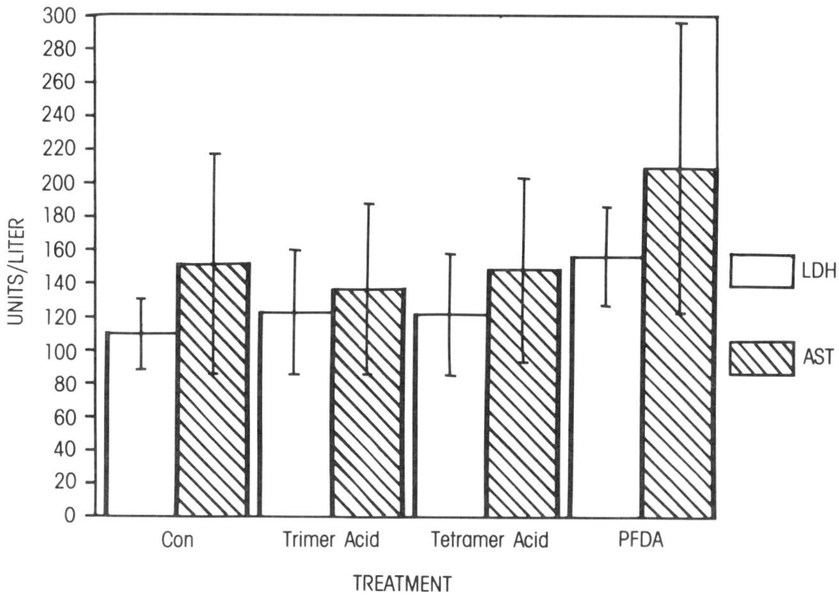

FIGURE 3. Leakage of LDH and AST from hepatocytes exposed to the halogenated fatty acids, C_6 chlorotrifluoroethylene oligomer acid (trimer acid), C_8 chlorotrifluoroethylene oligomer acid (tetramer acid), and perfluoro-*n*-decanoic acid (PFDA) at 50 μg/ml for 72 h.

The principle of trypan blue dye exclusion is that viable cells will exclude the dye, while nonviable cells take up the dye. To determine cell viability, 0.1 ml of cell suspension is added to 0.1 ml of trypan blue (0.08%) in a 12 × 75-mm test tube and mixed thoroughly. The test tube is then allowed to stand for 3 min. Cells should not be allowed to stand for extended periods of time because viable cells may begin to take up the dye. With a coverslip placed on a hemacytometer, a small amount of stained cell suspension is transferred to both chambers using a pasteur pipette. Care should be taken not to overfill or underfill the chambers. Beginning with the first chamber, all cells are counted in the center 1-mm square and four 1-mm corner squares. Cells touching the middle line of the top and left perimeter of each square should be counted. A separate count of viable and nonviable cells is noted. Counts should be repeated, with appropriate dilution factor, if greater than 10% of the cells appear clustered or if less than 20 or greater than 50 cells per square are observed. The number of cells per ml is calculated by multiplying the average total cell count per square by the reciprocal of the dilution factor. The resulting number is then multiplied by the reciprocal of the volume over each chamber ($1/10^{-4}$ cm^3 or 10^4). The final number is expressed as "x" number of cells per ml. The percent viability is determined by dividing the viable cell count by the total cell count and multiplying by 100.

2. Lactate Dehydrogenase Leakage

The LDH enzyme activity in suspension or plated cultures of primary hepatocytes can be determined by an automated method using a DuPont ACA clinical analyzer. This method is a modification of the enzymatic lactate to pyruvate procedure first reported by Wacker et al.[27] and later modified by Gay et al.[28] The principle of this procedure is that LDH catalyzes the oxidation of L-lactate to pyruvate with simultaneous reduction of nicotinamide adenine dinucleotide (NAD). The change in absorbance at 340 nm due to the appearance of reduced NAD (NADH) over time is directly proportional to the LDH activity.

One half milliliter of cell culture supernate is removed and placed into appropriately labeled 1.5-ml conical microcentrifuge tubes. These tubes are then centrifuged at 7000 × g for 5 min. After centrifugation, 0.4 ml of the supernate is removed and placed into a second set of 1.5-ml microcentrifuge tubes. Analysis of LDH activity must take place within 24 h of sampling. Stored sample must be at 4°C and not frozen. The LDH activity data are expressed as a percentage of total intracellular content. This is determined by lysing control cells using 0.6% Triton X-100 and then measuring the activity of the released LDH. The data are reported in international units per liter and are normalized by subtracting the average background LDH activity in the medium of control cells from the total intracellular value. It has generally been considered that only experiments in which the background LDH activity of control cells is ≤25% of the total available intracellular activity are valid.

3. Aspartate Aminotransferase Leakage

The AST activity in suspension or plated cultures of primary hepatocytes is determined by an automated method using a Kodak Ectachem clinical analyzer. The principle of this procedure is that in the presence of sodium pyridoxal-5-phosphate the amino group of L-aspartate is transferred to α-ketoglutarate to produce glutamate and oxaloacetate. Oxaloacetate is then converted to malate by malate dehydrogenase in the presence of NADH which is oxidized to NAD^+. The oxidation of NADH is monitored at 37°C by reflectance spectrophotometry at 340 nm and is used to measure AST activity. The activity of AST is reported in international units per liter and is derived by the conversion of the rate of change in reflectance density in the linear region.

Supernate sample preparation from hepatocyte suspension or plated cultures is the same as that described for LDH. Ten microliters of culture supernate is deposited on an Ektachem AST clinical chemistry multilayer slide and the sample is analyzed. Because a small amount of sample is required for this method, both LDH and AST activities can be determined from the same sample.

C. PHASE I METABOLIC REACTIONS

Metabolism of chemicals or drugs involves two sequential mechanisms known as phase I and phase II reactions. Phase I reactions involve the oxidation/reduction of chemicals or drugs to form more polar water soluble metabolites. Most of these reactions are carried out

TABLE 6
Reaction Mixture Reagents and Buffers Used to Assess Cytochrome P-450 Activity in Primary Hepatocytes

Buffers	
Tris-HCL	50 m*M*, pH 7.8
Glycine-NaOH	1.0 *M*, pH 10.6
Sodium chloride	0.1 *M*
Reagents	
7-Ethoxycoumarin	19.0 mg/ml
NADP	74.6 mg/ml
D-Isocitric acid	284.0 mg/ml
Magnesium sulfate (anhydrous)	120.0 mg/ml
Isocitrate dehydrogenase	100 U/ml

by the mixed function oxidase system, of which the various forms of cytochrome P_{450} are major components. Because of the many different isozyme forms of cytochrome P_{450}, and other phase I enzymatic reactions, the choice of assay will be dependent on the experimental question asked. However, the general overall activity of all the major forms of phase I reactions can be obtained by using a broad substrate. If a particular cytochrome P_{450} isozyme or other phase I enzyme activity is being studied, more specific substrates such as ^{14}C-laurate[29] (CYP4A1), benzo[a]pyrene[30] (aryl hydrocarbon hydroxylase; CYP1A1), and ethoxyresorufin[31] (polycyclic aromatic hydrocarbon dealkylation; CYP1A2) can be chosen. Due to the scope of this chapter, only the method for the general overall cytochrome P_{450} activity using the broad substrate 7-ethoxycoumarin (7-EC) will be discussed in detail below.

1. 7-Ethoxycourmarin-O-Deethylation (ECOD) Activity

A sensitive indicator of overall monooxygenase activity (phase I reactions) is the O-deethylation of 7-EC to the highly fluorescent product 7-hydroxycoumarin (7-HC). The formation of this product can be monitored directly[32] or indirectly by a series of extractions.[33] However, the indirect method is more sensitive and recent modifications have further increased this sensitivity.[34,35] Therefore, the fluorometric assay utilized by Gray et al.[35] for primary hepatocytes will be discussed below.

a. Buffer and Reagents

The composition of the buffers and a list of assay reagents is presented in Table 6. A working stock of 50-m*M* Tris-HCl buffer (pH 7.8) is made by adding 33.7 ml of 0.1 *N* HCl to 25 ml of 0.2-*M* Tris-base solution. The pH of the Tris-HCl buffer is adjusted to 7.8 with 1 *N* HCl or 1 *N* NaOH if needed, and the total volume of buffer is brought to 100 ml with distilled water. A 0.5-*M* glycine-NaOH buffer (pH 10.6) is made by adding 22 ml of 2.0 *N* NaOH to 50 ml of a 1-*M* glycine solution. The pH of the resulting buffer is adjusted to 10.6 with 2.0 *N* NaOH if necessary, and the final volume is brought to 100 ml with distilled water. Each of the reaction mixture components (NADP, DL-isocitric acid, isocitrate dehydrogenase, and magnesium sulfate) are made up in 2.0 ml of 50-m*M* Tris-HCl buffer, respectively. Each respective reaction mixture component is then aliquoted (100 μl) into 500-μl sample tubes and frozen at −20°C (ca. 20 tubes/reagent). The reaction mixture components are frozen in aliquots sufficient to run five assays with corresponding blanks. Complete reaction mixture is prepared by adding 1 tube of each of the 4 components indicated above into 19.4 ml of the Tris-HCl buffer.

b. Standards

A stock solution of 7-HC (25 m*M*; mol wt 162.14) is made by adding 4.1 mg to 10 ml of methanol. Four 10-fold serial dilutions of this 7-HC stock solution are then made in 0.1 ml of methanol, resulting in a range of standards from 25 m*M* to 2.5 μ*M*. Twenty-five μl of each standard is added to the reaction mixture, respectively, after the reaction mixture has been incubated for 30 min at 37°C and acidified by the addition of 4 *N* HCl. The reaction mixture is then extracted with chloroform and glycine NaOH buffer and read in a spectrofluorometer as described in the assay procedure below. The standards should be run two additional times on different days to account for technical and instrument variations. A standard curve can then be generated from the pooled fluorescence determinations made on each day. The equation used to define the resulting standard curve is used to determine unknown concentrations of 7-HC in test samples.

c. Assay Procedure

The methanolic 7-EC substrate solution is made the day the assay is to be run and is kept at 4°C until needed. Complete reaction mixture buffer is aliquoted (1.98 ml) into a sufficient number of acid cleaned 16 × 100-mm glass test tubes to accommodate all "test" samples, blanks, and three of the standards (25 m*M* and two others). Using cell sonicates prepared as described above (Section IV.A), 10 μl (ca. 100- to 150-μg cell protein) is added to both "test" and "blank" tubes. The 7-EC substrate (10 μl) is then added to only the "test" samples. All tubes are then incubated at 37°C with vigorous shaking in a vortex evaporator. After 30 min of incubation, the reaction is terminated by the addition of 0.5 ml of 4.0 *N* HCl to all tubes. The contents of the tubes are then transferred to a second set of acid-cleaned tubes with ground glass stoppers, and 6.0 ml of spectrophotometric grade chloroform is added to each tube. Prior to extraction, 10 μl of 7-EC is added to the "blank" tubes, and 25 μl of the three 7-HC standards are added to their respective tubes. Methanol (25 μl) is added to the standard "blank" tube. The tubes are then extracted by vigorous shaking for 1 min on a vortex. After vortexing, 4.0 ml of the chloroform layer is removed from each tube and placed into a third set of acid-cleaned glass tubes with ground glass stoppers. The chloroform containing the fluorescent 7-HC product is then extracted by the addition of 4.0 ml of glycine-NaOH buffer (pH 10.6) followed by vigorous vortexing for 1 min. Approximately 3.0 ml of the glycine-NaOH buffer is removed from each tube and placed into acid-cleaned quartz cuvettes. The fluorescence of the "test" samples, along with the 3 standards, are determined in a spectrofluorometer at an excitation wavelength of 380 nm and an emission maximum of 452 nm. The three standards are read along with the "test" samples to validate the previously determined standard curve. The molar concentration of 7-HC formed in test sample is derived from the equation of the standard curve. The resulting molar concentrations of 7-HC formed are converted to nmol amounts, normalized to mg of cell protein in the reaction mixture, and expressed as a rate of product formed per min (nmol/mg/min). An example of the effects of various halogenated fatty acids on cytochrome P450 activity in primary hepatocytes cultured for 96 h is presented in Table 7 and illustrates the usefullness of using primary hepatocytes to evaluate chemical or drug effects on phase I reactions.

D. PHASE II CONJUGATION REACTIONS

The products of phase I reactions of xenobiotics produced by the mixed function oxidase system are generally electrophilic metabolites. The detoxification of these metabolites, as well as peroxides, proceeds through conjugation reactions that convert these toxic nonpolar metabolites to more polar compounds that can be excreted via the bile or urine.[36] However, it should also be noted that the products of phase I metabolism may generate nontoxic metabolites that are bioactivated to toxic moieties by phase II conjugation reactions.[37] The

TABLE 7
Phase I and Phase II Reactions in Primary Rat Hepatocytes after Exposure to Various Halogenated Fatty Acids

Assay	Treatment[a]			
	Conc	Trimer acid	Tetramer acid	PFDA
7-ECOD (nmol/min/mg)	0.13 ± 0.10[b]	0.31 ± 0.18*	0.19 ± 0.15	0.08 ± 0.04
GSH (nmol/mg)	17.5 ± 10.3	23.7 ± 12.2	7.8 ± 2.4*	2.3 ± 1.5*
GST (nmol/min/mg)	609.0 ± 204.3	676.7 ± 114.2	539.2 ± 81.5	462.3 ± 133.3

[a] All treatment groups were dosed at 50 μg/ml in 0.5% DMSO for 96 h. Controls were dosed with DMSO at 0.5%.
[b] Values represent the mean and standard deviation from three experiments with triplicate plates for each treatment group.
* Significantly different from control as determined by a multifactorial ANOVA with Tukey post hoc comparisons of significant means at $p \leq 0.05$.

metabolites formed by phase I reactions can form conjugates with glucuronic acid, glycine, sulfates, glutathione (GSH), and others.[38] Because liver GSH plays an important role in the detoxification of xenobiotics, it will be discussed in more detail below. The conjugation of toxic intermediates with GSH is catalyzed by the enzyme glutathione *S*-transferase (GST) which also plays an important role in detoxification reactions. Therefore, this enzyme will also be discussed below. Chemical or drug treatment that results in depletion of GSH, or decreased GST activity, in hepatocytes makes them more susceptible to cell damage by increasing the probability of electrophilic metabolite interactions with cellular membranes and macromolecules. An example of using primary hepatocytes to rapidly screen chemical or drug effects on GSH level and GST activity is presented in Table 7.

1. Glutathione Determination

Glutathione is a small peptide containing only 3 amino acid residues (glutamic acid, glycine, and cysteine) and exists in the thiol-reduced (ca. 99%) and disulfide-oxidized (ca. 1%) forms. The enzymes GSH peroxidase and GST are highly specific for GSH and play key roles in detoxification reactions. The conjugation of GSH with activated metabolic electrophiles and oxygen-derived electrophiles protects against cell damage by scavenging these highly reactive free radicals that can interact with critical cellular components. Therefore, by monitoring changes in GSH homeostasis, an indication of the potential for cell injury can be determined. Additional information on the function and regulation of GSH can be found in a number of reviews.[39-43] The fluorescence assay described below for measuring GSH content in primary hepatocytes in an adaptation of the method developed by Hissin and Hilf.[44]

a. Buffer and Reagents

The composition of the buffer and a list of the reagents used in the assay to measure GSH levels in primary hepatocyte cultures are presented in Table 8. The sodium phosphate-ethylenediaminetetraacetic acid (EDTA) buffer (SPEB; pH 8.0) is made by dissolving 12.0 g of sodium phosphate (monobasic) and 1.47 g of EDTA (disodium) in 1 l of distilled water. The pH of SPEB is adjusted to 8.0 with 1 *N* NaOH if necessary. The metaphosphoric acid and *O*-phthalaldehyde solutions are made the day the assay is to be run. The 25% meta-

TABLE 8
Reaction Mixture Used in the Determination of Cellular GSH Levels

Buffer	
Sodium phosphate (monobasic)	0.1 *M*, pH 8.0
EDTA (disodium)	5.0 m*M*
Reagents	
Metaphosphoric acid	25% (wt/vol)
O-Phthalaldehyde	1.0 mg/ml, methanol

phosphoric acid solution is made by dissolving 2.5 g of the acid into 7.5 ml of distilled water in a 10-ml volumetric flask. After the acid has dissolved, the final volume is brought to 10.0 ml with distilled water. *O*-Phthalaldehyde is a nonfluorescent compound that becomes highly fluorescent when conjugated to GSH. A working solution of this compound is made by dissolving 2.0 mg in 2.0 ml of methanol.

b. Standards

A stock 130-μM GSH (mol wt 307.33) solution (40 μg/ml) is made in 5.0 ml of SPEB. Four serial dilutions of this GSH solution are made in 1.0 ml of SPEB resulting in final concentrations of 65 μ*M*, 6.5 μ*M*, 0.65 μ*M*, and 65 n*M*, respectively. These GSH standards are made up each time a standard curve is to be generated. The standards (0.1 ml) are added to 16 × 100-mm test tubes containing 1.8 ml of SPEB and 0.1 ml of *O*-phthalaldehyde. The "blank" tube is set up in the same manner except that GSH is omitted. The fluorescence of the standards is then determined in acid-cleaned quartz cuvettes using a spectrofluorometer as indicated in the GSH assay procedure below. The GSH standard curve is generated in the same manner as that described previously for the 7-ECOD assay.

c. Assay Procedure

Hepatocyte cell sonicates are prepared as previously described and 75 μl (ca. 0.5- to 1.0-mg cell protein) of each sonicate is added to 1.5 ml micro centrifuge tubes containing 0.5 ml of SPEB and 0.15 ml of 25% metaphosphoric acid for protein precipitation. These tubes are then placed in a freezer at −20°C for 10 to 15 min, without freezing, to enhance protein precipitation. Following this chilling period, the tubes are centrifuged at 20,000 × g for 30 min at 4°C in a microcentrifuge. After centrifugation, a 4-fold dilution of the supernate is made by removing 0.5 ml from each tube and adding them to appropriately labeled 16 × 100-mm test tubes containing 1.5 ml of SPEB. A subsequent 20-fold dilution is made by removing 0.1 ml from these tubes and adding them to a second set of appropriately labeled 16 × 100-mm test tubes containing 1.8 ml of SPEB and 0.1 ml of *O*-phthalaldehyde. The fluorescence of the "test" samples, along with 3 of the GSH standards, is determined in a spectrofluorometer at an excitation wavelength of 350 nm and an emission maximum of 420 nm. The "blank" tube used for the GSH standards is also used with the unknown "test" samples. The GSH concentration of the "test" samples is derived from the molar GSH standard curve and is then converted to a nmol amount. The sample dilutions are factored in and the nmol amount of GSH is normalized to mg cell protein. Results are typically reported in nmol GSH/mg protein.

2. Glutathione *S*-Transferase (GST) Activity

The critical role of SH in the detoxification of hydrophilic electrophiles generated by metabolism has been generally stated above. As previously mentioned, the enzyme that catalyzes the conjugation of GSH with these toxic intermediates of metabolism is GST. This

TABLE 9
Reaction Mixture Used in the Determination of GST Activity in Primary Hepatocytes

Buffer	
Potassium phosphate (monobasic)	0.1 *M*, pH 6.5
Reagents	
1-Chloro-2,4-dinitrobenzene	12.2 mg/ml, ethanol
Glutathione	6.2 mg/ml

enzyme exists as a group of at least eight cytosolic isozymes with multifunctional properties.[45,46] This group of isozymes is also capable of direct binding of toxic electrophilic metabolites[47] and detoxification of hydroperoxides resulting from cell membrane and DNA oxygen-free radical damage.[48,49] Therefore, measurements of GST activity may help explain decreased detoxification of electrophilic metabolites when it appears that GSH levels are unaffected. To acquire a general knowledge of the overall activity of GST, the substrate 1-chloro-2,4-dinitrobenzene (CDNB) with broad GST specificity is used. The procedure described below for GST activity is that of Ahmed et al.[50]

a. *Buffer and Reagents*

The composition of the buffer and a list of the reagents required to assess GST activity in primary hepatocyte cultures is presented in Table 9. After preparing the monobasic potassium phosphate buffer (PPB; 13.6 g/l), the pH is adjusted to 6.5 by the addition of 1 *N* HCl. The solutions of CDNB and GSH are prepared the day the assay is to be run.

b. *Assay Procedure*

Prior to initiating the GST activity assay, 1.4 ml of PPB is placed into appropriately labeled 12 × 75-mm test tubes. A 5-μl sample of hepatocyte cell sonicate (ca. 10 μg protein) is added to both "test" and corresponding "blank" tubes. The tubes are then allowed to stand at room temperature for 10 min. Following this 10 min incubation, 25 μl of CDNB is added to both "test" and "blank" tubes and the tubes are mixed by vortexing. The "test" sample, along with its corresponding "blank", is read at 25°C on a dual beam spectrophotometer. The "test" sample (without GSH) and "blank" are placed in 1-cm path length cuvettes, and the background absorbance rate is determined at a wavelength of 340 nm. After determining the background activity, 50 μl of GSH is added to the "test" sample only, and the "test" sample and "blank" are read again in the spectrophotometer. Cellular GST activity is determined from the spectrophotometric measurement at 340 nm of the rate of formation of NADH resulting from the conjugation reaction of GSH with CDNB. Based on the linear absorbance rate per minute for the assay, and assuming an extinction coefficient of 4.906 cm^{-1} mM^{-1}, GSH activity is expressed as nmol of NADH formed per minute. Typically, the data are normalized to the amount of cell protein (mg) in the reaction mixture and are reported as the amount of NADH formed per min/mg protein.

E. PEROXISOMAL β-OXIDATION

Peroxisomes are cytoplasmic organelles that possess numerous enzymes involved in alternate routes of metabolism of fatty acids. Liver enlargement and induction of peroxisomal fatty acid β-oxidation have been shown to be produced by a wide variety of chemicals in rodents.[51,52] There has been mounting evidence that there is a positive correlation between exposure to peroxisome proliferators and liver tumor formation in rodents.[53-55] It has been proposed that nongenotoxic hepatocarcinogenesis develops as a result of hydroperoxides generated from the induction of peroxisomal β-oxidation enzyme activities.[53] Whether the

TABLE 10
Species Response Differences of Hepatocytes Exposed to Two Chlortrifluoroethylene Oligomer Acid Peroxisome Proliferators *In Vitro*

		Assay (nmol/min/mg)	
Treatment[a]	Species	Palmitoyl CoA β-Oxidation[b]	Carnitine acetyltransferase[b]
Control	Rat	0	3.5 ± 1.4[c]
	Primate	0	5.4 ± 1.3[d]
Trimer acid	Rat	13.2 ± 7.7	28.7 ± 13.6*
	Primate	0	12.6 ± 1.3*
Tetramer acid	Rat	11.3 ± 5.3	23.7 ± 11.1*
	Primate	0	7.2 ± 3.3

[a] Rat and primate treatment groups were dosed at 50 μg/ml in 0.5% DMSO for 96 and 120 h, respectively. Controls were dosed with DMSO at 0.5%.
[b] Values represent the mean and standard deviation from three experiments (rat) or one experiment (primate) in triplicate plates.
* Significantly different from control as determined by a multifactorial ANOVA with Tukey post hoc comparisons of significant means at $p \leq 0.05$.

relationship between peroxisomal peroxisome proliferation and hepatocarcinogenesis is a casual or causal one remains unclear. While induction of peroxisomal β-oxidation has been associated with carcinogenesis, several studies have shown species[56-60] and compound potency[51,61] response differences. However, these response differences have been demonstrated *in vitro* (Table 10.)[35,62-65] Although peroxisome proliferation has been suggested to be only a rodent response, some studies have indicated that it does occur in primates[66] and man[67] at lower rates. Therefore, by correlating *in vivo/in vitro* studies and appropriate human hepatocyte studies, the potential carcinogenic risk of peroxisome proliferators in humans can be assessed. Two commonly measured fatty acid β-oxidation enzymes *in vitro*, acyl-CoA oxidase (ACO) and carnitine acetyltransferase (CAT), will be discussed in detail below. A number of reviews on peroxisomal enzymes and their biology can be consulted for further information.[68-70]

1. Cyanide-Insensitive Acyl-CoA Oxidase

Peroxisomal ACO is assessed by the cyanide-insensitive oxidation of palmitoyl-CoA as described by Gray et al.[35] This method is based on the spectrophotometric assay of peroxisomal β-oxidation described by Lazarow.[71] The principle of this assay is that in the presence of palmitoyl CoA, NAD is reduced to NADH during the β-oxidation spiral reaction. The reduction of NAD in the absence of substrate is subtracted from the total measured activity. Therefore, peroxisomal β-oxidation is described as acyl-CoA-dependent NAD reduction. Because cyanide does not inhibit peroxisomal β-oxidation *in vitro,* it can be used in crude subcellular fractions to inhibit reoxidation of the NADH formed. The spectrophotometric procedure for measuring peroxisomal β-oxidation in primary hepatocyte cultures is discussed below.

a. Buffer and Reagents

The composition of the buffer and a list of reagents required to assess peroxisomal β-oxidation in primary hepatocyte cultures is presented in Table 11. The 50-m*M* Tris-HCl (pH 7.8) used in the assay reaction mixture is the same as that used in the 7-ECOD assay described above (Section IV.C.1.a). The reaction mixture components are made up in

TABLE 11
Reaction Mixture Used to Determine the Rate of Peroxisomal β-Oxidation in Primary Hepatocyte Cultures

Buffer	
Tris-HCl	50 m*M*, pH 7.8
Reagents	
Bovine serum albumin (fraction V)	30.0 mg/ml
Triton X-100	2% (wt/vol)
Potassium cyanide (KCN)	10.0 mg/ml
Dithiothreitol (DTT)	321.0 mg/ml
Coenzyme A	10.0 mg/ml
Nicotinamide adenine dinucleotide (NAD)	16.6 mg/ml
Palmitoyl CoA-potassium	25.2 mg/ml

1.0 ml volumes. All of these components, except dithiothreitol (DDT), palmitoyl-CoA, and potassium cyanide (KCN), are aliquoted into 250-μl Eppendorf tubes (100 μl) and frozen at −20°C. Palmitoyl-CoA and DDT are added to 250-μl Eppendorf tubes in 20- and 30-μl aliquots, respectively. These tubes are then also frozen at −20°C. Addition of one tube each of the reaction mixture components to 9.5 ml of the 50-m*M* Tris-HCl buffer is sufficient to run 5 assays with corresponding blanks. The KCN solution is made by dissolving 10.0 mg in 1.0 ml of distilled water and is used the day the assay is to be run by adding 100 μl to the reaction mixture.

b. Assay Procedure

After adding the reaction mixture components and KCN to the 50-m*M* Tris-HCl buffer, the complete reaction mixture is incubated at 37°C for 30 min. Spectrophotometric cuvettes (1-cm path length)are kept at 37°C in a water bath. Prior to initiating the assay, 988 μl of reaction mixture and 10 μl of cell sonicate (100 to 150 μg protein) are added to paired cuvettes, and the background activity over 5 min is determined using a dual beam spectrophotometer at a wavelength of 340 nm. The rate of peroxisomal β-oxidation is then determined after the addition of 2 μl of palmitoyl-CoA to the "test" cuvette only; both the "test" and "blank" cuvettes are mixed by inversion prior to reading. Using the linear absorbance rate calculated by the instrument, and assuming an extinction coefficient of 6.22 cm^{-1} mM^{-1}, the rate of peroxisomal β-oxidation of palmitoyl-CoA is determined. If background activity was determined, it must be subtracted from the total rate. The resulting rate is then normalized per mg of cell protein in the cuvette and is typically reported in nmol of NADH formed per min/mg protein.

2. Carnitine Acetyltransferase

The fatty acid β-oxidation enzyme CAT is found predominantly in the mitochondria (54% total enzyme activity) and in lower concentrations in peroxisomes (14% total enzyme activity).[72] This enzyme is responsible for catalyzing the acylation of carnitine (a stimulator of mitochondrial fatty acid oxidation) with fatty acids and plays an important role in fatty acid oxidation in mitochondria. In contrast to peroxisomal β-oxidation, mitochondrial fatty acid oxidation is dependent on an active electron transport system. Therefore, this enzyme is sensitive to cytochrome inhibitors such as KCN. Increased levels of palmitoyl-CoA oxidation and CAT activity seen *in vitro,* with concomitant increase in peroxisome number, have been previously shown to correlate very well with *in vivo* results.[35,73–76] The assay for CAT activity is based on the colorimetric method described by Ellman.[77] This activity is measured spectrophotometrically and is described below.

TABLE 12
Reaction Mixture Used to Measure Carnitine Acetyltransferase Activity in Primary Hepatocyte Cultures

Buffer	
Tris-HCl	50 m*M*, pH 8.0
Reagents	
Acetyl CoA-sodium	20.0 mg/ml
EDTA (disodium)	46.5 mg/ml
DL-Carnitine	123.5 mg/ml
Dithio-(2-nitrobenzoic acid (DTNB)	3.1 mg/ml

a. Buffer and Reagents

The composition of the buffer and a list of the reagents required to assess the activity of CAT in primary hepatocyte cultures is presented in Table 12. The 50-m*M* Tris-HCl buffer (pH 8.0) is made by adding 25 ml of 200-m*M* Tris-base to 27.9 ml of 0.1 *N* HCl and bringing the total volume to 100 ml with distilled water. The acetyl-CoA component of the reaction mixture is made by dissolving 25 mg in 1.25 ml of this Tris-HCl buffer. The EDTA and DL-carnitine reaction mixture components are made by dissolving 93.0 mg and 247.0 mg in 2.0 ml of Tris-HCl buffer (pH 8.0), respectively. The substrate 5,5-dithiobis(2-nitrobenzoic)acid (DTNB) is made the day the assay is to be run and 12.4 mg is dissolved in 4.0 ml of Tris-HCl buffer (pH 8.0). The acetyl-CoA and EDTA reaction mixture components are aliquoted (100 μl) into 250-μl Eppendorf tubes and frozen at −20°C, respectively. The DL-carnitine is added to 250-μl Eppendorf tubes in 50-μl aliquots and frozen as above. The addition of each tube of reaction mixture component, except DL-carnitine, to 9.4 ml of Tris-HCl buffer (pH 8.0) is sufficient to run 5 assays with corresponding "blanks".

b. Assay Procedure

Complete reaction mixture and paired cuvettes (1-cm path length) are maintained in a water bath at 37°C. Using a micropipetter, 985 μl of reaction mixture and 10 μl of cell sonicate (100 to 150 μg protein) are added to paired cuvettes. The cuvettes are then mixed by inversion and the background activity determined in a dual beam spectrophotometer at a wavelength of 412 nm for 5 min. After determining the background activity, 5 μl of DL-carnitine is added to the "test" cuvette only. The "test" and "blank" cuvettes are then mixed by inversion and the CAT activity is measured. The rate of CAT activity is determined, after subtracting the background rate, using the instrument-calculated linear absorbance rate of the formation of acyl carnitine DTNB derivatives and an assumed extinction coefficient of 13.6 cm^{-1} mM^{-1}. This activity is then normalized to mg cell protein in the cuvette by dividing the activity rate per min by the measured protein. The rate of CAT activity measured in primary hepatocyte cultures is typically reported in nmol/min/mg protein.

V. METABOLISM

A. INTRODUCTION

Whole animal studies have been traditionally used to study the biotransformation of chemicals and drugs. Technical problems involved with preservation, separation, and isolation of metabolites and nonmetabolized parent compounds from tissues and biological fluids limit their use in such studies. The value of using primary hepatocytes that maintain their *in vivo* functions in culture to study chemical or drug toxicity has been discussed above. Furthermore, primary hepatocytes that maintain their differentiated functions are extremely useful for studying relationships between normal cell metabolism and chemical or drug biotransformation. The maintenance of the cytochrome P450 family of isoenzymes and metabolic activities at *in vivo* levels has been found to be dependent on specific media supplementations and other media components.[78–80] Because the activity of a number of the cytochrome P450 isozymes can be detected in primary hepatocyte cultures using specific xenobiotic substrates, primary hepatocytes can also be used in metabolic studies to determine which isozyme of cytochrome P450 contributes to the metabolism in cultured cells. While hepatic microsomes from isolated hepatocytes or liver tissue can also be used in *in vitro* metabolic studies, they may not accurately reflect the *in vivo* or intact cell situation.[81] Because microsome preparations lack cytosolic enzymes and cofactors, metabolites formed in the cytosol of intact cells may go undetected. Recently, it has been shown that some of the metabolites of 1,3-diaminobenzene identified *in vivo* and in primary hepatocyte cultures were not formed using the microsomal system.[82] The use of isolated cells for toxicity studies,[83] and analytical methods for metabolite isolation and identification,[84] have been reviewed.

B. EXAMPLE

2,3,4-Trimethylpentane (2,3,4-TMP), a principal constituent of gasoline that is used in assigning "octane rating", has been shown to induce a hydrocarbon nephropathy in male rats.[85] The metabolites of 2,3,4-TMP have previously been identified *in vivo* in the urine of male rats.[86] An *in vitro* study was conducted to determine if these metabolites could be identified in 4-h suspension cultures of primary hepatocytes. Replicate culture flasks containing 4.0 ml of cell suspension, at a cell density of 1×10^6 hepatocytes/ml, were dosed with a nonlethal concentration of 2,3,4-TMP. After 4 h of exposure, the replicate flasks were pooled and centrifuged at $50 \times g$ for 3 min. Both the supernate and washed cells were saved for metabolite extraction. Supernate and/or cells were first acidified to a pH of 4.4 and then hydrolyzed with glucuronidase-sulfatase at 37°C for 16 h. The samples were then poured onto Clin ELUT disposable columns (Analytichem International, Harbor City, CA), and the metabolites were eluted with methylene chloride. The methylene chloride-extracted metaboliteswere concentrated under nitrogen and then analyzed by GC and GC/mass spectrometry (GC/MS). Supernate and/or cell metabolites were identified by comparing sample GC retention times and GC/MS fragmentation patterns with authentic metabolite standards. Results from this study indicated that the 3 metabolites of 2,3,4-TMP previously identified *in vivo* were identified in 4-h primary hepatocyte suspension cultures (Figure 4).[87] This evidence further supports the use of primary hepatocytes for screening chemical or drug metabolism.

VI. CONCLUSION

Primary hepatocytes provide a valuable research tool for studying chemical/drug metabolism and toxicity that conserves laboratory resources and reduces whole animal use. However, primary cells from other various target organs can also be obtained. Although these cells offer an important tool in assessing toxic mechanisms, many researchers do not utilize them due to perceived difficulties and ambiguities in primary cell isolation and culture techniques. This has hampered the development of primary cell types as *in vitro* screens for toxicity and metabolism. Most researchers tend to choose cell lines that are easier to work with. Although hepatocyte cell lines can be valuable research tools for certain types of toxicity and genotoxicity studies, these cells possess low levels of the cytochrome P450 metabolizing enzymes and do not readily lend themselves to studies of chemical or drug metabolism. Although compounds such as phenobarbital can be used to induce cytochrome

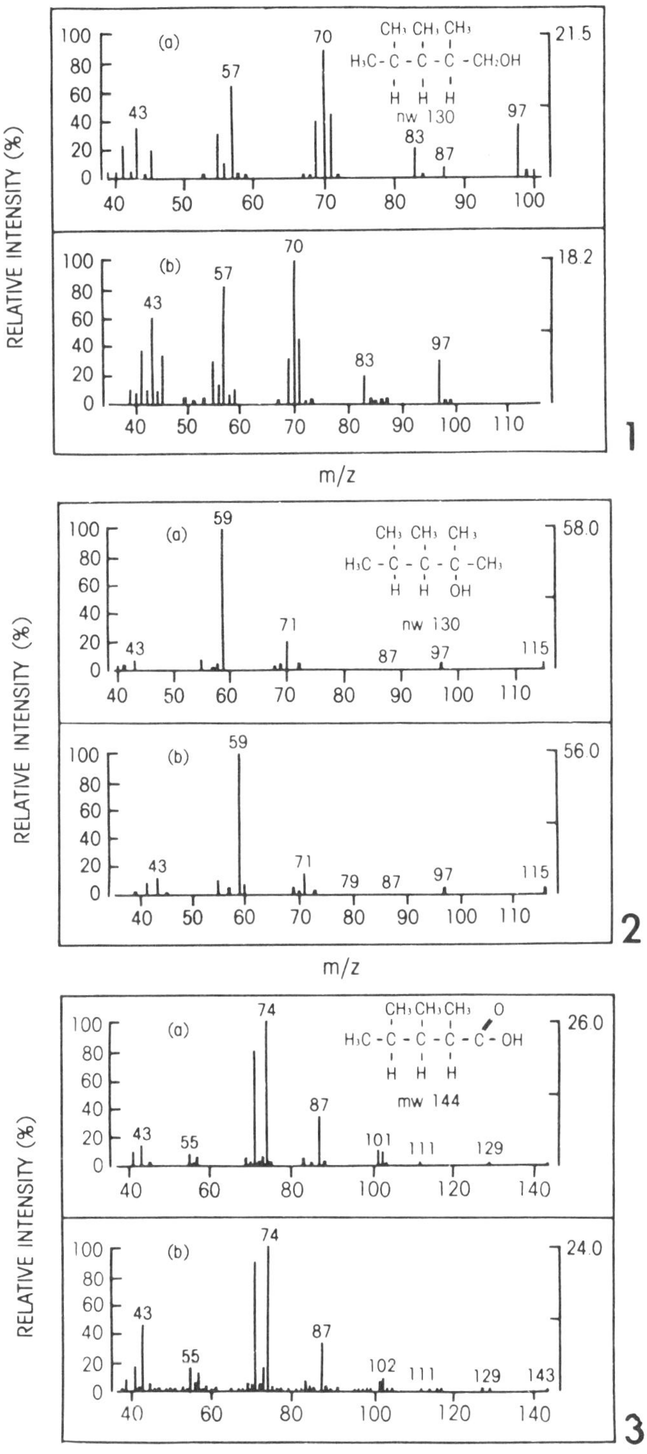

FIGURE 4. Mass spectra of authentic 2,3,4-TMP metabolites and metabolites identified in 4-h suspension cultures of hepatocytes exposed to 2,3,4-TMP: 1 (a) 2,3,4-trimethyl-1-pentanol, (b) culture medium extract; 2 (a) 2,3,4-trimethyl-2-pentanol, (b) culture medium extract; 3 (a) 2,3,4-trimethyl-1-pentanoic acid, (b) culture medium extract (modified from DelRaso et al.[87]).

P450 activity, it is still lower than that found in primary cells. Therefore, it is important to establish cell culture systems that maintain their *in vivo* functions so that correlations of cytotoxic indices between *in vitro* and *in vivo* test systems can be made. A number of reviews on the use of cell cultures as alternatives to whole animal testing have been written.[88–94]

REFERENCES

1. **Berry, M. N. and Friend, D. S.,** High-yield preparation of isolated rat liver parenchymal cells, *J. Cell Biol.*, 43, 506, 1969.
2. **Bonney, R. J.,** Adult liver parenchymal cells in primary culture: characteristics and cell recognition, *In Vitro*, 10, 130, 1974.
3. **Oldam, J. W., Casciano, D. A., and Farr, J. A.,** The isolation and primary culture of viable nonproliferating rat hepatocytes, *TCA Manual*, 5, 1047, 1979.
4. **Kreamer, B. L., Staecker, J. L., Sawada, N., Sattler, G. L., Hsia, M. T. S., and Pitot, H. C.,** Use of a low-speed iso-density Percoll centrifugation method to increase the viability of isolated hepatocyte preparations, *In Vitro*, 22, 201, 1986.
5. **Jones, D. P., Orrenius, S., and Mason, H. S.,** Hemoprotein quantitation in isolated hepatocytes, *Biochem. Biophys. Acta*, 576, 17, 1979.
6. **Acosta, D. and Sorensen, E. M. B.,** Role of calcium in cytotoxic injury of cultured hepatocytes, *Ann. N.Y. Acad. Sci.*, 407, 78, 1983.
7. **Nelson, K. F. D., Acosta, D., and Bruckner, J. V.,** Long-term maintenance and induction of cytochrome P-450 in primary cultures of rat hepatocytes, *Biochem. Pharmacol.*, 31, 2211, 1982.
8. **Paine, A. J., Hockin, L. J., and Allen, C. M.,** Long term maintenance and induction of cytochrome P-450 in rat liver cell culture, *Biochem. Pharmacol.*, 31, 1175, 1982.
9. **Landry, J., Bernier, D., Ouellet, C., Goyette, R., and Marceau, N.,** Spheroidal aggregate culture of rat liver cells: histotypic reorganization, biomatrix disposition, and maintenance of functional activities, *J. Cell Biol.*, 101, 914, 1985.
10. **Jauregui, H. A., McMillan, P. N., Driscoll, J., and Naik, S.,** Attachment and long term survival of adult rat hepatocytes in primary monolayer cultures: comparison of different substrata and tissue culture media formulations, *In Vitro*, 22, 13, 1986.
11. **Guguen-Guillouzo, C., Clement, C. B., Baffet, G., Beaumont, C., Morel-Chany, E., Glaise, D., and Guillouzo, A.,** Maintenance and reversibility of active albumin secretion by adult rat hepatocytes co-cultured with another liver epithelial cell type, *Exp. Cell Res.*, 143, 47, 1983.
12. **Martinez-Hernandez, A.,** The hepatic extracellular matrix. I. Electron immunohistochemical studies in normal rat liver, *Lab. Invest.*, 51, 57, 1984.
13. **Sawada, N., Tomomura, A., Sattler, C. A., Satller, G. L., Kleinman, H. K., and Pitot, H. C.,** Extracellular matrix components influence DNA synthesis of rat hepatocytes in primary culture, *Exp. Cell Res.*, 167, 458, 1986.
14. **Sawada, N., Tomomura, A., Satller, C. A., Satller, G. L., Kleinman, H. K., and Pitot, H. C.,** Effects of extracellular matrix components on growth and differentiation of cultured rat hepatocytes, *In Vitro*, 23, 267, 1987.
15. **Guguen-Guillouzo, C. and Guillouzo, A.,** Modulation of functional activities in cultured rat hepatocytes, *Mol. Cell Biochem.*, 53/54, 35, 1983.
16. **Rojkind, M., Gatmaitan, Z., Mackensen, S., Giambrone, M. A., Ponce, P., and Reid, L.,** Connective tissue biomatrix. Its isolation and utilization for long-term culture of normal rat hepatocytes, *J. Cell Biol.*, 87, 255, 1980.
17. **Hadley, M. A., Byers, S. W., Suarez-Quian, C. A., Kleinman, H. K., and Dym, M.,** Extracellular matrix regulates sertoli cell differentiation, testicular cord formation, and germ cell development *in vitro*, *J. Cell Biol.*, 101, 1511, 1985.
18. **Acosta, D., Anufuro, D., Mitchell, D. B. Santone, K. S., and Nelson, K. F.,** A primary cell culture system for hepatotoxic assessment, *Lab. Anim.*, 14, 31, 1985.
19. **Tyson, C. A. and Green, C. E.,** Cytotoxicity Measures: choices and methods, in *The Isolated Hepatocyte: Use in Toxicology and Xenobiotic Biotransformations*, Rauckman, E. J. and Padilla, G. M., Eds., Academic Press, Orlando, 1987, 119.
20. **Bridges, J. W., Benford, D. J., and Hubbard, S. A.,** Mechanisms of toxic injury, *Ann. N.Y. Acad. Sci.*, 407, 42, 1983.

21. **Grishham, J. W.,** Use of hepatic cell cultures to detect and evaluate the mechanisms of action of toxic chemicals, *Int. Rev. Exp. Pathol.*, 20, 123, 1979.
22. **Jeejeehoy, K. H. and Phillips, M. T.,** Isolated mammalian hepatocytes in culture, *Gastroenterology*, 71, 1086, 1986.
23. **Krebs, H. A., Cornell, N. W., Lund, P., and Hems, E.,** Isolated liver cells as experimental material, in *Regulation of Hepatic Metabolism*, Lundquist, F. and Tygstrup, N., Eds., Munksgaard, Copenhagen, 1973, 726.
24. **Bradford, M. M.,** A rapid and sensitive method for the quantitation of protein utilizing the principle of protein-dye binding, *Anal. Biochem.*, 72, 248, 1976.
25. **Pappas, N. J., Jr.,** Increased rat liver homogenate mitochondrial, and cytosolic aspartate aminotransferase activity in acute carbon tetrachloride poisoning, *Clin. Chim. Acta*, 106, 223, 1980.
26. **Green, C. E., Dabbs, J. E., and Tyson, C. A.,** Metabolism and cytotoxicity of acetaminophen in hepatocytes isolated from resistant and susceptible species, *Toxicol. Appl. Pharmacol.*, 76, 139, 1984.
27. **Wacker, W. E. C., Ulmer, D. D., and Vallee, B. L.,** Metaloenzymes and myocardial infarction. II. Malic and lactic dehydrogenase activities and the zinc concentration in serum, *N. Engl. J. Med.*, 255, 449, 1956.
28. **Gay, R. J., McComb, R. B., and Bowers, G. N., Jr.,** Optimum reaction conditions for human lactate dehydrogenase activity, *Clin. Chem.*, 14, 740, 1968.
29. **Fan, L. L., Masters, B. S. S., and Prough, R. A.,** Microsomal lauric 11- and 12-hydroxylation: a new assay utilizing high pressure liquid chromatography, *Anal. Biochem.*, 71, 265, 1976.
30. **Dehnen, W., Tomingas, R., and Ross, J.,** A modified method for the assay of benzo(*a*)pyrene hydroxylase, *Anal. Biochem.*, 53, 373, 1973.
31. **Burke, M. D. and Meyer, R. T.,** Ethoxyresorufin: direct fluorometric assay of a microsomal O-dealkylation which is preferentially inducible by 3-methylcholanthrene, *Drug Metab. Dispos.*, 2, 583, 1974.
32. **Ullrich, V. and Weber, P.,** The *O*-deethylation of 7-ethoxycourmarin by liver microsomes, *Hoppe Seyler's Z. Physiol. Chem.*, 353, 1171, 1972.
33. **Jacobson, M., Levin, W., Popper, P. J., Wood, A. W., and Conney, A. H.,** Comparison of the *O*-deethylation of 7-ethoxycoumarin and the hydroxylation of benzo(a)pyrene in human placenta, *Clin. Pharmacol. Ther.*, 16, 701, 1974.
34. **Greenlee, W. F. and Poland, A.,** An improved assay of 7-ethoxycoumarin *O*-deethylase activity: induction of hepatic enzyme activity in C57BL/6J and DBA/2J mice by phenobarbital, 3-methylcholanthrene, and 2,3,7,8-tetrachlorodibenzo-p-dioxin, *J. Pharmacol. Exp. Ther.*, 205, 596, 1978.
35. **Gray, T. J. B., Lake, B. G., Beamand, J. A., Foster, J. R., and Gangolli, S. D.,** Peroxisome proliferation in primary cultures of rat hepatocytes, *Toxicol.Appl. Pharmacol.*, 67, 15, 1983.
36. **Gillette, J. R., Mitchell, J. R., and Brodie, B. B.,** Biochemical mechanisms of drug toxicity, *Annu. Rev. Pharmacol.*, 14, 271, 1974.
37. **Monks, T. J., Anders, M. W., Dekant, W., Stevens, J. L., Lau, S. S., and van Bladeren, P. J.,** Glutathione conjugate mediated toxicities, *Toxicol. Appl. Pharmacol.*, 106, 1, 1990.
38. **Vessey, D. A.,** Hepatic metabolism of drugs and toxins, in *Hepatology. A Textbook of Liver Disease*, Zakim, D. and Boyer, T., Eds., W.B. Saunders, Philadelphia, 1982, 197.
39. **Kaplowitz, N., Aw, T. Y., and Ookhtens, M.,** The regulation of hepatic glutathione, *Annu. Rev. Pharmacol.*, 25, 715, 1985.
40. **Meister, A. and Anderson, M. E.,** Glutathione, *Annu. Rev. Biochem.*, 52, 117, 1983.
41. **Meister, A.,** Metabolism and function of glutathione, *TIBS-Sept.*, 231, 1981.
42. **Orrenius, S., Ormstad, K., Thor, H., and Jewell, S. A.,** Turnover and functions of glutathione studied with isolated hepatic and renal cells, *Fed. Proc.*, 42, 3177, 1983.
43. **Larsson, A., Orrenius, S., Holmgren, A., and Mannervik, B., Eds.,** *Functions of Glutathione: Biochemical, Physiological, Toxicological, and Clinical Aspects*, Raven Press, New York, 1983.
44. **Hissin, P. J. and Hilf, R.,** A fluorometric method for determination of oxidized and reduced glutathione in tisuses, *Anal. Biochem.*, 74, 77, 1976.
45. **Ketterer, B., Beale, D., and Meyer, D. J.,** The structure and multiple functions of glutathione transferases, *Biochem. Soc. Trans.*, 10, 82, 1982.
46. **Jakoby, W. B., Ketterer, B., and Mannervik, B.,** Glutathione S-transferases: nomenclature, *Biochem. Pharmacol.*, 33, 2539, 1984.
47. **Smith, G. J. and Litwack, G.,** Roles of ligandin and the glutathione S-transferases in binding steroi metabolites, carcinogens and other compounds, *Rev. Biochem. Toxicol.*, 2, 1, 1980.
48. **Tan, K. H., Meyer, D. J., Belin, J., and Ketterer, B.,** Inhibition of microsomal lipid peroxidation by glutathione and glutathione S-transferases B and AA. Roles of endogenous phospholipase A2, *Biochem. J.*, 220, 243, 1984.
49. **Ketterer, B., Tan, K. H., Meyer, D. J., and Coles, B.,** Glutathione transferases: a possible role in the detoxification of DNA and lipid hydroperoxides, in *Glutathione Transferases and Carcinogenesis*, Mantle, T., Picket, C. B., and Hayes, J. D., Eds., Taylor & Francis, London, 1986, 149.

50. **Ahmed, A. E., Soliman, S. A., Loh, J-P., Hussein, G. I.,** Studies on the mechanism of haloacetonitriles toxicity: inhibition of rat hepatic glutathione S-transferases *in vitro, Toxicol. Appl. Pharmacol.*, 100, 271, 1989.
51. **Cohen, A. J. and Grasso, P.,** Review of the hepatic response to hypolipidemic drugs in rodents and assessment of its toxicological significance to man, *Food Cosmet. Toxicol.*, 19, 585, 1983.
52. **Orton, T. C. and Parker, G. L.,** The effect of hypolipidemic agents on the hepatic microsomal drug-metabolizing enzyme system of the rat. Induction of cytochrome(s) P-450 with specificity toward terminal hydroxylation of lauric acid, *Drug Metab. Dispos.*, 10, 110, 1982.
53. **Reddy, J. K. and Lalwani, N. D.,** Carcinogenesis by hepatic peroxisome proliferators: evaluation of the risk of hypolipidemic drugs and industrial plasticizers to humans, *CRC Crit. Rev. Toxicol.*, 12, 1, 1983.
54. **Reddy, J. K., Azarnoff, D. L., and Hignite, C. E.,** Hypolipidemic peroxisome proliferators form a novel class of chemical carcinogens, *Nature*, 283, 397, 1980.
55. **Elcombe, C. R.,** Species differences in carcinogenicity and peroxisome proliferation due to trichloroethylene: a biochemical human hazard assessment, *Arch. Toxicol.*, 8, 6, 1985.
56. **Lake, B. G., Evans, J. G., Gray, T. J. B., Korosi, S. A., and North, C. J.,** Comparative studies on nafenopin-induced hepatic peroxisome proliferation in the rat, syrian hamster, guinea pig, and marmoset, *Toxicol. Appl. Pharmacol.*, 99, 148, 1989.
57. **Lake, B. G. and Gray, T. J. B.,** Species differences in hepatic peroxisome proliferation, *Biochem. Soc. Trans.*, 13, 859, 1985.
58. **Lake, B. G., Gray, T. J. B., Foster, J. R., Stubberfield, C. R., and Gangolli, S. D.,** Comparative studies on di(2-ethylhexyl)phthalate-induced hepatic peroxisome proliferation in the rat and hamster, *Toxicol. Appl. Pharmacol.*, 72, 46, 1984.
59. **Holloway, B. R., Bentley, M., and Thorp, J. M.,** Species differences in the effect of ICI-55897 on the plasma lipids and hepatic peroxisomes, *Ann. N.Y. Acad. Sci.*, 386, 439, 1982.
60. **Orton, T. C., Adam, H. K., Bentley, M., Holloway, B., and Tucker, M. J.,** Clobuzarit: species differences in the morphological and biochemical response of the liver following chronic administration, *Toxicol. Appl. Pharmacol.*, 73, 138, 1984.
61. **Reddy, J. K., Reddy, M. K., Usman, M. I., Lalwani, N. D., and Rao, M. S.,** Comparison of hepatic peroxisome proliferative effect and its implication for hepatocarcinogenicity relationship (SAR) studies, in *Molecular and Quantum Pharmacology*, Bergmann, E. and Pullman, B., Eds., D. Reidel, Holland, 1986, 457.
62. **Bichet, N., Cahard, D., Fabre, G., Remandet, B., Gouy, D., and Cano, J-P.,** Toxicological studies on a benzofuran derivative. III. Comparison of peroxisome proliferation in rat and human hepatocytes in primary culture, *Toxicol. Appl. Pharmacol.*, 106, 509, 1990.
63. **Lake, B. G., Gray, T. J. B., Lewis, D. F. V., Beamand, J. A., Hodder, K. D., Purchase, R., and Gangolli, S. D.,** Structure-activity relationships for induction of peroxisomal enzyme activities by phthalate monoesters in primary rat hepatocyte cultures, *Toxicol. Ind. Health*, 3, 165, 1987.
64. **Lake, B. G., Gray, T. J. B., Pels Rijcken, W. R., Beamand, J. A., and Gangolli, S. D.,** The effect of hypolipidemic agents on peroxisomal β-oxidation and MFO activities in primary cultures of rat hepatocytes: relationship between induction of palmitoyl-CoA oxidation and lauric acid hydroxylation, *Xenobiotics*, 14, 269, 1984.
65. **Gray, T. J. B., Beamand, J. A., Lake, B. G., Foster, J. R., and Gangolli, S. D.,** Peroxisome proliferation in cultured rat hepatocytes produced by clofibrate and phthalate ester metabolites, *Toxicol. Lett.*, 10, 273, 1982.
66. **Reddy, J. K., Lalwani, N. D., Qureshi, S. A., Reddy, M. K., and Moehle, C. M.,** Induction of hepatic peroxisome proliferation in non-rodent species including primates, *Am. J. Pathol.*, 114, 171, 1984.
67. **Hanefeld, M., Kemmer, C., and Kadner, E.,** Relationship between morphological changes and lipid lowering action of p-chlorophenoxyisobutyric acid (CPIB) on hepatic mitochondria and peroxisomes in man, *Atherosclerosis*, 46, 239, 1983.
68. **Lock, E. A., Mitchell, A. M., and Elcombe, C. R.,** Biochemical mechanisms of induction of hepatic peroxisome proliferation, *Annu. Rev. Pharmacol. Toxicol.*, 29, 145, 1989.
69. **Stott, W. T.,** Chemicall induced proliferation of peroxisomes: implications for risk assessment, *Regul. Toxicol. Pharmacol.*, 8, 125, 1988.
70. **Hawkins, J. M., Jones, W. E., Bonner, F. W., and Gibson, G. G.,** The effect of peroxisome proliferators on microsomal, peroxisomal, and mitochondrial enzyme activities in the liver and kidney, *Drug Metab. Rev.*, 18, 441, 1987.
71. **Lazarow, P. B.,** Assay of peroxisomal β-oxidation of fatty acids, *Methods Enzymol.*, 72, 315, 1981.
72. **Markwell, M. A. K., McGroarty, E. J., Bieber, L. L., and Tulbert, N. E.,** The subcellular distribution of carnitine acetyltransferases in mammalian liver and kidney, *J. Biol. Chem.*, 43, 506, 1973.
73. **Lazarow, P. B. and DeDuve, C.,** A fatty acyl-CoA oxidizing system in rat liver peroxisomes: enhancement by clofibrate, a hypolipidemic drug, *Proc. Nat. Acad. Sci. U.S.A.*, 73, 2043, 1976.

74. **Moody, D. E. and Reddy, J. K.,** Increase in hepatic carnitine acetyltransferase activity associated with peroxisomal (microbody) proliferation induced by the hypolipidemic drug clofibrate, nafenopin and methyl clofenapate, *Res. Commun. Chem. Pathol. Pharmacol.*, 9, 501, 1974.
75. **Osumi, T. and Hashimoto, T.,** Subcellualr distribution of the enzymes of the fatty acyl-CoA β-oxidation system and their induction by di-(2-ethyl-hexyl)phthalate in rat liver, *J. Biochem.*, 85, 131, 1979.
76. **Berge, R. K. and Bakke, O. M.,** Changes in lipid metabolizing enzymes of hepatic subcellular fractions from rats treated with tiadenol and clofibrate, *Biochem. Pharmacol.*, 30, 2251, 1981.
77. **Ellman, G. L.,** A colorimetric method for determining low concentrations of mercaptans, *Arch. Biochem. Biophys.*, 74, 443, 1958.
78. **Dickins, M. and Petersen, R. E.,** Effects of a hormone-supplemented medium on cytochrome P-450 content and mono-oxygenase activities of rat hepatocytes in primary culture, *Biochem. Pharmacol.*, 29, 1231, 1980.
79. **Grant, M. H., Melvin, M. A. L., Shaw, P., Melvin, W. T., and Burke, M. D.,** Studies on the maintenance of cytochrome reductases in primary cultures of rat hepatocytes, *FEBS Lett.*, 190, 99, 1985.
80. **Turner, N. A. and Pitot, H. C.,** Dependence of the induction of cytochrome P-450 by phenobarbital in primary cultures of adult rat hepatocytes on the composition of the culture medium, *Biochem. Pharmacol.*, 38, 2247, 1989.
81. **Benford, D. J.,** Biological models as alternatives to animal experimentation, *ATLA*, 14, 318, 1987.
82. **Bisgaard, H. C. and Lam, H. R.,** *In vitro* and *in vivo* studies on the metabolism of 1,3-diaminobenzene: comparison of the metabolites formed by the perfused rat liver, primary hepatocyte culture, hepatic microsomes and the whole rat, *Toxicol. In Vitro*, 3, 167, 1989.
83. **Smith, M. T. and Orrenius, S.,** Studies on drug metabolism and drug toxicity in isolated mammalian cells, in *Drug Metabolism and Drug Toxicity*, Mitchell, J. R. and Horning, M. G., Eds., Raven Press, New York, 1984.
84. **Wilson, I. D.,** Analytical procedures for metabolites: metabolite profiling and the isolation and identification of metabolites, in *Xenobiotic Metabolism and Disposition: The Design of Studies on Novel Compounds*, Illing, H. P. A., Ed., CRC Press, Boca Raton, FL, 1989, 149.
85. **Hobson, D. W., D'Addario, A. P., Uddin, D. E., Olson, C. T., and Serve, M. P.,** Use of a rapid urine screening procedure to determine the relative nephrotoxicity of trimethylpentane isomers in the male F-344 rat, *Toxicologist*, 5, 58, 1985.
86. **Yu, K., Olson, C. T., Hobson, D. W., and Serve, M. P.,** Identification of urinary metabolites in rats exposed to the nephrotoxic agent 2,3,4-trimethylpentane, *Biomed. Environ. Mass Spectrom.*, 14, 639, 1987.
87. **DelRaso, N. J., Mattie, D. R., and Godin, C. S.,** *In vitro* toxicity of solubilized 2,3,4-trimethylpentane. I. Cytotoxicity and metabolism of TMP using primary hepatocytes, *In Vitro*, 25, 1031, 1989.
88. **Tyson, C. A. and Stacey, N. H.,** *In vitro* screens from CNS, liver and kidney for systemic toxicity, *Toxicol. Indust. Health*, 5, 107, 1989.
89. **Gad, S. C.,** Recent developments in replacing, reducing, and refining animal use in toxicological research and testing, *Fund. Appl. Toxicol.*, 15, 8, 1990.
90. **Klausner, A.,** Tissue culture for improved toxicology, *Biotechnology*, 5, 779, 1987.
91. **Bradlaw, J. A.,** Evaluation of drug and chemical toxicity with cell culture systems, *Fundam. Appl. Toxicol.*, 6, 598, 1986.
92. **Goldberg, L.,** Charting a course for cell culture alternatives to animal testing, *Fundam. Appl. Toxicol.*, 6, 607, 1986.
93. **Rauckman, E. J. and Padillia, G. M. (Eds.),** *The Isolated Hepatocyte: Use in Toxicology and Xenobiotic Biotransformations*, Academic Press, Orlando, FL. 1987.
94. **Grisham, J. W. and Smith, G. J.,** Predictive and mechanistic evaluation of toxic responses in mammalian cell culture systems, *Pharmacol. Rev.*, 36, 151, 1984.

Chapter 15

IN VITRO DETECTION OF CHROMOSOMAL ABERRATIONS

Toshio Sofuni

TABLE OF CONTENTS

I. INTRODUCTION

The alteration of chromosomes carrying DNA (genes) morphologically and numerically, resulting in a quantitative alteration or rearrangement of genes, has been substantially studied in a variety of fields. One major reason for this is that a considerable number of congenital abnormalities in humans are found to be directly related to chromosomal aberrations; for example, Down's syndrome with mental retardation and multiple anomalies has a numerical aberration, that is, an extra chromosome (trisomy) of chromosome 21.

Another important reason is the relationship to human carcinogenesis. Several chromosomal rearrangements detected in some leukemias, lymphomas, and solid tumors have been discussed with regard to the activation of some cellular oncogenes.[2]

Various types of chemical, physical, or biological agents can cause chromosomal aberrations,[3] and many of those are considered to contribute to carcinogenesis or genetic burden in the human population. Therefore, it is significantly important to detect agents that have clastogenic potential and to avoid human exposure to them.

The safety of a variety of environmental chemicals has been evaluated by toxicology and mutagenicity tests, which have included chromosomal aberration tests. As shown in Table 1, there are several types of chromosomal aberration tests, of which that using mammalian cells in culture has several advantages: (1) higher mammalian cells including human materials such as peripheral blood can be used; (2) when established cell lines are used, identical cells are always available owing to cryopreservation; and (3) experimental conditions (concentration of test articles, treatment time, and so on) can be critically controlled, and relatively high concentrations of test substances can be investigated. A methodology of chromosomal aberration testing using cultured mammalian cells is introduced here.

II. EXPERIMENTAL PROCEDURES

Procedures varied according to the test purpose or the type of cells. For the chromosomal aberration test, we used a Chinese hamster cell line (CHL/IU) established from the lung of a female newborn, and the cells were cultured with Eagle's minimum essential medium (MEM; Gibco) supplemented with 10% heat-inactivated calf serum.[4] We have examined over 800 chemicals during the past 15 years, using CHL cells with a fixed experimental protocol[5] (Figure 1).

A. CELLS

According to the review of about 250 publications on chromosomal aberration tests in cultured mammalian cells, 61 types of cultured cells have been used.[6] Several cell lines derived from Chinese hamsters, such as CHL, CHO, and V79, were used most frequently, followed by cultured human lymphocytes (Table 2).

When cells derived from human, mice, and rats were cultured successively, polyploid cells with double the chromosome number or more appeared frequently after long periods and finally all cells became polyploid. These cells were generally inadequate for detailed chromosomal examination. On the other hand, Chinese hamster cells mostly retained the chromosome number within diploid range (around 22) even after long-term culture, and the chromosome size was relatively large. These were practical advantages for chromosome observation under the microscope and provided the major rationale for using Chinese hamster cells so frequently in chromosomal aberration tests.

Cultured human lymphocytes from peripheral blood had several advantages, such as more reliable extrapolation of test results and a eudiploid chromosome constitution indicating the identical human genetic background.

TABLE 1
Major Chromosomal Aberration Tests

a. Chromosomal aberration test using mammalian cells in culture
b. Micronucleus test using mammalian cells in culture
c. Chromosomal aberration test using rodent bone marrow cells
d. Micronucleus test using rodent bone marrow and peripheral blood cells
e. Chromosomal aberration test using rodent germinal cells
f. Dominant lethal test using rodents
g. Heritable translocation test using mice
h. Chromosome aberration test using plants
i. Chromosome aberration (aneuploidy) test using *Saccharomyces cerevisiae*

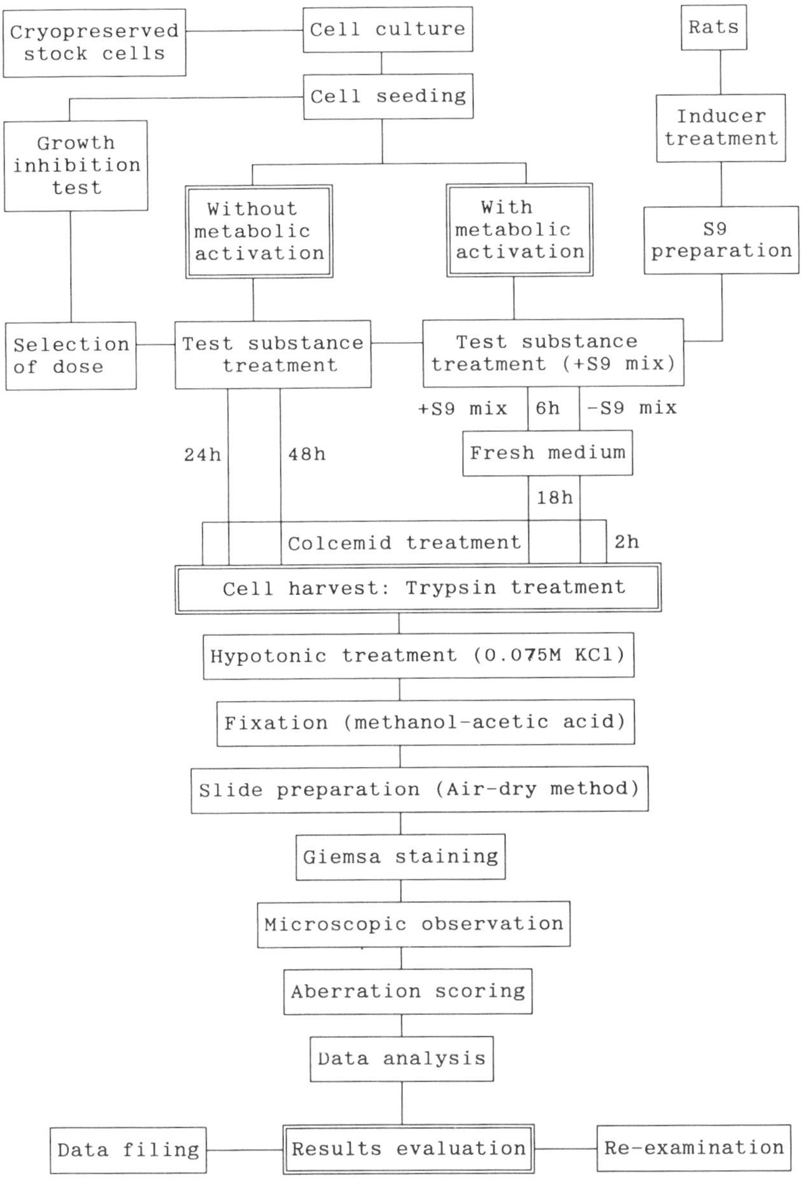

FIGURE 1. Flow chart of chromosomal aberration test using CHL cells.

TABLE 2
Representative Types of Cultured Mammalian Cells Used for Chromosomal Aberration Tests

Cell types	Origin	Culture medium	Doubling time (h)	MCN*
Chinese hamster cells: CHL(IU)	Female newborn lung	Eagle's MEM with 10% heat-inactivated calf serum	15–17	25
Chinese hamster cells: CHO-K1 (a clone of CHO)	Female ovary	Ham F-12 with 10% fetal calf serum	12–14	20
Chinese hamster cells: V79	Male lung	Eagle's MEM with 10% fetal calf serum	10–12	22
Chinese hamster cells: Don D-6 (a clone of Don)	8-month male lung	Eagle's MEM with 10% fetal calf serum	12	22
Human lymphocytes	Peripheral blood of healthy young male	RPMI1640 with 10–15% fetal calf serum	12–18	46

* MCN: Modal chromosome number.

B. SOLVENT OR VEHICLE OF TEST CHEMICALS

The test chemical was dissolved in an appropriate solvent then added to the culture. Water-soluble chemicals were dissolved in sterilized physiological saline. Insoluble test chemicals were dissolved in dimethylsulfoxide (DMSO). When the test chemical was insoluble in DMSO, it was suspended in 1% carboxymethylcellulose sodium salt (CMC), and a fine and uniform suspension was added into culture medium. The amount of solvent used did not exceed 10% in saline or CMC and 1% in DMSO.

C. EXOGENOUS METABOLIC ACTIVATION METHOD

Some chemicals exhibited mutagenic potential by the conversion to activating forms due to metabolic enzymes. However, the activity of metabolic enzymes in established cell lines was frequently lacking or extremely decreased, so exogenous metabolic activation methods should be adopted in such cell lines. The most representative method was the use of a postmitochondrial fraction (S9) obtained from liver homogenate of rats pretreated with inducers.[7] Originally polychlorinated biphenyls were used as inducers, but recently phenobarbital and 5,6-benzoflavone were used concurrently. S9 has been mixed with cofactors, but the constituents varied among researchers. The constitution of 10 ml of our S9 mix was as follows: 3 ml of S9 fraction, 2 ml of 20-m*M* HEPES buffer (pH 7.2), 1 ml each of 50-m*M* $MgCl_2$, 330 m*M* KCl, 50 m*M* glucose 6-phosphate, 40 m*M* NADP, and distilled water. The constituents except for the S9 fraction were sterilized by filtration and S9 mix was prepared just before use.

D. TREATMENT TIME

Since chromosomal aberrations induced by clastogenic chemicals were generally thought to appear throughout the DNA synthesis period (S phase), the treatment of a test chemical should cover over one cell-cycle. The duration of the cell-cycle varied among cell lines (Table 2); so, the treatment or harvest times should be adjusted to the cell types.

We have two different treatment systems: one is without S9 mix (nonactivated) and the other is with S9 mix (activated). Both systems had two different procedures: 24- and 48-h continuous exposure, and 6-h exposure with and without S9 mix, for the nonactivated and activated methods, respectively.

In the nonactivated method, 2.2×10^4 cells were seeded in a plastic dish (diameter 60 mm) with 5 ml of culture medium. On the third day, the cells were treated with test substances for the next 24 or 48 h continuously and then harvested. As the duration of one cell-cycle of CHL cells was 15 to 17 h, and the treatment with a test chemical especially at the high concentration frequently caused cell-cycle delay, a 1.5 cell-cycle treatment, that is, 24 h, was used in our protocol. Some metabolic inhibitors or base analogues induced chromosomal aberrations at extremely late periods after the treatment, and polyploidy, a numerical aberration, appeared in the second division or later. Therefore, we also adopted a 48-h in addition to a 24-h treatment.

In the activated method, the cells were treated for 6 h with 0.5 ml of S9 mix and 2.5 ml of culture medium together with a test solution (amount depending upon the solvent as mentioned in Section B). The final concentration of S9 was 5%.

The protocol in which cells were incubated only with the test substance (without S9 mix) for 6 h was also adopted. The results from this protocol were not always identical to those obtained from the nonactivated method, because of different concentrations of test chemicals and different lengths of the treatments. Therefore, whether clastogenic potential of a test substance appeared by the activation of the S9 mix or not could be judged only by comparing the data set from both experiments with and without the S9 mix (Figure 1). Occasionally, inactivation of the clastogenic potential by the S9 mix was demonstrated by this comparison.

After 6 h treatment, the reaction mixture was replaced with fresh culture medium, and the cells were cultured for another 18 h. Colcemid (0.2 μg/ml final concentration) was added 2 h prior to the termination of culture.

E. TEST SUBSTANCE CONCENTRATION

The concentrations of test substances were generally determined based on preliminary tests in which the 50% growth inhibitory concentration was estimated. The appearance of chromosomal aberrations was frequently accompanied with cell growth or division inhibition. The preliminary tests in our laboratory were performed as follows.

1.2×10^4 cells were seeded in 35-mm culture dishes with 2 ml of culture medium and cultured for 3 days. In the nonactivated system, the cells were treated with the test substance at over 5 concentrations (usually diluted at a ratio of 1:2) for 24 or 48 h. The cells were washed with saline, fixed with 10% formalin, and stained with 0.1% crystal violet. The relative values of the staining intensity, being 100% for the control culture and 0% for the blank dish, were measured optically (Monocellator, Olympus), and the concentration required for 50% cell growth inhibition was approximated.

There were two alternative methods: the first was to estimate the concentration which resulted in a 50% decrease of the cell number after trypsinization, and the second was to estimate the concentration that caused a 50% decrease of the mitotic index by microscopic observation of chromosome slides.

A concentration over the 50% cell growth inhibitory concentration was selected as the maximum, and this determination was generally reliable for the chromosomal aberration test. However, at the maximum concentration selected by this method, chromosome observation was occasionally impossible due to insufficient mitoses. On the other hand, chromosomes could be observed in some instances by the sufficient mitoses even at distinctly cytotoxic concentrations. Therefore, the highest concentration in which chromosomes could be observed was basically the maximum concentration to be tested.

The maximum concentration was usually diluted at a ratio of 1:2, and three or more concentrations were selected. Single or duplicate cultures were used for each treatment.

Of the test chemicals showing almost no cytotoxicity, the maximum concentration was increased to the point that pH, osmolarity, ion balance, and nutrient conditions would be drastically changed, which may affect chromosomal aberration induction or induce chro-

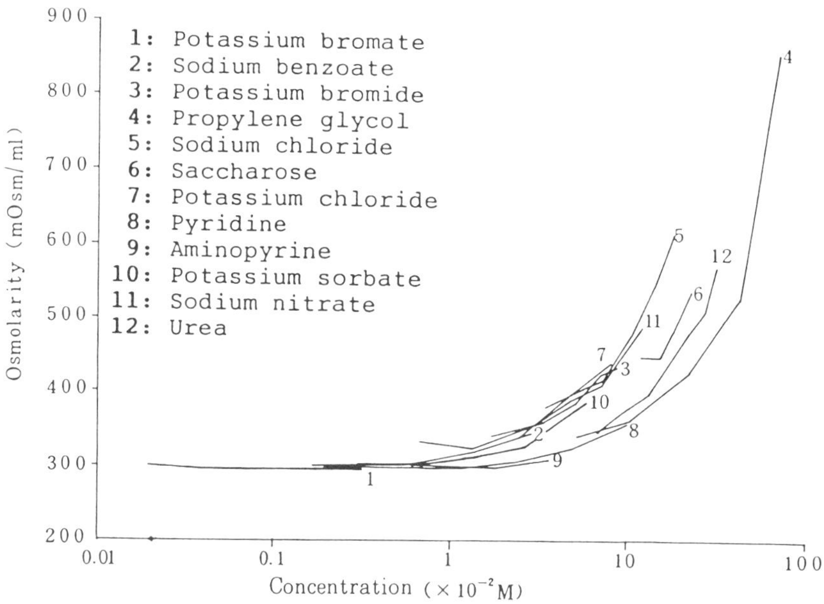

FIGURE 2. Osmotic pressure vs. concentration of test chemicals in culture medium determined by a freezing-point technique.

mosomal aberrations secondarily. We measured the osmolarity at extremely high concentrations of several chemicals, and the increase in osmolarity was demonstrated at about 10 m*M* (Figure 2). Therefore, we suggested that the maximum concentration in the chromosomal aberration test should be limited to 10 m*M*.[8] In natural products or mixed compounds in which molecular weights were unclear, the maximum concentration was limited to 5 mg/ml. Recently interaction between chromosome aberration induction and the high concentration of test chemicals has been studied and several publications[9–11] can be referred to for detailed information.

F. CONTROL SUBSTANCES

Solvents or vehicles for dissolving or suspending the test substances were used as negative controls. Untreated controls were included in the test as required.

Positive controls consisted of well-known clastogenic chemicals. In the CHL cells, the following were used:

1. The nonactivated system
   - Mitomycin C
   - *N*-Methyl-*N'*-nitro-*N*-nitrosoguanidine
   - Methyl methanesulfonate
2. The activated system
   - Benzo[a]pyrene
   - Cyclophosphamide
   - Dimethylnitrosamine

G. CHROMOSOME PREPARATION

Chromosome preparations are usually made by the air-drying technique, but this is often modified in each laboratory. The method used in our laboratory was as follows.

Culture medium was poured into a centrifuge tube, and 2 ml of 0.25% trypsin solution prewarmed at 37°C was added to the culture. After several minutes, the cells were resuspended by pipetting, and trypsin treatment was stopped by the addition of the culture medium kept in a centrifuge tube. The cell suspension was centrifuged at approximately 1000 rpm for 5 min, and the supernatant was decanted. The cells were thoroughly dissociated by shaking and were swollen in approximately 5 ml of hypotonic solution (0.075 *M* KCl). The cell suspension was incubated in a water bath at 37°C for 10 to 15 min. About 1 ml of freshly prepared fixative (cooled methanol mixed with glacial acetic acid 3:1 v/v) was slowly added to the cell suspension and gently mixed. The cells were centrifuged and resuspended in the fixative. This process was repeated at least three times. A slightly turbid cell suspension was prepared, and two drops of it were placed on a clean glass slide. Two or more slides per culture were prepared. After air drying, the slides were stained with 1 to 3% Giemsa solution (pH 6.8) for 15 to 20 min, rinsed with tap water, and allowed to dry.

III. MICROSCOPIC OBSERVATION

One hundred well-spread metaphases per culture were analyzed under the light microscope. Well-spread metaphases were first selected under low magnitude (10 × 10 or 10 × 20) according to the following criteria. Early metaphases with extremely long and slender chromosomes and late metaphases with extremely short and condensed chromosomes were excluded. Metaphases spreading in a circle were predominantly selected, but those in which several chromosomes were scattered outside of metaphase were excluded. Metaphases with many overlapped chromosomes, indistinct shape, those covered with cell debris, or staining precipitate were also excluded.

At the observation under high magnitude, metaphases lacking three or more chromosomes from the modal chromosome number were excluded. Metaphases in which chromosome analysis was disturbed by chromosome overlapping, indisticnt shape, cell debris, or staining precipitate, were rejected. Otherwise, all metaphases selected by low magnitude were analyzed regardless of aberrations.

IV. CLASSIFICATION OF CHROMOSOMAL ABERRATIONS

Chromosomal aberrations have been classified in detail[12] and an international nomenclature established.[13] Chromosomal aberrations are classified into two major groups: one is structural aberrations, and the other is numerical aberrations (Table 3).

A. STRUCTURAL ABERRATIONS

The structural aberrations are further divided into two, chromatid- and chromosome-type aberrations. Both types of aberrations included gaps, breaks, and exchanges; so, structural aberrations are classified into six different types.

When chromosomal aberrations were induced by ionizing irradiation, the type of aberration induced was dependent on the phase of the cell-cycle. If the cells were irradiated at the G1-phase, only chromosome-type aberrations were induced, whereas if the cells were irradiated at the G2-phase, chromatid-type aberrations were induced. The irradiation of the cells in the S-phase produced both chromatid- or chromosome-type aberrations depending on the status of the DNA synthesis of each chromosome. On the other hand, most clastogenic chemicals induced only chromatid-type aberrations, even though the cells were treated at G1-phase. This may be caused by a different reaction to DNA between radiation and clastogenic chemicals: the former directly causes DNA double strand breaks, and the latter

TABLE 3
Classification of Chromosomal Aberrations

A. Structural aberration
  1. Chromatid-type aberration
    a. Chromatid gap: ctg
    b. Chromatid break: ctb
    c. Chromatid exchange: cte (complete and incomplete)
      Intrachange
        Intraarm exchange
          Asymmetric; acentric chromatid ring
          Symmetric; paracentric chromatid inversion
          Sister union: SU
            (Not union distal: NUd; Not union proximal: NUp)
        Interarm exchange
          Asymmetric; chromatid ring (accompanying with a ctb)
          Symmetric; pericentric chromatid inversion
      Interchange
        Quadriradial: qr (asymmetric and symmetric)
        Triradial: tr
      Complex: cs
    d. Other: fragmentation: frg
  2. Chromosome-type aberration
    a. Chromosome gap: csg
    b. Chromosome break: csb
      (acentric fragment: ace, terminal deletion: del)
      (minute or double minute: min or dmin)
    c. Chromosome exchange: cse
      Intrachange
        Intraarm exchange
          Asymmetric; acentric ring: ace-r
            (interstitial deletion: del)
          Symmetric; paracentric inversion: inv
        Interarm exchange
          Asymmetric; ring: r (accompanying with an ace)
          Symmetric; pericentric inversion: inv
      Interchange
          Asymmetric; dicentric: dic (accompanying with an ace)
          Symmetric; reciprocal translocation: t
          Complex: cx
            Tricentric: tri, insertion: ins, and others
B. Numerical aberration
  1. Aneuploidy
    Hypodipoloidy and hyperdiploidy
  2. Polyploidy
    Triploidy, tetraploidy and others
    Endoreduplication: end
C. Others
  1. Ill-defined chromosome abnormality: attenuation, stickiness, ruffling, haziness, erosion, and others
  2. Pulverization: pvz
    Premature chromosome condensation: pcc (G1-pcc, S-pcc, and G2-pcc)
  3. C-mitosis: ski-pair

causes only modification of DNA following the appearance of aberrations throughout S-phase.

Six major aberrations were defined as follows (Figures 3, 4, and 5).

- Chromatid gap (ctg): a nonstaining region in one chromatid showing a clear discontinuity (the size of which is almost equal to or more than the width of the chromatid),

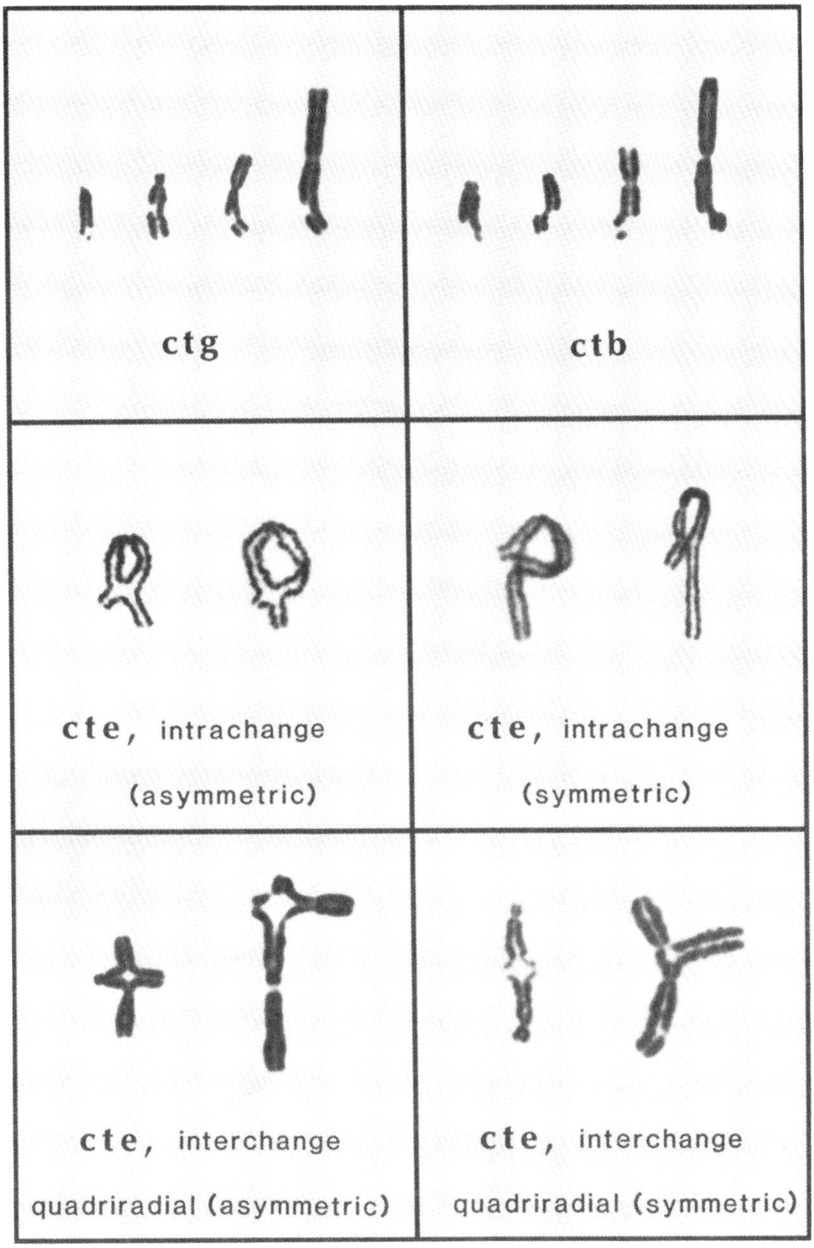

FIGURE 3. Representatives of chromatid-type aberrations: ctg, chromatid gaps; ctb; chromatid breaks; and cte, chromatid exchanges.

but the distal part of the chromatid showing no distinct dislocation or misalignment.

- Chromatid break (ctb): the complete severance of the distal part of one chromatid with a distinct dislocation or misalignment.
- Chromatid exchange (cte): rearrangements as a consequence of misreunion between two or more chromatid breaks, including interchromosomal exchanges such as triradials and quadriradials and intrachromosomal exchanges such as chromatid rings and inversions. Complex chromatid exchanges involving three or more chromosomes are also included in this category.

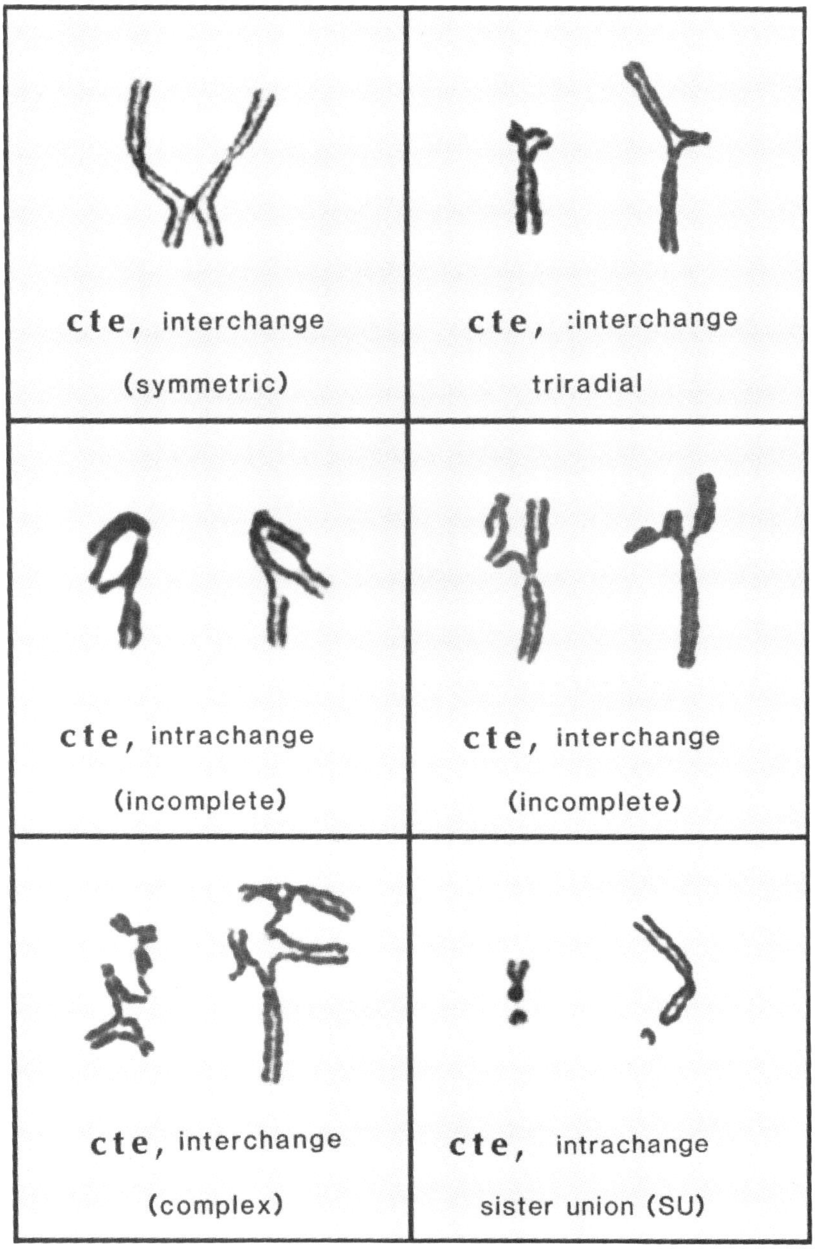

FIGURE 4. Representatives of chromatid-type aberrations: cte; chromatid exchanges.

Chromatid exchanges were not always completely connected and sometimes the morphological configuration changed from the original (see the middle [''incomplete''] of Figure 4). In this case the disconnected part was not counted as a chromatid break. Chromatid aberrations include so-called ''isochromatid breaks (gaps)'' that two chromatid breaks (gaps) cause accidentally at the same locus in both sister chromatids. These are indistinguishable from chromosome breaks (gaps) under a microscope, and are usually scored as chromosome breaks (gaps). These can be classified depending only upon the type of exchange aberrations induced simultaneously or the consideration of induction mechanism.

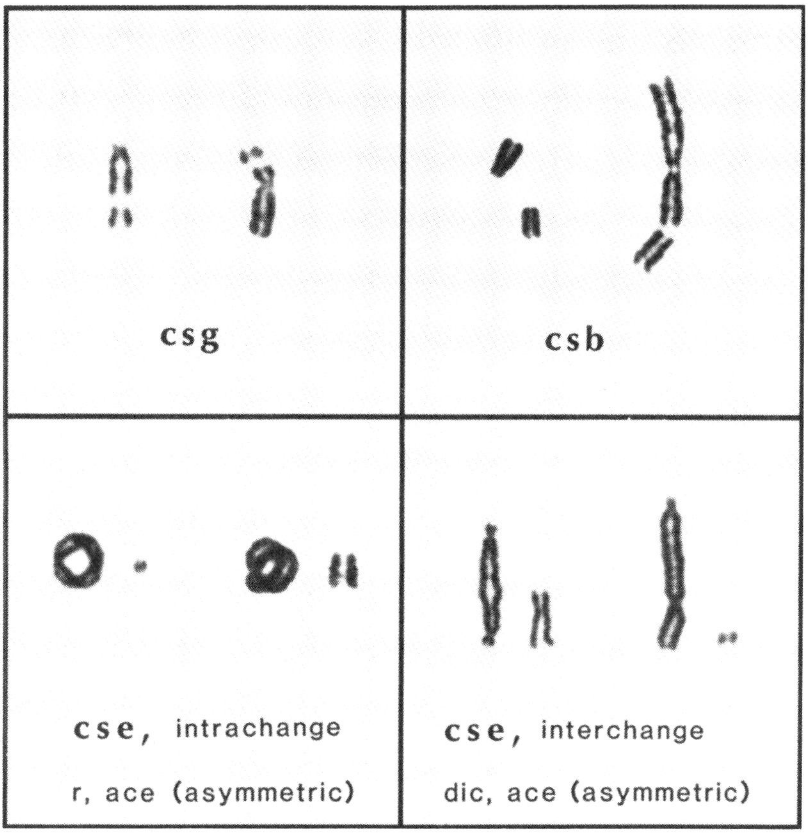

FIGURE 5. Representatives of chromosome-type aberrations: csg; chromosome gaps; csb; chromosome breaks; and cse; chromosome exchanges.

In relation to isochromatid breaks, there are so-called sister unions (SU), in which sister chromatid reunion occurs at an isochromatid break, resulting in a U-shape configuration (bottom right of Figure 4). In addition to this complete type, incomplete types including no union of the proximal (NUp) and distal parts (NUd) are occasionally observed. As these three types are caused by reunion of chromatid breaks, we classify them as chromatid exchanges (Table 3).

- Chromosome gap (csg): same as chromatid gaps, but occurring at the same locus in both sister chromatids.
- Chromosome break (csb): the complete severance of the terminal region of a chromosome arm which gives rise to a shortened chromosome and an acentric chromosome fragment, and which is not associated with any obvious exchange process.
- Chromosome exchange (cse): rearrangements as a consequence of misreunion between two or more chromosome breaks include dicentrics and rings (these are associated with an acentric fragment, and it is scored as one aberration, but not as two independent aberrations). Acentric rings derived from interstitial deletions are included in this type aberrations. Complex chromosome exchanges such as tricentrics are also included in this category.

As peculiar aberrations, fragmentation (frg) is defined as metaphases with a large number of ctg and ctb, but without ctc. This type of aberration is occasionally observed at higher concentrations of the test chemicals which induce predominantly ctg and/or ctb.

Minute chromosome fragments or double minute fragments (min or dmin) are another type of peculiar aberrations. These are small double dots; the size of a dot is almost equal to or smaller than the width of a chromatid, and those which are larger than the chromatid width are scored as acentric rings. Routinely, this type aberration is included in chromosome breaks when scoring.

Both chromatid and chromosome gaps could be combined and scored simply as gaps. Exchange aberrations of both chromatid- and chromosome-types are further classified, if necessary, into several subgroups (Table 3).

Chromatid-type convert to chromosome-type aberrations through cell division and these are called derived chromosome-type aberrations. Chromosome breaks are derived from chromatid breaks, rings from chromatid intrachange (asymmetrics), inversions from chromatid intrachange (symmetrics), dicentrics from asymmetrical quadriradials and sister unions, and reciprocal translocations from symmetrical quadriradials. When chromosome-type aberrations are observed at the late sampling time, it should be considered whether these are real chromosome-type aberrations or derived types from chromatid-type aberrations.

There are two ways to express the frequency of chromosome aberrations: the number of aberrations per cell, and the number (%) of cells with aberrations per total of cells observed. The former was suitable for expressing a dose-dependent relationship, but inconvenient in cells with uncountable and complicated aberrations frequently induced at the high concentration of the test chemicals. The latter was useful practically, but types of aberrations observed in each cell should be recorded according to the six or more basic classes described above, and any cell with one or more aberrations was counted as one aberrant cell.

B. NUMERICAL ABERRATIONS

The numerical aberrations are classified into two types: aneuploidy and polyploidy. Aneuploidy included hyperdiploidy and hypodiploidy, the latter being usually indistinguishable from cells lacking several chromosomes artificially in the process of slide preparation. Since the chromosome number of established cell lines somehow varied, it was inadequate to detect aneuploid cells. Therefore, only polyploid cells were scored as the numerical aberrations in established cell lines. Though the polyploidy included triploidy, tetraploidy, pentaploidy, hexaploidy, etc., the cells were practically divided into only two types, diploid and tetraploid range, and then the polyploid cells were defined as having a chromosome number in the tetraploid range or more. In the CHL cells, polyploid cells were defined as metaphases having chromosomes in approximate multiples of the modal chromosome number (25), and, practically, metaphases with more than 38 chromosomes were scored as polyploid cells. The structural aberrations observed in polyploid cells were also scored.

Endoreduplication (metaphases with paired duplicated chromosomes [diplochromosomes]) observed less frequently is included in polyploidy, but the frequency may be recorded separately.

C. OTHER ABNORMALITIES

Other abnormalities such as pulverization (pvz), in which one or several chromosomes in diploid cells or a half set of chromosomes in polyploid cells showed a mass of minute fragments or small dots, were not included in the structural aberration, but recorded separately as the occasion demanded. This phenomenon occurred in multi- or micronucleated cells formed spontaneously or induced by viral or nonviral agents, when one nucleus underwent an asynchronous entry into mitosis (when both nuclei entered synchronously into mitosis, pvz did not occur). Morphological features of pvz were variable depending on the cell-cycle of the affected interphase nucleus, and they were called G1-, S-, or G2-PCC (premature chromosome condensation). This type of aberration was recorded but not scored as an aberration, since pvz was an indirect phenomenon which occurred incidentally in multi- or micronucleated cells.

In addition, there was so-called ill-defined abnormalities, such as attenuation, stickiness, ruffling, haziness, and erosion. These were thought to be alterations or partial distortion of high-dimensional construction of DNA and protein composing of chromosomes, and to have no DNA modification or DNA strand breaks resulting in structural aberrations. Therefore, these were in principle negligible for chromosomal aberration scoring.

Recently, we published *The Atlas of Chromosomal Aberrations Induced by Chemicals*[14] including about 200 microscopic photographs in which many examples of aberrations described in Table 3 were presented. This atlas is useful as a reference to understand the identification of a variety of chromosomal aberrations.

V. EVALUATION OF TEST RESULTS

At the evaluation of test results, the frequency of chromosomal aberrations in the negative (solvent) control was important, though this value varied among the cell lines. If the frequency of chromosomal aberrations in the negative control is unusually deviated from the historical data of the negative control, the experiment should be judged technically inadequate and a reexamination performed. In CHL cells, our historical data base showed that the frequency of cells with aberrations (including gaps) or polyploidy in untreated and solvent-treated negative controls did not exceed 4%. When the frequency of aberrant cells in the negative control was 5% or more, a reexamination was made. When a substantial number of subcultures are to be passaged, it is better to use cryopreserved stock cells.

The final judgement of each test, for structural aberrations or polyploid cells, was made separately. We called it negative (−) if the frequency of aberrant cells (including gaps for structural aberrations) or polyploidy in treatment groups was less than 5%. The result was judged positive (+) when the frequency of aberrant cells or polyploidy was about 2-fold greater than that of the upper limit of the historical control, that is over 10%. The suspicious range between negative and positive, that is 5 to 10%, we called inconclusive (±). Overall evaluation for each chemical was made after the individual results were evaluated among different dose groups. If the outcome was evaluated as inconclusive or showed no dose-related response, the experiment was repeated. No statistical procedures were applied to the judgement of chromosomal aberrations in the CHL cells.

VI. PROBLEMS IN JUDGEMENT OF CHROMOSOMAL ABERRATIONS

One of the major problems in the chromosomal aberration test is that the definition of aberrations, especially of gaps, varied among researchers. Though gaps are defined as achromatic lesions or nonstaining regions, faintly stained regions were frequently judged to be gaps, and these were seen to be connected between both distal parts. Therefore, these gaps were not thought to be real discontinuity and were excluded from the structural aberrations. Many researchers, however, had scored these gaps but finally excluded them from the aberrations at the evaluation of the results. Chromatid size was used as a standard to measure the size of the nonstaining region, and any nonstaining region smaller than the chromatid width was defined as a gap, and a break was defined as when the nonstaining region was more than the chromatid width even without misalignment.[15]

Our criteria of gaps and breaks were different from that described above. The discrimination of gaps and breaks has been made by the absence or presence of dislocation or misalignment of the distal region as described in Section IV. When the size of a nonstaining region was almost equal to or more than the chromatid width and there was no distinct dislocation or misalignment, these were classified into gaps. This indicated that nonstaining regions less than the chromatid width (gaps in the former criteria) were not recorded as aberrations at microscopic observation. When the nonstaining region without misalignment was distinctly wide and looked to be discontinuous, these were likely to be classified as breaks. The gaps in our criteria were identical to some part of the breaks in the former criteria and were included as aberrations. Therefore, both scoring systems were finally comparable at the evaluation of the results.

Chromatid width was not always used as the standard but only as a reference, because this parameter varied according to the chromosome condensation in each metaphase. To judge gaps or breaks, discontinuity is more important than the size of a nonstaining region: when the size of a nonstaining region is more than the chromatid width but the continuity is suspected morphologically, this should not be included in aberrations. On the other hand, when the size of the nonstaining region is slightly narrower than the chromatid width but a clear discontinuity is recognizable, this should be included within aberrations for evaluation.

Our criteria of gaps and breaks described above were made with the intention of applying them to routine screening to detect clastogenic potential of environmental chemicals, but in research works in which more detailed analyses are needed, more precise definition of each aberration should be made.

REFERENCES

1. **Hamerton, J. L., Canning, N., Ray, M., and Smith, S.,** A cytogenetic survey of 14,069 newborn infants. I. Incidence of chromosome abnormalities, *Clin. Genet.*, 8, 223, 1975.
2. **Klein, G.,** The role of gene dosage and genetic transpositions in carcinogenesis, *Nature*, 294, 313, 1981.
3. **German, J.,** *Chromosomes and Cancer*, John Wiley & Sons, New York, 1974.
4. **Ishidate, M., Jr. and Odashima, S.,** Chromosome tests with 134 compounds on Chinese hamster cells *in vitro* — A screening for chemical carcinogens, *Mutat. Res.*, 48, 337, 1977.
5. **Ishidate, M., Jr.,** *Data Book of Chromosomal Aberration Test In Vitro*, rev. ed., Life-Science Information Center, Tokyo, 1987.
6. **Ishidate, M., Jr., Harnois, M. C., and Sofuni, T.,** A comparative analysis of data on the clastogenicity of 951 chemical substances tested in mammalian cell cultures, *Mutat. Res.*, 195, 151, 1988.
7. **Matsuoka, A., Hayashi, M., and Ishidate, M., Jr.,** Chromosomal aberration tests on 29 chemicals combined with S9 mix *in vitro*, *Mutat. Res.*, 66, 277, 1979.
8. **Ishidate, M., Jr., Sofuni, T., Yoshikawa, K., Hayashi, M., Nohmi, T., Sawada, M., and Matsuoka, S.,** Primary mutagenicity screening of food additives currently used in Japan, *Food. Chem. Toxic.*, 22, 623, 1984.
9. **Ashby, J. and Ishidate, M., Jr.,** Clastogenicity *in vitro* of the Na, K, Ca and Mg salts of saccharin; and of magnesium chloride; consideration of significance, *Mutat. Res.*, 163, 63, 1986.
10. **Brusick, D.,** Genotoxic effects in cultured mammalian cells produced by low pH treatment conditions and increased ion concentration, *Environ. Mutagen.*, 8, 879, 1986.
11. **Morita, T., Watanabe, Y., Takeda, K., and Okumura, K.,** Effects of pH in the *in vitro* chromosomal aberration test, *Mutat. Res.*, 225, 55, 1989.
12. **Savage, J. R. K.,** Classification and relationships of induced chromosomal structural changes, *J. Med. Genet.*, 13, 103, 1976.
13. An international system for human cytogenetic nomenclature, *Cytogenet. Cell Genet.*, 21, 309, 1978.
14. The Mammalian Mutagenesis Study Group of the Environmental Mutagen Society of Japan (JEMS-MMS), *The Atlas of Chromosomal Aberrations Induced by Chemicals*, Asakura Publishing Co., Tokyo, 1988.
15. **Schinzel, A. and Shimid, W.,** Lymphocyte chromosome studies in human exposed to chemical mutagens. The validity of the method in 67 patients under cytostatic therapy, *Mutat. Res.*, 40, 139, 1976.

Chapter 16

MEASUREMENT OF INTRACELLULAR Ca^{2+} AND pH^{in} IN CULTURED CELLS BY FLUORESCENCE SPECTROSCOPY*

Raul Martínez-Zaguilán

TABLE OF CONTENTS

* The abbreviations used are pH^{in}, intracellular pH; $[Ca^{2+}]_i$, intracellular calcium; R, ratio; R_{max}, maximum ratio; R_{min}, minimum ratio; BCECF, 2′,7′-bis-(2-carboxyethyl)-5(and-6)carboxyfluorescein; Pyranine, 8-hydroxypyrene-1,3,6-trisulfonate; SNARF-1, carboxy-seminaphtorhodafluor; X-AM, acetoxymethylester form of fluoroprobe X; Fura-2, 5-oxazolecarboxylic acid, 2-(6-(bis(carboxymethyl)amino)5-5(2-(2-bis(carboxymethyl)amino)-5-methylphenoxy-2-benzofuranyl); HEPES, 25 m*M* *N*-2-hydroxyethylpiperazine-*N*′-2-ethanesulfonic acid; MOPS, 3-(*N*-morpholino)propanesulfonic acid; EGTA, ethylene glycol-bis(β-aminoethyl ether)-*N,N,N′,N′*,-tetraacetic acid; MES, 2-(*N*-morpholino)ethanesulfonic acid.

I. BACKGROUND

Responses to a variety of hormones and mitogenic agents include turnover of inositol phospholipids,[1-3] activation of protein kinase C,[1,4,5] kinase A,[3,6] calmodulin kinase,[2,7] and tyrosine kinase.[8] These responses are often associated with changes in pH^{in} (References 9 to 12) and $[Ca^{2+}]_i$ (References 6, 13 to 16). Although the precise roles for these $[Ca^{2+}]_i$ changes are unclear, they afford a useful tool for cataloging and distinguishing the signal transduction pathway used by different mitogens and hormones in phenomena as diverse as secretion, neurotransmission, proliferation, and differentiation. The understanding of these processes often involves the use of a variety of pharmacological agents that affect $[Ca^{2+}]_i$ regulation. Interference of any of these pathways with pharmacological agents to halt specific physiological and biochemical responses can affect pH^{in} and/or $[Ca^{2+}]_i$, and such evidence is often used to ascribe cause-effect relationships.

There are several techniques to measure $[Ca^{2+}]_i$ including microelectrodes, nuclear magnetic resonance (NMR) spectroscopy, and fluorescence spectroscopy. Fluorescence spectroscopy is the least biologically disruptive technique, since it is extremely sensitive. An advantage of fluorescence spectroscopy over other techniques is that it permits very fast tracking of changes in intracellular ions, even at millisecond sampling rates. An important drawback when using fluorescence spectroscopy is that all of the the currently available Ca^{2+} fluoroprobes (e.g., Quin-2, BAPTA, Indo-1, Fura-2, Fluo-2, Fluo-3, Rhod-1, Rhod-2) are affected to various degrees by pH.[17-21] This is generally due to the presence of protonatable groups in these Ca^{2+} fluoroprobes. The binding of H^+ to these dyes results in changes in both their spectral properties and their affinity for Ca^{2+} (Kd_a). Since changes in both pH^{in} and $[Ca^{2+}]_i$ are among the most common responses to cell treatment with hormones or other pharmacological agents, and the interrelationship between these ions is largely unclear, it is therefore desirable to simultaneously monitor these two ions in order to quantitate and understand the changes which may take place.

There are several fluorescent indicators for measuring pH^{in} and $[Ca^{2+}]_i$ (References 22, 23). Most of these are commercially available in acetoxymethyl ester forms, allowing passive loading of cells without the need for microinjection, scrape loading, glass bead loading, and electroporation. Although these latter manipulations are capable of disrupting the cell physiology,[24] they can have the advantage of loading a quantitative amount of dye into a known compartment (e.g., cytosol).[25]

The use of excitation or emission ratios to estimate pH^{in} and $[Ca^{2+}]_i$ reduces artifacts that result from uneven dye distribution, dye leakage, and photobleaching. In the ratio method, one selects for ion-sensitive excitation or emission wavelengths which increase or decrease upon cation binding. An isoexcitation or isoemissive point (which is ion-insensitive) is greatly desirable, since it allows one to simultaneously determine efficiency of dye loading, dye leaking, and quenching effects. After correcting for autofluorescence, the ratio of the fluorescence at these two ion-sensitive wavelengths can be used to determine the extent of dye bound and, hence, the free ion concentration by the equations:[19,26]

$$pH = pK_a + \log(S_{f2}/S_{b2}) + \log[(R - R_{min})/(R_{max} - R)] \quad (1)$$

$$[Ca^{2+}] = Kd_a(S_{f2}/S_{b2})[(R - R_{min})/(R_{max} - R)] \quad (2)$$

where R, R_{min}, and R_{max} are the measured minimum and maximum ratios, respectively. In the case of pH indicators, R increases with deprotonation, so R_{max} represents the ratio of fully deprotonated dye, while R_{min} is the ratio for fully protonated dye. In the case of Ca^{2+} indicators, R increases with increasing Ca^{2+}, so R_{min} represents a fully free Ca^{2+} indicator while R_{max} represents the Ca^{2+}-dye chelate. S_{f2} and S_{b2} are the fluorescence values for the free and bound forms of the dye, respectively, at the denominator wavelength. The quantities S_{f2}/S_{b2} are used to correct for the fact that the denominator wavelength is ion-sensitive.

A number of fluorescent Ca^{2+} indicators have been described in the literature, since the introduction of Quin-2 by Tsien et al.[27] Even with its documented pitfalls, the most informative Ca^{2+} fluorescent probe has been Fura-2.[23] Some of the problems in using this dye are incomplete hydrolysis of the acetoxymethylester form,[28] compartmentalization into organelles,[29,30] photobleaching,[31] extrusion from the cell by anion transport mechanisms,[32] and effects of temperature[33] and pH[17-21] on its Kd_a. Notwithstanding these problems, by using appropriate controls, quantitative measurements using Fura-2 can be made.[19,23] Most recently, a new set of Ca^{2+} indicators was generated by coupling the Ca^{2+}-chelator BAPTA to derivatives of fluorescein (Fluo-1, -2, and -3) and rhodamine (rhod-1 and -2).[20] These new indicators should prove useful in monitoring Ca^{2+} by fluorescence microscopy and flow cytometry since they can be excited at 488 nm with an argon-ion laser for fluorescein derivatives, or the 531-nm line of a krypton-ion laser, or the 546-nm line of a mercury arc for the rhodamine derivatives. Furthermore, the new dyes can be used in conjunction with the currently available photolabile "caged" compounds (nucleotides, IP_3, and Ca^{2+}), whereas with Fura-2 and Indo-1, the excitation wavelengths photolyze the "caged" compounds, thus complicating the interpretation of the results. An important disadvantage of these new dyes is that they cannot be used in ratio mode, and therefore are much more difficult to use quantitatively.

The most popular family of pH indicators has been the fluorescein-derivatives such as BCECF (Figure 1A). These indicators generally have pK_a values near 7.0. However, they lack a definitive isoexcitation point[22,23] and can compartmentalize into acidic organelles.[34] Pyranine has also been used with certain success: it has a clear isoemissive point and therefore it is possible to determine pH by ratio.[35-37] Furthermore, the recent availability of pyranine in an esterified form should eliminate most of the problems of dye loading. Its major drawback is a relatively high pK_a. Recently, a new family of pH-fluorescent indicators has been developed.[23,38] Carboxy SNARF-1 is an example: it has dual emission wavelengths, a clear isoemissive point, and a good *in situ* pK_a (Figure 1B).[19,39]

Attempts to simultaneously measure pH^{in} and $[Ca^{2+}]_i$ by fluorescence spectroscopy have been made earlier by Simpson and Rink,[40] using human platelets coloaded with Fura-2 and BCECF. The fluorescence spectra of these two dyes are so close that fluorescence energy transfer is feasible (cf. Figure 1). Fluorescence energy transfer is primarily a result of dipole-dipole interactions between two fluorophores (i.e., the donor and the acceptor) and therefore both their relative orientation and the relative distance between them (usually <100 Å) dominate this phenomenon.[41] This effect occurs when (1) the emission spectrum of one fluoroprobe overlaps the excitation spectrum of the other; (2) there is little direct excitation of the acceptor at the excitation maximum of the donor; and (3) there is emission overlap between the two fluoroprobes. As shown in Figure 1, these conditions are met by both pH probes in combination with Fura-2. It is not known whether energy tranfer occurs between Fura-2 and BCECF. It does not occur between Fura-2 and SNARF-1, however. Recently, we have reported the simultaneous measurement of pH^{in} and $[Ca^{2+}]_i$ by using the fluorescence of SNARF-1 and Fura-2 (Figure 1). The versatility of different excitation and emission wavelengths offered by SNARF-1 allowed us to specifically select those excitation and emission wavelenghts far away from those of Fura-2, further minimizing the possibility of fluorescence energy transfer. The results of such analysis allowed us to conclude that, under our experimental conditions, Fura-2 does not interfere with the fluorescence of SNARF-1 or vice versa.[19] The judicious use of this technique should allow one to distinguish changes in the spectral properties of Fura-2 due to binding of H^+ from those changes due to the

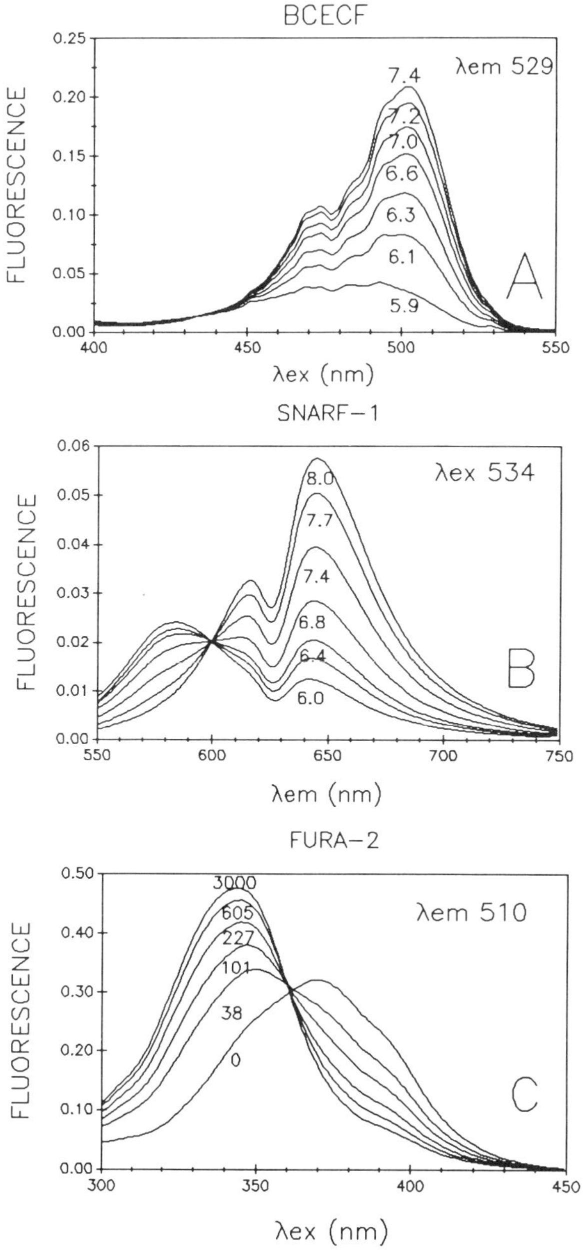

FIGURE 1. (A) *In vitro* fluorescence excitation spectra of BCECF in nigericin buffer at various pH values. Two μM BCECF (free acid) was dissolved in nigericin buffer at various pH values. Excitation spectra were collected using an emission wavelength of 529. Notice the "isoexcitation point" at 440 and the peak at 500 which increase as the solution pH increaes. The ratio 500/440 or 500/450 is traditionally used to measure pH; (B) *in vitro* fluorescence emission spectra of SNARF-1 in nigericin buffer at various pH values. Two μM SNARF-1 (free acid) was dissolved in nigericin buffer at various pH values. Emission spectra were collected using an excitation wavelength of 534. Notice the isoemissive point at 560 and peaks at 584 and 644 nm which decrease and increase, respectively, as the solution pH increases; (C) *in vitro* fluorescence excitation spectra of Fura-2 at various concentrations of free Ca^{2+}. One μM Fura-2 (free acid) was dissolved in Ca^{2+}-EGTA buffer, at the indicated free Ca^{2+} concentrations (nM). Excitation spectra were collected using an emission wavelength of 510. The remarkable features are the isoexcitation point at 360 and peaks at 340 and 380 nm which increase and decrease, respectively, as Ca^{2+} increases. (B and C from Martínez-Zaguiln̆, R. et al., *Am. J. Physiol.*, 260, C297, 1991. With permission.)

binding of Ca^{2+} and should enhance our knowledge of the interrelationship between these two ions in the signal transduction pathway leading to particular physiological responses. More recently, a report in abstract form has appeared in the literature which suggests the possibility of using Indo-1 and SNARF-1 to simultaneously measure $[Ca^{2+}]_i$ and pH^{in} (Reference 42).

II. MEASUREMENT OF pH^{in} AND $[Ca^{2+}]_i$

Buffers — Cell suspension buffer (CSB) contained 1.3 m*M* $CaCl_2$, 1 m*M* $MgSO_4$, 5.4 m*M* KCl, 0.44 m*M* KH_2PO_4, 110 m*M* NaCl, 0.35 m*M* NaH_2PO_4, 5 m*M* glucose, 2 m*M* glutamine, and 25 m*M* HEPES, at a pH of 7.15 at 37°C. 0 Ca^{2+} buffer (KEGTA) contained 110 m*M* KCl, 20 m*M* MOPS, 20 m*M* NaCl, 10 m*M* K_2H_2EGTA. Calcium-saturated buffer (CaEGTA) contained 110 m*M* KCl, 20 m*M* MOPS, 20 m*M* NaCl, 10 m*M* K_2CaEGTA. High K^+ buffer (High K^+) contained 146 m*M* KCl, 5 m*M* glucose, 2 m*M* glutamine, 10 m*M* HEPES, 10 m*M* MES, 10 m*M* Bicine. All chemicals were obtained from Sigma Chemical (St. Louis, MO), unless otherwise stated.

III. CELL CULTURE PREPARATION FOR FLUORESCENCE MEASUREMENTS

A. ANCHORAGE-DEPENDENT CELL LINES

For these experiments a number of anchorage-dependent cell lines were used. BALB/c-3T3 embryo fibroblasts were obtained from American Type Cell Culture Collection, Rockville, MD (ATTCC CCL 163). Primary human leiomyosarcoma cells were provided by Dr. Albert Liebowitz at the Arizona Cancer Center. These cells were cultured as fully described elsewhere.[19,39] For $[Ca^{2+}]_i$ and pH^{in} measurements, cells were subcultured on glass coverslips (9 × 22 mm), in 100-mm dish at 1 × 10^5 cells per dish and used after 48 to 72 h. These cells were washed three times with CSB. Subsequently, two coverslips (containing cells) were incubated for 45 min at 37°C, in a 5% CO_2 atmosphere with 3 ml of CSB containing 0.2% (v/v) Nu-serum (0.2% CSB) plus 7 μ*M* SNARF-1 (AM) and 2 μ*M* of Fura-2 (AM) and placed onto a rocker platform (Bellco Biotech, Vineland, NJ). These dyes were obtained from Molecular Probes (Eugene, OR). The AM forms of these dyes are lipophilic and cell permeant. Cellular esterases cleave the ester groups of these acetoxymethyl esters to yield the free acids which are more impermeant, and, therefore, "trapped" within cells.[23] After the 45-min incubation, buffer was removed by aspiration and the cells were washed 3 times with 0.2% CSB, followed by a second incubation in 0.2% CSB for 30 min at 37°C, to allow the complete hydrolysis of these dyes. After this time, two coverslips were placed back-to-back in a holder/perfusion device,[43] which was subsequently inserted into the fluorometer cuvette. All fluorescence measurements were performed in a temperature-controlled stirring cuvette unit housed in an SLM8000C (SLM, Urbana, IL), using 4-nm slits and an external rhodamine standard as a reference. Sample temperature was maintained at 37°C by keeping both the water jacket and the perfusion buffer at 37°C using a circulator water bath (Lauda Mod. RM20, Brinkmann Instruments Co.).

B. SUSPENSION CELL LINES

A variety of suspension cell lines were used in the present study. EPO8A7A6F12 hybridoma (EPO) cells were obtained from Amgen, Boulder, CO. These cells were cultured as fully described elsewhere.[19] For experiments, cells were seeded at 2 × 10^5 in a 1-l spinner flask. As needed, cells were centrifuged at 350 × g for 5 min. The pellet was resuspended in the appropriate buffer. Large luteal cells were obtained from superovulated western range ewes, separated by elutriation as described elsewhere.[44] Aliquots of 2 × 10^6 cells per 3.0 ml (fluorometer cuvette) were used for $[Ca^{2+}]_i$ and pH^{in} measurements. Cell loading with SNARF-1 and Fura-2 was performed essentially as described for anchorage-dependent cells,[19] except that after the second incubation, cells were washed again at 350 × g for 5 min, to remove excess dye. Fluorescence measurements were performed in a temperature-controlled, continuously stirred cuvette, at 37°C.

C. *IN VITRO* pH MEASUREMENTS

SNARF-1 in its free acid from was dissolved in "high K^+" buffer without nigericin, pH was varied between 6.0 to 8.0, and emission spectra were recorded at various excitation wavelengths. Although SNARF-1 offers a wide variety of possible combinations of excitations or emission wavelengths, the highest dynamic range for pH measurement was obtained at an excitation wavelength of 534, with emission wavelengths of 584 and 644 nm. The prominent features of these spectra are the isoemissive point at 600 and the peaks at 584 and 644 nm, which decrease and increase, respectively, as the solution pH is increased (Figure 1B). The ratio of fluorescence intensities at emissions of 644 and 584 nm can be used to generate calibration curves for pH (cf. Fig 2A). The fitting of these data into Equation 1 allowed us to obtain the following *in vitro* parameters for SNARF-1: $pK_a = 7.30$; $R_{min} = 0.44$; and $R_{max} = 1.86$. *In vitro* pH values used for calibration were obtained with a Beckman model 71 pH meter, using a Beckman gel-filled combination electrode. The electrode was calibrated at two known pH values, using commercially prepared standards from VWR Scientific (San Francisco, CA).

D. *IN VITRO* Ca^{2+} DETERMINATIONS

Ca^{2+}-EGTA buffers of defined compositions were used to generate both *in vitro* and *in situ* calibration curves with Fura-2. Corrections of Ca^{2+}/EGTA associations constants for pH, temperature, and ionic strength were performed as described by Harrison and Bers.[45] An alternative method to calculate the association constants for Ca^{2+}/EGTA is the computer method developed by Fabiato.[46] There is a very good agreement when using either method. Once these association constants are calculated, the *in vitro* and *in situ* calibration curves with Fura-2 are performed as described elsewhere.[19,47] Briefly, the titration was performed starting with 30 ml of KEGTA plus 1 μM Fura-2 (free acid), adjusting the pH at 7.10, at 37°C. An aliquot of 3.0 ml from this solution was removed and used to record its spectrum. Then, 3.0 ml of CaEGTA containing 1 μM Fura-2 was added to the remaining 27 ml, giving 9 m*M* KEGTA/1 m*M* CaEGTA. The pH was readjusted to 7.10, an aliquot of 3.0 ml was removed, and its spectrum recorded. Subsequent iterations were performed by removing 3.0 ml and replacing with equal volumes of the Ca^{2+}-containing solution. An alternative method to generate *in vitro* calibration curves for Fura-2 is to vary $[Ca^{2+}]$ using Chelex (Sigma Chemical) in the presence of trace $^{45}Ca^{2+}$, as described by Lattanzio.[17] Fluorescence of Fura-2 was monitored at 510-nm emission wavelength. The prominent features of these spectra are the isoexcitation point at 360 nm and the increase in fluorescence upon Ca^{2+} binding at 340 nm with a decrease in intensity at 380 nm (Figure 1C). Fluorescence at 360 nm (isoexcitation point) is proportional to the total amount of intracellular Fura-2 and can be used to evaluate possible quenching. The ratio of intensities at excitations of 340 and 380 nm can be used to generate calibration curves for Ca^{2+} (cf. Figure 2B). The fitting of these data into Equation 2 allowed us to obtain the *in vitro* Kd_a, R_{min}, and R_{max} for Fura-2 as a function of pH (Figure 4) (*vide supra*). It is worthwhile to mention that the effect of pH on Fura-2 fluorescence occurs not only at the 340 and 380 nm, but also in the fluorescence at the isoemissive point. These phenomena are inherent to Fura-2 and independent of the presence of SNARF-1 in the solution.

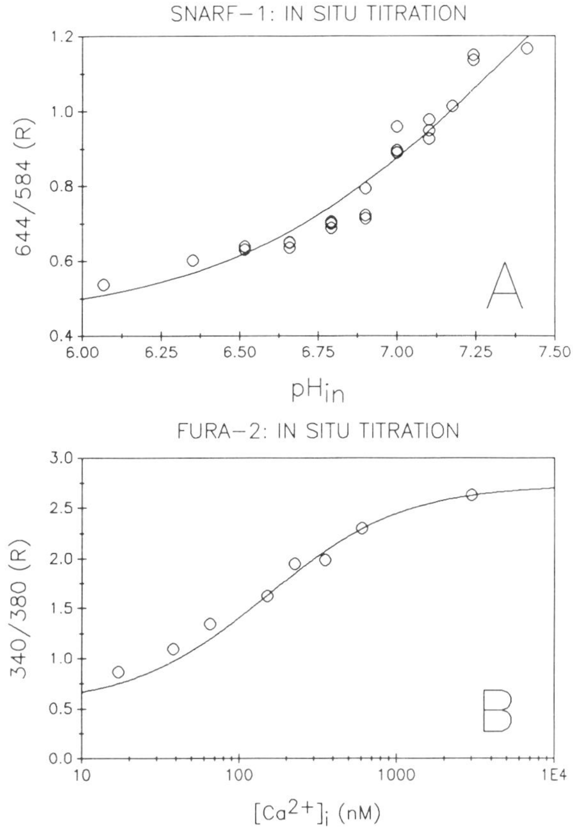

FIGURE 2. (A) *In situ* calibration of SNARF-1 in anchorage-dependent 3T3 cells. (B) *In situ* calibration of Fura-2 in anchorage-dependent 3T3 cells. BALB/c-3T3 cells grown onto coverslips were loaded with either 7 μM SNARF-1 (A), or 2 μM Fura-2 (B) (*vide infra*). Subsequently, two coverslips back to back were inserted into the fluorometer cuvette using a holder device[43] and their fluorescence spectra were recorded. Data were fitted using Equations 1 and 2. (From Martínez-Zaguilán, R., Martínez, G. M., Lattanzio, G., and Gillies, R. J., *Am. J. Physiol.*, 260, C297, 1991. With permission.)

E. EFFECT OF DYE CONCENTRATION

A complication shared by SNARF-1 and Fura-2 is the effect of dye concentration on their respective ratio (Figure 3). It is commonly assumed that fluorescence ratio corrects for variations in dye concentrations. This is true only for low dye concentrations or short pathlengths. In the case of SNARF-1, the ratio of 644/584 increases as the concentration of the dye increases (Figure 3A, solid line). This effect is much greater on the R_{max} than the R_{min}. This is not an exclusive problem of SNARF-1, since increases or decreases in ratio as a function of dye-concentration have been observed in other pH fluorescent dyes (Reference 22, unpublished observations). The ratio 340/380 for Fura-2 is also affected by the dye concentration. The effect is in the opposite direction to that displayed by SNARF-1, because the lower wavelength is in the numerator in this case (Figure 3B, solid line). Similar to our findings with SNARF-1, this effect is also greater on the R_{max} than on the R_{min} (Figure 3B).

The effect of dye concentration on the fluorescence ratios is mostly due to inner filters, since they can be corrected by fitting the fluorescence data into the following equation:

$$F_{corr} = F_{obs}\{\text{antilog}[A_{ex} + A_{em})/2]\} \quad (3)$$

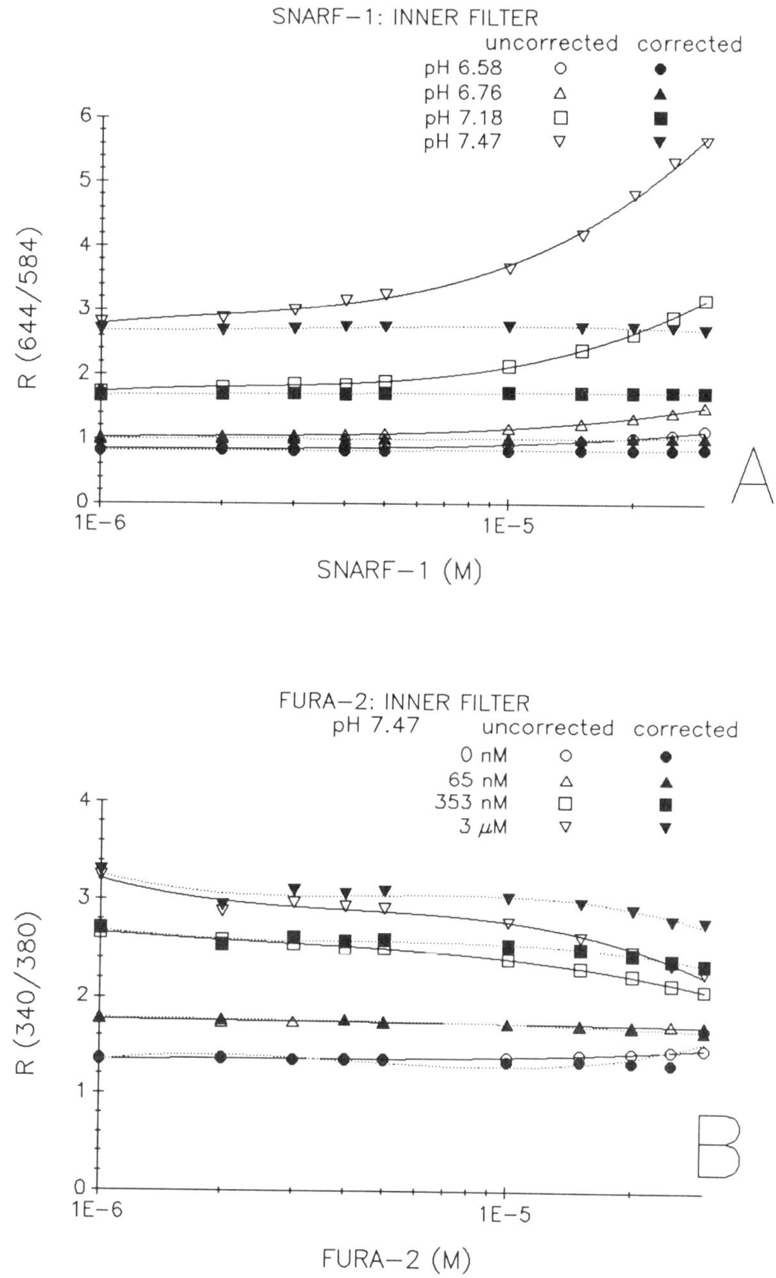

FIGURE 3. (A) Effect of Fura-2 concentration on the 340/380 fluorescence ratio at different free Ca^{2+} concentrations at pH 7.40. Fura-2 (free acid) was dissolved at various concentrations in Ca^{2+}-EGTA buffers at the indicated free Ca^{2+} concentrations and their spectra were recorded. The dotted line represents data that has been corrected for inner filter whereas the solid line represents data uncorrected for inner filter; (B) Effect of SNARF-1 concentration on the 644/584 fluorescence ratio at different pHs. SNARF-1 was dissolved at the indicated dye concentrations in high K^+ buffer at various pHs, and their spectra were recorded as described in the legend to Figure 1. The dotted line represents data that has been corrected for inner filters whereas the solid line represents data uncorrected for inner filters.

where F_{corr} is the corrected fluorescence value, F_{obs} is the fluorescence obtained at the particular wavelength of interest, and A_{ex} and A_{em} are the absorbances at excitation and emission wavelengths, respectively.

The dotted lines in Figure 3A and 3B represent data corrected for inner filter using Equation 3. These indicate that corrections for inner filter of SNARF-1 ratios totally abolish the effect of dye concentration on the estimated R values of SNARF-1 (Figure 3A, dotted lines). In contrast, the effect of dye concentration on the Fura-2 fluorescence cannot fully be explained by the inner filter, since corrections for the inner filter do not abolish such anomalous behavior and may involve self-quenching effects (cf. Figure 3B, dotted lines). Although inner filter effects cannot be neglected *in vitro,* cells are so thin that this does not likely represent a serious problem *in situ*. This is especially true when dealing with anchorage-dependent cells, where the pathlength is limited to a few μm (i.e., a single monolayer of cells). However, the inner filter could represent a significant problem in suspension cell cultures and in tissues where the pathlength used is variable, i.e., proportional to the concentration of cells in the cuvette or to the tissue thickness, respectively. Therefore, differences in cell number and dye-loading would result in significant differences in the Fura-2 ratio. This problem can be minimized by using a microcuvette or a cuvette with a front phase geometry[41] and by carefully controlling experimental variables such as cell number and dye-loading conditions. In tissues, this problem is essentially intractable.

F. FLUOROMETRIC DATA COLLECTION AND DATA ANALYSIS

For simultaneous pH^{in} and $[Ca^{2+}]_i$ measurements using SNARF-1 and Fura-2, data were collected in a continuous acquisition mode where the emission and excitation mode was alternated as follows: emission at 510 nm with excitations wavelengths of 340, 360, and 380 nm (Fura-2 conditions); followed by excitation at 534 nm with acquisitions of the emissions at 584, 600, and 644 nm (SNARF-1 conditions). Experiments in our lab have shown that the fluroescence of SNARF-1 do not interfere with the Fura-2 fluorescence, and vice versa[19]. This cycle lasts 0.266 min and is repeated as many times as necessary. Data were translated to ASCII format. Conversions of ratio values to both pH^{in} and Ca^{2+} were performed with Lotus 1-2-3 (Lotus Development Corp.) using Equations 1 and 2 and plotted using commercial graphics software (Sigmaplot, Scientific Graph System by Jandel, Sci.). Analysis of both *in vitro* and *in situ* calibration curves as well as the estimation of Kd_a, R_{max}, and R_{min} values were performed using the simplex method (MINSQ, MicroMath Scientific Software, Salt Lake, UT). An alternative method to obtain these parameters has been described by Eidelman and Cabantchik[26] and is based in the linearization of the data by using the following equation:

$$R = R_{max} - (\alpha.Kd_a)(R - R_{min})/[Ca^{2+}] \quad (4)$$

where α represents the S_{f2}/S_{b2} ratio (*vide infra*). Thus, by plotting R vs. $(R - R_{min})/[Ca^{2+}]$ for the range of Ca^{2+}-concentration used (i.e., submicromolar to micromolar), one can obtain the $\alpha \cdot Kd_a$ from the slope and R_{max} from the Y intercept.

Although similar results are obtained by using either method, Equation 4 allows one to use a relatively discrete number of calibration points and, most important, avoids the use of relatively high concentrations of Ca^{2+} for the determination of R_{max}, which in some cases is troublesome since it induces cell clumping (in suspension cells) or contraction in attached cells.[48] In contrast, when using the simplex method, we must use higher $[Ca^{2+}]$ in our titrations and the goodness of the fit depends on the number of calibration points available.

G. *IN SITU* CALIBRATION OF SNARF-1

Since the pK_a, R_{max}, and R_{min} of a dye may vary from cell to cell, possibly due to inherent differences in intracellular environment, we emphasize the need to perform *in situ* calibration curves for each of the cell lines of interest. Calibration of intracellular SNARF-1 in both anchorage-dependent and suspension cells was performed as described previously.[19] Briefly, in the case of anchorage-dependent cells, SNARF-1 loaded cells were perfused with high K^+ buffer containing 6.8 μM of the K^+/H^+ ionophore nigericin and 2 μM valinomycin. The K^+ concentration in high K^+ buffer is equal to that present in their respective cells.[19,35,36,44] Nigericin sets the H^+ gradient equal to the K^+ gradient, and valinomycin completes the collapse of the K^+ gradient without significant effects on cell volume. Under these conditions, the pH^{in} of the cells is equal to the extracellular pH (pH^{ex}). By varying pH^{ex} between pH 5.5 to 8.0, one can obtain the pK_a of SNARF-1 from these *in situ* calibration curves, using Equation 1. In the case of suspension cell lines, an aliquot of SNARF-1 loaded cells were resuspended in 3.0 ml of high K^+ buffer containing 6.8 μM nigericin and 2 μM valinomycin, and the pH in the solution was increased stepwise by adding 3 μM of 1 M NaOH directly into the fluorometer cuvette. The ratio of 644/584 fluorescence of SNARF-1 was used to generate the *in situ* calibration curves for each of the cell lines being used (Figure 2A).

H. *IN SITU* CALIBRATION OF FURA-2

For calibration of intracellular Fura-2 in anchorage-dependent and suspension cell lines, we included in the Ca^{2+}-EGTA buffer the nonfluorescent analog of the Ca^{2+} ionophore A23187, 4Br-A23187 (5 μM) (Molecular Probes), to collapse the Ca^{2+} gradient[49] and 6.8 μM nigericin plus 2 μM valinomycin to set $pH^{ex} = pH^{in}$ (Reference 19). For anchorage-dependent cells, FURA-2 loaded cells were perfused with high K^+/CaEGTA buffers containing 4Br-A23187, nigericin, and valinomycin at selected pH values, with variable free Ca^{2+} concentrations ranging from 0 to 3 μM (*vide supra*). Alternately, FURA-2 loaded cells were incubated for 10 min in high K^+/CaEGTA buffers in the presence of 4Br-A23187, nigericin, and valinomycin, with selected Ca^{2+} concentrations. Subsequently, coverslips containing cells were transferred to the fluorometer cuvette and perfused continuously with their respective high K^+/CaEGTA buffer containing ionophores. For the *in situ* titration of suspension cells, aliquots of Fura-2 loaded cells were allowed to equilibrate for 10 min in the presence of 4Br-A23187, valinomycin, and nigericin at the above-mentioned concentrations, centrifuged at 350 × g for 5 min, resuspended in their respective high K^+/CaEGTA buffer containing ionophores, and the 340/380 fluorescence ratio of Fura-2 was used to generate the *in situ* titration curves. We have selected these conditions to do *in situ* calibration curves of anchorage-dependent and suspension cell lines,[19,44] since the Kd_a of Fura-2 is significantly affected by pH in the physiological range (Figures 4 and 5), and important changes in pH^{in} may occur in some cell types upon 4Br-A23187 treatment (Figure 6). Therefore it can be anticipated that calibration of those "A23187-responsive" cells is not a trivial matter. Indeed, we have observed that it is very straightforward to calibrate cells *in situ* that do not increase their pH^{in} upon 4Br-A23187 treatment, such as small and large ovine luteal cells and hybridoma (EPO) cells. In contrast, the calibration of 3T3 cells, which do respond with an increase in pH^{in} upon A23187 treatment, is extremely difficult. A partial solution to this problem is to set both $pH^{ex} = pH^{in}$ and $[Ca^{2+}]^{ex} = [Ca^{2+}]_i$ by using both nigericin, valinomycin, and 4Br-A23187, in order to obtain an *in situ* Kd_a for Fura-2 at various pHs. Since it is difficult to predict which cell types would respond with pH^{in} changes upon A23187 treatment, we recommend using this approach to calibrate all cells *in situ*.

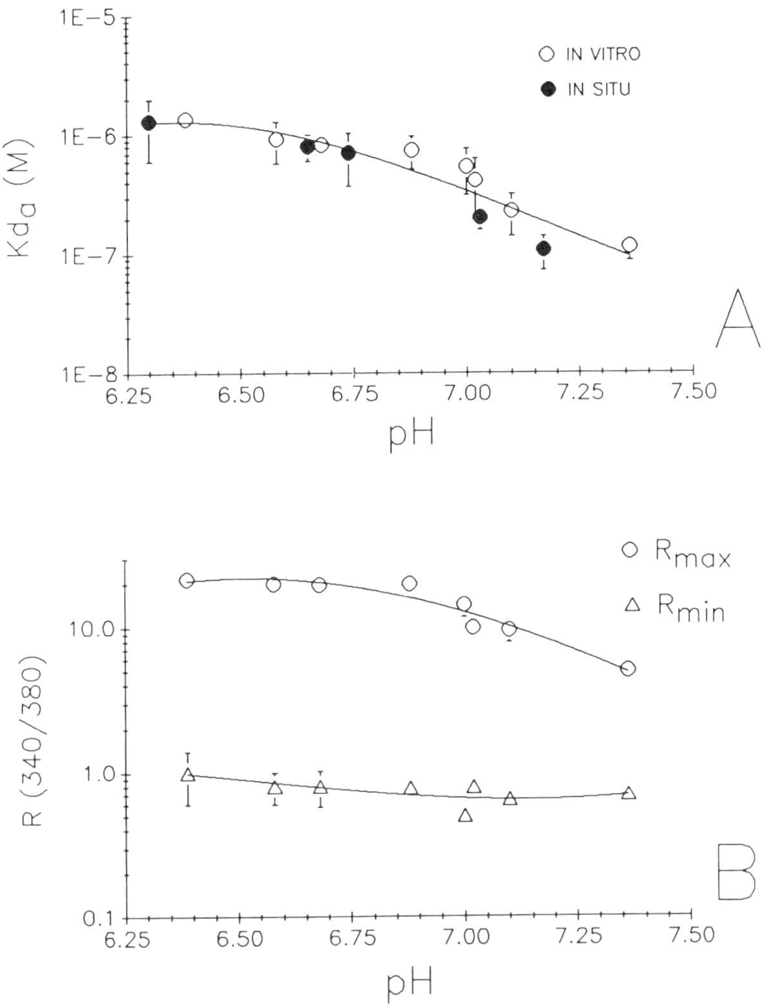

FIGURE 4. (A) Effect of pH on the Kd_a of Ca^{2+} binding to Fura-2 *in vitro* (solid line) and *in situ* (dashed line). Titration curves similar to that shown in Figure 2B at various pHs were generated both *in vitro* and in 3T3 cells growth onto coverslips. Each point represents the mean ± S.D. of 9 to 11 different Ca^{2+} concentrations, at the indicated pH value. H^+ and Ca^{2+} association constants for EGTA were calculated as described elsewhere.[45,46] Fitting of the curve was done using Equation 5; (B) effect of pH on the *in vitro* R_{max} and R_{min} of Fura-2. Values of R_{max} and R_{min} were obtained by fitting the experimental values from curves similar to that shown in Figure 2B (Equation 2) and therefore represent the mean ± S.D. of 9 to 11 data points per indicated pH value. These curves were fitted into Equation 6 to obtain the parameters that describe the effect of pH on R_{max} and R_{min} (*vide infra*).

We have generated a number of titration curves similar to that shown in Figure 2B at a variety of pHs and have fit these data into Equation 2 to obtain the Kd_a, R_{max}, and R_{min}. The results of such analyses are summarized in Figure 4. Figure 4A shows that the *in vitro* Fura-2 Kd_a decreases as pH is increased. Superimposable curves are obtained when 3T3 cells are used to generate the *in situ* titrations. We have used similar experimental protocols for the *in situ* calibration of Fura-2 in other cell lines and have determined similar behavior regarding the effect of pH on Kd_a.[19,44] Since the Kd_a values of Fura-2 are so affected by

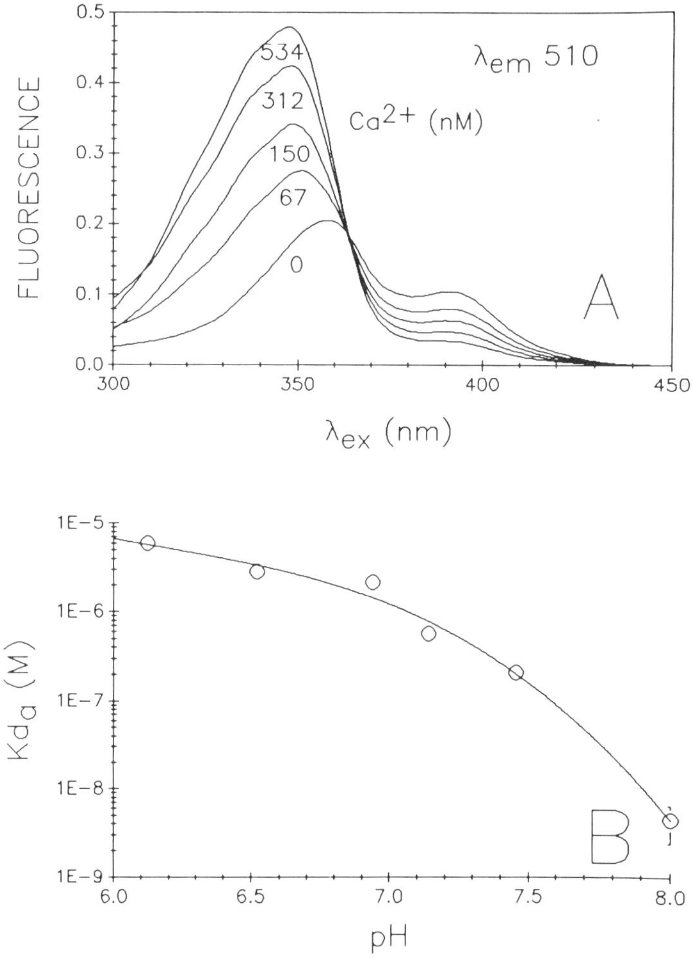

FIGURE 5. An atypical form of Fura-2 is present in some Fura-2 batches. (A) *In vitro* fluorescence excitation spectra of Fura-2 at various concentrations of free Ca^{2+}. One μM Fura-2 (free acid) was dissolved in a Ca^{2+}-EGTA buffer at the indicated free Ca^{2+} concentrations (nM). Excitation spectra were collected using an emission wavelength of 510 nm. The remarkable features of these spectra include the isoexcitation point at 360, the peaks at 340 and 380 nm which increase and decrease, respectively, as Ca^{2+} is increased, and the shoulder at 390 nm (cf. Figure 1C); (B) effect of pH on the Kd_a of the atypical form of Fura-2. Titration curves similar to that shown in Figure 5A at various pHs were generated *in vitro*. From such calibration curves, Kd_a values were obtained using Equation 2. Each point is the result of 11 different free Ca^{2+} concentrations at the indicated pH value (cf. Figure 4A).

pH, the Kd_a must be adjusted throughout an experiment to reflect changes in pH values. This requires simultaneous measurement of both pH^{in} and $[Ca^{2+}]_i$.

The effect of pH on the FURA-2 Kd_a can be described by the following equation:

$$Kd_{a,pHcorr} = [Kd_{a,max} + 10(pH^{in} - pK_a) \cdot Kd_{a,min}]/[10(pH^{in} - pK_a) + 1] \qquad (5)$$

where $Kd_{a,\,pHcorr}$ is the pH corrected Kd_a, and $Kd_{a,\,max}$ and $Kd_{a,\,min}$ are the maximum and minimum Kd_a, respectively. By fitting the data shown in Figure 4A into Equation 5, we obtain the following parameters: $Kd_{a,\,max}$ = 3,586 nM; $Kd_{a,\,min}$ = 116 nM; pK_a = 5.12.

During the course of our *in vitro* experiments we also noticed that the Fura-2 R_{max} and

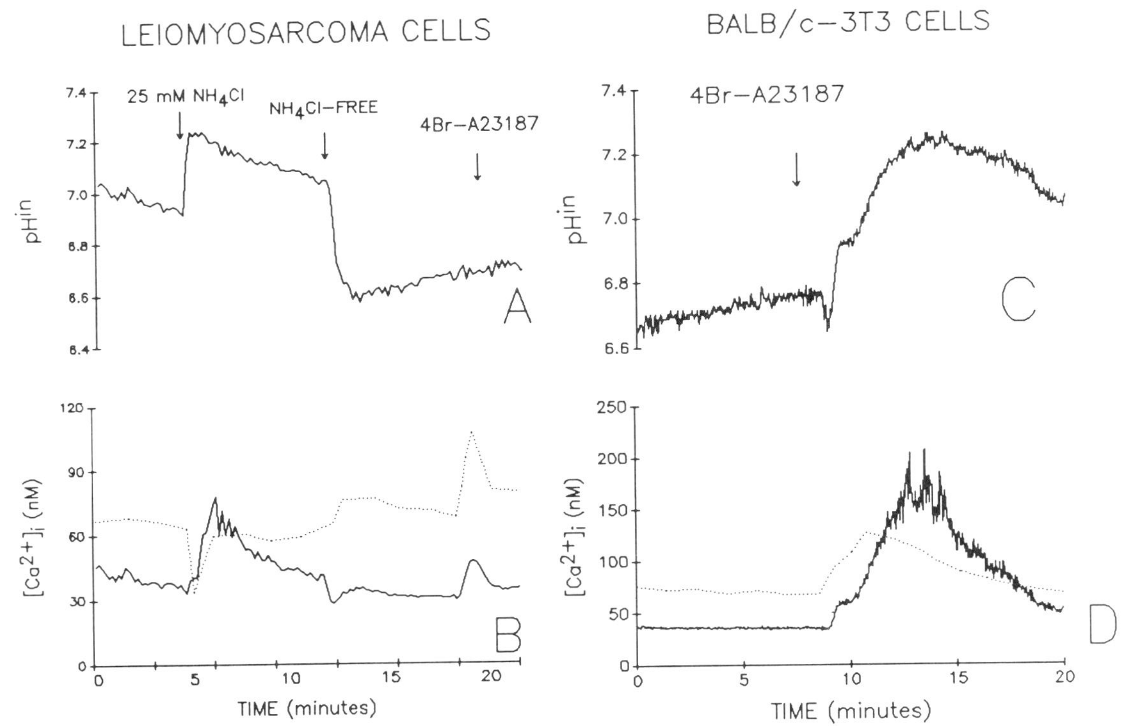

FIGURE 6. Left: simultaneous evaluation of the effect of NH_4Cl and 4Br-A23187 on pH^{in} (A) and $[Ca^{2+}]_i$ (B) in primary human leiomyosarcoma cells. Leiomyosarcoma cells were grown onto coverslips, coloaded with Fura-2 and SNARF-1, and their fluorescence was recorded. Perfusion was begun with CSB, HCO_3^--free. At the time indicated, media was exchanged for CSB containing 25 m*M* NH_4Cl. Subsequently, media was exchanged for NH_4Cl-free. At the time indicated, media was exchanged for CSB containing 5 μ*M* 4Br-A23187. Right: simultaneous evaluation of the effect of 4Br-A23187 on pH^{in} (C) and $[Ca^{2+}]_i$ (D) in BALB/c-3T3 cells. BALB/c-3T3 cells were grown onto coverslips and coloaded with Fura-2 and SNARF-1. Perfusion was begun with CSB, HCO_3^--free. At the times indicated by arrows, perfusate was exchanged by CSB containing 4Br-A23187 at the concentration of 10 μ*M*. In panels B and D, the solid line represents the estimated $[Ca^{2+}]_i$ using the pH-corrected Fura-2 Kd_a, R_{max} and R_{min}. The dotted lines represent the estimated $[Ca^{2+}]_i$ using pH-uncorrected parameters of Kd_a obtained from the literature (i.e., 224 n*M*).[47] (C and D from Martínez-Zaguilán, R. et al., *Am. J. Physiol.*, 260, C297, 1991. With permission.)

R_{min} values were also affected by pH. As shown in Figure 4B, increasing pH causes a decrease in both R_{max} and R_{min} *in vitro* and *in situ*. The magnitude of these effects of pH are similar between *in vitro* and *in situ* data for R_{min}, but not in the case of R_{max} (data not shown). The reasons for this anomalous behavior of the dye are unknown. The effect of pH on the R_{max} and R_{min} can be fit to a polynomial equation:

$$[R = k_1(pH)^3 + k_2(pH)^2 + k_3(pH) + k_4] \tag{6}$$

The fitting of the *in vitro* data shown in Figure 4B into Equation 6 produced the following results: For R_{max}, ($k_1 = 30.32$; $k_2 = -640.27$; $k_3 = 4479.6$; $k_4 = -10372$); for R_{min}, ($k_1 = 1.057$; $k_2 = -21.486$; $k_3 = 144.99$; $k_4 = -324.03$).

Therefore, the effect of pH on the Kd_a, R_{min}, and R_{max} of Fura-2 can be predicted by Equations 5 and 6 with the fitting parameters discussed above. By using these equations with simultaneous measurement of pH^{in}, the Kd_a, R_{min}, and R_{max} of Fura-2 can be calculated at any pH and at any time and used to calculate the $[Ca^{2+}]_i$. These corrections are probably not cell-type specific, given the coincidence of *in vitro* and *in situ* curves (Figure 3B and 4A). An important drawback when using these corrections is that they are only valid within the boundary condition of $6.3 > pH \leq 7.4$.

A further consideration when applying this technique is that during the course of our experiments we noticed that certain batches of Fura-2 exhibited a shoulder at ca. 390 nm (Figure 5A; cf. Figure 1B). The presence of this shoulder at ca. 390 nm is reported to represent a dye that has undergone decomposition or that has been incompletely hydrolyzed when loaded into cells as Fura-2(AM).[50,51] Furthermore, it has been suggested that this form of Fura-2 represents a Ca^{2+}-insensitive form of Fura-2.[51] The data shown in Figure 5A were obtained using the free-acid form of Fura-2 and indicates that this dye with a shoulder at 390 nm is as Ca^{2+}-sensitive as the parental form (cf. Figure 1B). We have generated a number of calibration curves, at various pHs, and have found that this form of "Fura-2" is more pH sensitive that the parental compound. We have also found this form of "Fura-2" in cells loaded with Fura-2(AM) in a number of different batches from Molecular Probes. The presence of this contaminant further complicates any correction for pH on the Kd_a, R_{max}, and R_{min}. Therefore, caution must be exercised when using the commercial form of this dye, since it is possible that a number of other intermediate forms of Fura-2, with different sensitivity for both Ca^{2+} and pH exist. We strongly emphasize the need to routinely acquire a full spectrum of Fura-2 at the beginning and at the end of each experiment, to check for the absence of such a shoulder. If such a shoulder is present, quantitative measurements of Ca^{2+} using Fura-2 should be avoided. Then, alternatives dyes such as Indo-1 should be considered. Recently, Weigmann et al.[42] have performed simultaneous measurements of pH^{in} and $[Ca^{2+}]^{in}$ using the fluorescence of SNARF-1 and Indo-1. Corrections for pH on the Kd_a of Indo-1 should be straightforward, using the methods described here.

I. SIMULTANEOUS MEASUREMENTS OF pH^{in} AND $[Ca^{2+}]_i$ IN ANCHORAGE-DEPENDENT AND SUSPENSION CELL LINES

Once the optimal experimental conditions for the simultaneous measurement of pH^{in} and $[Ca^{2+}]_i$ were established, we next tested for the usefulness of this system to monitor changes in pH^{in} and $[Ca^{2+}]_i$ in anchorage-dependent and suspension cell lines. Figure 6 shows the effect of NH_4Cl in anchorage-dependent primary human leiomyosarcoma cells, coloaded with Fura-2 and SNARF-1. Perfusion was started with CSB, HCO_3^--free media, at a $pH^{ex} = 7.15$. At the time indicated by the arrow, the perfusate was exchanged for CSB containing

25 mM NH_4Cl. This induced a rapid increase in pH^{in} (Figure 6A).[14] The increase in pH^{in} is associated with a decrease in the pH-uncorrected Fura-2 fluroescence (Figure 6B, dotted lines). This is expected since the Fura-2 Kd_a decreases with increasing pH (cf. Figure 4A). Subsequently, the NH_4Cl solution was exchanged for HCO_3^--free CSB, to wash out the NH_4Cl. This induced a rapid acidification of the cytosol that is associated with an increase in the pH-uncorrected Fura-2 signal (Figure 6A; Figure 6B, dotted lines). The pH-uncorrected Ca^{2+} values were obtained by using Kd_a = 224 nM[47] and pH-uncorrected values for R_{max} and R_{min}. In order to make quantitative measurements of Ca^{2+}, we have corrected for the effect of pH on the Kd_a, R_{max}, and R_{min} using Equations 5 and 6. The solid lines indicate the pH-corrected Ca^{2+} values and indicate that after NH_4Cl treatment there is a significant increase in $[Ca^{2+}]_i$ (Figure 6B, solid line) which slowly relaxes back to the baseline. Removal of the NH_4Cl results in an insignificant decrease in $[Ca^{2+}]_i$ (Figure 6B, solid line).Further addition of 4Br-A23187 resulted in a transient increase in $[Ca^{2+}]_i$ with no changes in pH^{in}.

Figures 6C and 6D show the effect of 4Br-A23187 on pH^{in} and $[Ca^{2+}]_i$ in serum-deprived quiescent 3T3 cells. The treatment of these cells with the ionophore in bicarbonate-free CSB, at a pH^{ex} of 7.10, results in increases in both $[Ca^{2+}]_i$ and pH^{in}. These changes in both pH^{in} and Ca^{2+} occur simultaneously with a half time of approximately 3 min. (Figures 6C and 6D) In a nominally Ca^{2+}-free media, addition of 4Br-A23187 does not induce a significant increase in pH^{in} and Ca^{2+} (cf. Reference 19).

Summarizing, in human leiomyosarcoma cells and in 3T3 cells, we have shown that an increase in both pH^{in} and Ca^{2+} occurs upon treatment of cells with NH_4Cl, to increase pH^{in} or, with A23187, to increase Ca^{2+} (Figure 6). Similar suggestions that an increase in pH^{in} is associated with an increase in Ca^{2+}, and that an increase in Ca^{2+} seems to be associated with increases in pH^{in}, have been reported in the literature in different cell types, through nonsimultaneous analysis of pH^{in} and Ca^{2+} (References 3, 12, 14, 21, 52). However, our results are discrepant with those of others that have shown no relationship between increases in pH^{in} and $[Ca^{2+}]_i$ or vice versa.[40,53,54] Although changes in pH^{in} and/or $[Ca^{2+}]_i$ have been reported in a variety of cell types, most of those studies provide only circumstantial evidence for the relatedness of such changes. Reasons for these apparent discrepancies between labs are multiple and might involve artifactual effects of pH on the Kd_a of the Ca^{2+} fluoroprobes being used. Therefore, simultaneous measurements of these parameters associated with corrections for the effect of pH on the Kd_a, R_{max}, and R_{min} are necessary to understand the temporal relationship, if any, between pH^{in} and $[Ca^{2+}]_i$.

We emphasize corrections for pH effects on the parameters Kd_a, R_{max}, and R_{min} in those cases where changes in Ca^{2+} are associated with changes in pH^{in}. This is further supported by our observations in suspension cells (Figure 7). Treatment of EPO hybridoma cells with 4Br-A23187 induced a large increase in $[Ca^{2+}]_i$ with no change in pH^{in} (Figures 7A and 7B). Treatment of large ovarian luteal cells with 500 nM $PGF_{2\alpha}$ induced a small, but significant increase in $[Ca^{2+}]_i$ with no changes in pH^{in} (cf. Reference 44). Further addition of 4Br-A23187 results in a large increase in $[Ca^{2+}]_i$ with no changes in pH^{in} (Figures 7C and 7D). Under these conditions, notice that both the uncorrected (dotted lines) and pH-corrected (solid line) data are practically superimposable in both cell types (cf. Figure 6). This is due to the fact that the pH^{in} is ca. 7.3 in these cells, and the effect of pH on the Fura-2 Kd_a, R_{max}, and R_{min} is minor under these conditions (cf. Figures 4A and 4B). These data strongly support our assertion that if the pH^{in} is $\geq$7.2 and changes in pH^{in} do not occur upon cell-treatment with hormones or drug, quantitation of changes in $[Ca^{2+}]_i$ does not require simultaneous pH measurement. However, if treatment induces changes in pH^{in}, interpretation of the Fura-2 fluorescence data could be erroneous, unless corrections for pH on the Kd_a, R_{max}, and R_{min} are performed (cf. Figure 6).

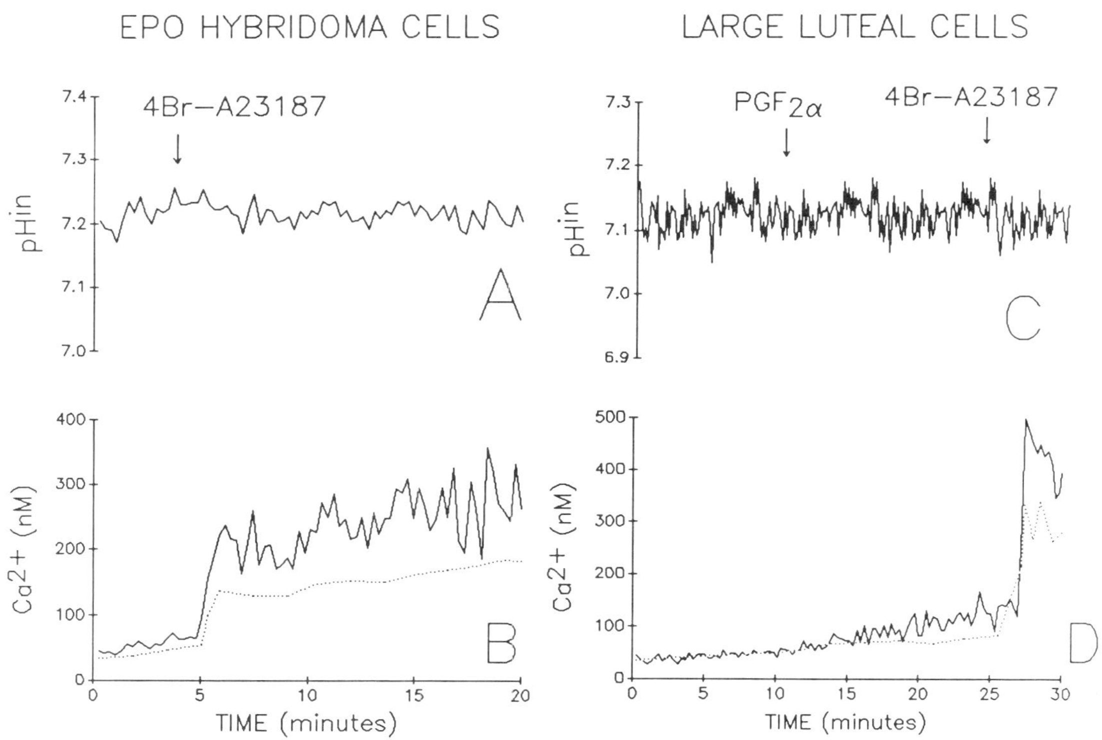

FIGURE 7. Simultaneous measurement of pH^{in} and $[Ca^{2+}]_i$ in suspension cell cultures. Left: simultaneous measurement of pH^{in} (A) and $[Ca^{2+}]_i$ (B) in EPO hybridoma cell line. The EPO hybridoma cell line was cultured as described elsewhere.[19] These cells were coloaded with Fura-2 and SNARF-1 and their fluorescence was recorded. At the time indicated, 5 μM 4Br-A23187 was added directly into the fluorometer cuvette. Right: effect of $PGF_{2\alpha}$ on pH^{in} (C) and $[Ca^{2+}]_i$ (D) in ovarian large luteal cells. Ovarian large luteal cells were obtained from corpora lutea of superovulated ewes as described elsewhere[44] and handled for fluorescence experiments as described for EPO cells. At the time indicated by the arrow, 500 nM $PGF_{2\alpha}$ was added directly into the fluorometer cuvette. Subsequently 5 μM 4Br-A23187 was added directly into the fluorometer cuvette. In panels B and D, the solid line represents the estimated $[Ca^{2+}]_i$ using the pH-corrected Fura-2 Kd_a, R_{max} and R_{min}. The dotted lines represent the estimated $[Ca^{2+}]_i$ using pH-uncorrected parameters of Kd_a obtained from the literature (i.e., 224 nM).[47] (A and B from Martínez-Zaguilán, R. et al., *Am. J. Physiol.*, 260, C297, 1991. With permission.)

IV. LIMITATIONS AND FUTURE PROSPECTS

Fluorescent spectroscopy is a powerful technique for studying dynamic changes in ions such as $[Ca^{2+}]_i$ and pH^{in} in a number of cellular processes such as secretion, neurotransmission, and cell proliferation upon treatment with hormones and other factors, as well as with pharmacological agents. Our understanding of the sequence of ionic events that occur upon cell stimulation or drug-treatment should be critical to elucidate the signal transduction mechanisms that underlie a particular effector.

As with any other technique, fluorescence spectroscopy is not free of drawbacks. If the fluorescence indicators were solely located at the compartment(s) that one wants to monitor, the cell population were homogenous, and the response of the cells were synchronous, then fluorescence spectroscopy would be the technique of choice. However, it has been found that some fluorescent ion-indicators do compartmentalize into organelles, and cell populations, although apparently morphologically homogeneous, exhibit heterogeneity in their physiological responses when assessed at a single cell level.[27,34,48,50,51,55] Further complications in using fluorescence spectroscopy arise from dye leakage or active extrusion of the dye, which impairs any measurement in those cells.[32] This represents a minor problem when dealing with attached cells, but represents a major problem when using suspension cells. In some cases this can be blocked by the use of anion transport inhibitors such as probenecid.[32] However, in some cases this hinders changes in the ion being measured.[44] The development of new drugs that block the export of these dyes without affecting physiological responses is one possibility to solve this problem. Antibodies against the fluoroprobe under study is another possibility. Most of the above problems can be theoretically solved using digital fluorescence microscopy. This is an extremely powerful technique. As a consequence, it is extremely sophisticated and prone to artifact in the hands of inexperienced investigators.

Another problem when using the AM form of the fluorescent indicators is that this form of the dye is cytotoxic. Fortunately, cytotoxicity is only observed after several hours. Cell viability is maintained for up to 4 h; however, incubation of cells with the AM form of the dye for as little as the normal time required for cell loading (i.e., 30 min at 37°C) at concentrations as low as 1 μM, followed by wash out of the dye, results in arrest of the cell proliferation within the first 24 h, possibly due to ATP depletion or to aldehyde formation upon cleavage of the AM form of these dyes.[19,56,57] Further studies are required to understand the molecular mechanisms that underlie the cytotoxicity of these dyes. The recent availability of Ca^{2+} fluoroprobes coupled to dextran should minimize problems associated with dye compartmentalization, dye leakage, and cytotoxicity. One of the most urgent needs is to develop new Ca^{2+} indicators with a much lower affinity for H^+s than the currently available. Until then, we will have to contend with corrections for effects of pH on Kd_a of Ca^{2+} indicators to obtain quantitative measurements, if pH^{in} changes occur concomitantly with $[Ca^{2+}]_i$ changes.

CONCLUSION

Intracellularly trapped pH and Ca^{2+} indicators such as SNARF-1 and Fura-2 have some distinct advantages over other techniques used for measuring ionic changes: unsurpassed time resolution in a continuous record, high sensitivity to small changes in pH and Ca^{2+}, relatively small number of cells required, and compatibility with almost any extracellular medium. Known limitations include a small but definite leakage, dye uptake into mitochondria and other organelles, pH effects on the Kd_a, R_{max}, and R_{min} of the Ca^{2+} indicators, and deleterious effects on cell proliferation in the long term. By using appropriate controls and by simultaneous measurements of pH^{in} and $[Ca^{2+}]_i$, quantitative $[Ca^{2+}]_i$ measurements can be made. We strongly recommend that simultaneous measurements of these two ions should be made when fluorescent Ca^{2+} indicators are being used. Our results indicate that, if important changes in pH occur upon stimulation of the cell, this would result in changes in Kd_a of these Ca^{2+}-fluoroprobes that would under- or overestimate the $[Ca^{2+}]_i$ concentration. The use of simultaneous pH^{in} and Ca^{2+} measurements should prove to be a useful tool not only for the measurement of ion movements in cell populations, but also to point out the location of site-specific biochemical events within a cell through image analysis. This should allow one to distinguish the heterogeneous behavior of cells in apparently uniform cell samples. The development of new and more versatile Ca^{2+} indicators, not affected by pH, should expand our capabilities in measuring Ca^{2+} movements in conjunction with other physiologically relevant ions. Furthermore, with the advent of new fluorescent probes it is possible to measure not only Ca^{2+} and H^+, but also other physiologically important ions such as Mg^{2+}, Cl^-, Na^+, and K^+ (for a review, see Reference 23).

ACKNOWLEDGMENTS

I would like to thank to Dr. Robert J. Gillies for critically reviewing this manuscript, Gloria M. Martínez and David Camacho for their technical assistance; Dr. Patricia B. Hoyer and Dr. Julie A. Wegner for providing ovine luteal cells; and Dr. Alexander Fabiato for providing me with a copy of his computer program SPECS to calculate Ca^{2+}/EGTA association constants. This work was supported by National Institutes of Health Grant R01 GM43046.

REFERENCES

1. **Williamson, J. R. and Monck, J. R.,** Hormone effects on cellular Ca^{2+} fluxes, *Annu. Rev. Physiol.*, 51, 107, 1989.
2. **Berridge, M. J.,** Inositol triphosphate and diacylglycerol: two interacting second messengers, *Annu. Rev. Biochem.*, 56, 156, 1987.
3. **Vincentini, L. M. and Villarreal, M. L.,** Inositol phosphate turnover, cytosolic Ca^{2+} and pH: putative signals for the control of cell growth, *Life Sci.*, 38, 2269, 1986.
4. **Nishizuka, Y.,** The role of protein kinase C in cell surface signal transduction and tumor promotion, *Nature (London)*, 308, 693, 1984.
5. **Smith, B. N. and Colburn, N. H.,** Protein kinase C and it substrates in tumor promoter-sensitive and -resistant cell, *J. Biol. Chem.*, 263, 6424, 1988.
6. **Rozengurt, E.,** Early signals in the mitogenic response, *Science*, 234, 161, 1986.
7. **Pietrobon, D., DiVirgilio, F., and Pozzan, T.,** Structural and functional aspects of calcium homeostasis in eukaryotic cells, *Eur. J. Biochem.*, 193, 599, 1990.
8. **Yarden, Y. and Ullrich, A.,** Growth factor receptor tyrosine kinases, *Annu. Rev. Biochem.*, 57, 443, 1988.
9. **Busa, W. B.,** Mechanisms and consequences of pH-mediated cell regulation, *Annu. Rev. Physiol.*, 48, 389, 1986.
10. **Moolenaar, W. H.,** Effects of growth factors on intracellular pH regulation, *Annu. Rev. Physiol.*, 48, 363, 1986.
11. **Roos, A. and Boron, W. F.,** Intracellular pH, *Physiol. Rev.*, 61, 296, 1981.
12. **Ives, H. E. and Daniel, T. O.,** Interrelationship between growth factor-induced pH changes and intracellular Ca^{2+}, *Proc. Natl. Acad. Sci. U.S.A.*, 84, 1950, 1987.
13. **Rasmussen, H. and Barret, P. Q.,** Calcium messenger system: an integrated view, *Physiol. Rev.*, 64, 934, 1984.
14. **Grinstein, S. and Cohen, S.,** Cytoplasmic $[Ca^{2+}]$ and intracellular pH in lymphocytes. Role of membrane potential and volume-activated Na^+/H^+ exchange, *J. Gen. Physiol.*, 89, 185, 1987.
15. **Akkon, D. L. and Rasmussen, H.,** A spatial-temporal model of cell activation, *Science*, 239, 998, 1988.

16. **Carafoli, E.,** Intracellular calcium homeostasis, *Annu. Rev. Biochem.,* 56, 395, 1987.
17. **Lattanzio, F.,** The effects of pH and temperature on fluorescent calcium indicators as determined with chelex-100 and EDTA buffer systems, *Biochim. Biophys. Res. Commun.,* 171, 102, 1990.
18. **Lattanzio, F.,** The effect of pH on rate constant, ion selectivity and thermodynamic properties of fluorescent calcium and magnesium indicators, *Biochim. Biophys. Res. Commun.,* 177, 184, 1990.
19. **Martínez-Zaguilán, R., Martínez, G. M., Lattanzio, F., and Gillies, R. J.,** Simultaneous measurements of intracellular pH and Ca^{2+} using the fluorescence of SNARF-1 and fura-2, *Am. J. Physiol.,* 260, C297, 1991.
20. **Minta, A., Kao, J. P. Y., and Tsien, R. Y.,** Fluroescent indicators for cytosolic calcium based on rhodamine and fluorescein chromophores, *J. Biol. Chem.,* 264, 8171, 1989.
21. **Ganz, M. B., Rasmussen, J., Bollag, W. B., and Rasmussen, H.,** Effect of buffer systems and pH_i on the measurement of $[Ca^{2+}]_i$ with fura-2, *FASEB J.,* 4, 1638, 1990.
22. **Graber, M. L., DiLilo, D. C., Friedman, B. L., and Pastoriza-Munoz, E.,** Characteristics of fluoroprobes for measuring intracellular pH, *Anal. Biochem.,* 156, 202, 1986.
23. **Tsien, R. Y.,** Fluorescent indicators of ion concentrations, *Methods Cell. Biol.,* 30, 127, 1989.
24. **McNeil, L. P.,** Incorporation of macromolecules into living cells, *Methods Cell. Biol.,* 29, 153, 1989.
25. **Wier, W. G.,** Cytoplasmic $[Ca^{2+}]$ in mammalian ventricle: dynamic control by cellular processes, *Annu. Rev. Physiol.,* 52, 467, 1990.
26. **Eidelman, O. and Cabantchik, I. Z.,** Continuous monitoring of transport by fluorescence on cells and vesicles, *Biochim. Biophys. Acta,* 988, 319, 1989.
27. **Tsien, R. Y., Pozzan, T.,and Rink, T. J.,** Calcium homeostasis in intact lymphocytes: cytoplasmic free calcium monitored with a new intracellularly trapped fluorescent indicator, *J. Cell. Biol.,* 94, 325, 1982.
28. **Oakes, S. G., Martini, W. J., Lisek, C. A., and Powis, G.,** Incomplete hydrolysis of the calcium indicator precursor FURA-2 pentaacetoxymethyl ester (FURA-2 AM) by cells, *Anal. Biochem.,* 169, 159, 1988.
29. **Davies, M. H., Altschuld, R. A., Jung, D. W., and Brierley, G. P.,** Estimation of intramitochondrial pCa and pH by FURA-2 and 2,7 biscarboxyethyl-5(6)-carboxyfluorescein (BCECF) fluorescence, *Biochem. Biophys. Res. Commun.,* 149, 40, 1987.
30. **McCormack, J. G., Browne, H. M., and Dawes, N. J.,** Studies on mitochondrial Ca^{2+} transport and matrix Ca^{2+} using FURA-2-loaded rat heart mitochondria, *Biochim. Biophys. Acta.,* 973, 420, 1989.
31. **Becker, P. L. and Fay, F. S.,** Photobleaching of FURA-2 and its effect on determination of calcium concentrations, *Am. J. Physiol.,* 253, C613, 1987.
32. **McDonough, P. M. and Button, D. C.,** Measurement of cytoplasmic calcium concentrations in cell suspensions: corrections for extracellular FURA-2 trough use of Mn^{2+} and probenecid, *Cell Calcium,* 10, 171, 1989.
33. **Shuttleworth, T. J. and Thompson, J. L.,** Effect of temperature on receptor-activated changes in $[Ca^{2+}]_i$ and their determination using fluorescent probes, *J. Biol. Chem.,* 266, 1410, 1991.
34. **Mozingo, N. M. and Chandler, D. E.,** The fluorescent probe BCECF has a heterogeneous distribution in sea urchin eggs, *Cell. Biol. Int. Rep.,* 14, 689, 1990.
35. **Giuliano, K. A. and Gillies, R. J.,** Determination of intracellular pH of BALB/c-3T3 cells using the fluorescence of pyranine, *Anal. Biochem.,* 167, 362, 1987.
36. **Gillies, R. J., Martinez, R., Sneider, J. M., and Hoyer, P. B.,** Sphingosine inhibits 12-myristate 13-acetate-, but not serum-induced, activation of Na^+/H^+ exchange in mammalian cells, *J. Cell. Physiol.,* 139, 125, 1989.
37. **Gillies, R. J. and Martínez-Zaguilán, R.,** Regulation of intracellular pH in BALB/c-3T3 cells: Bicarbonate raises pH via $NaHCO_3$/HCl exchange and attenuates the activation of Na^+/H^+ exchange by serum, *J. Biol. Chem.,* 266, 1551, 1991.
38. **Whitaker, J. E., Haugland, R. P., and Prendergast, F. G.,** Spectral and photophysical studies of benzo[*c*]xanthene dyes: dual emission pH sensors, *Anal. Biochem.,* 194, 330, 1991.
39. **Gillies, R. J., Martínez-Zaguilán, R., Martínez, R., Serrano, R., and Perona, R.,** Tumorigenic 3T3 cells maintain an alkaline intracellular pH under physiological conditions, *Proc. Natl. Acad. Sci. U.S.A.,* 87, 7414, 1990.
40. **Simpson, A. W. M. and Rink, T. J.,** Elevation of pH_i is not an essential step in calcium mobilization in FURA-2-loaded human platelets, *FEBS Lett.,* 222, 144, 1987.
41. **Lakowicz, J. R.,** *Principles of Fluorescence Spectroscopy,* Plenum Press, New York, 1986, 43.
42. **Weigmann, D. M., Welling, B. L. L., and Morris, S. J.,** Simultaneous analysis with fluorescent dyes of calcium and pH in living single kidney glomerular epithelial cells, *FASEB J.,* 5, A670a, 1991.
43. **Ohkuma, S. and Poole, B.,** Fluorescence probe measurement of the intralysosomal pH in living cells and the perturbation of pH by various agents, *Proc. Natl. Acad. Sci. U.S.A.,* 75, 3327, 1978.
44. **Wegner, J. A., Martínez-Zaguilán, R., Wise, M. E., Gillies, R. J., and Hoyer, P. B.,** Prostaglandin $F_{2\alpha}$-induced calcium transient in ovine large luteal cells. I. Alterations in cytosolic-free calcium levels and calcium flux, *Endocrinology,* 127, 3029, 1990.

45. **Harrison, S. M. and Bers, D. M.,** Correction of proton and Ca^{2+} association constants of EGTA for temperature and ionic strength, *Am. J. Physiol.,* 256, C1250, 1989.
46. **Fabiato, A.,** Computer programs for calculating total from specified free or free from specified total ionic concentrations in aqueous solution containing multiple metal and ligands, *Methods Enzymol.,* 157, 378, 1988.
47. **Grynkiewicz, G., Poenie, M., and Tsien, R. Y.,** A new generation of Ca^{2+} indicators with greatly improved fluorescence properties, *J. Biol. Chem.,* 260, 3440, 1985.
48. **Williams, D. A., Fogarty, K. E., Tsien, R. Y., and Fay, F. S.,** Calcium gradients in single smooth muscle cells revealed by the digital imaging microscope using FURA-2, *Nature (London),* 318, 558, 1985.
49. **Deber, C. M., Tom-Kun, J., Mack, E., and Grinstein, S.,** Bromo-A23187: a nonfluorescent calcium ionophore for use with fluorescent probes, *Anal. Biochem.,* 146, 349, 1985.
50. **Malgaroli, A., Milani, D., Meldolesi, J., and Pozzan, T.,** Fura-2 measurement of free Ca^{2+} in monolayers and suspensions of various types of animal cells, *J. Cell. Biol.,* 105, 2145, 1987.
51. **Scanlon, M., Williams, D. A., and Fay, F. S.,** A Ca^{2+} insensitive form of Fura-2 associated with polymorphonuclear leukocytes: assessment and accurate Ca^{2+} measurement, *J. Biol. Chem.,* 262, 6308, 1978.
52. **Siffert, W. and Akkermann, J. W. N.,** Activation of sodium-proton exchange is a prerequisite for Ca^{2+} mobilization in human platelets, *Nature (London),* 325, 456, 1987.
53. **Sage, S. O. and Rink, T. J.,** Effects of ionic substitutions on $[Ca^{2+}]_i$ rises evoked by thrombin and PAF in human platelets, *Eur. J. Pharmacol.,* 128, 99, 1987.
54. **Zavoico, G. B., Cragoe, E. L., and Feinstein, M. B.,** Regulation of intracellular pH in human platelets: effects of thrombin, A23187, and ionomycin and evidence for activation of Na^+/H^+ exchange and its inhibition by amiloride analogs, *J. Biol. Chem.,* 261, 13160, 1986.
55. **Tsien, R. Y. and Poenie, M.,** Fluorescence ratio imaging: a new window into intracellular ionic signalling, *Trends Biochem. Sci.,* 11, 450, 1986.
56. **Garcia-Sancho, J.,** Pyruvate prevents the ATP depletion caused by formaldehyde or calcium chelator esters in the human red cell, *Biochim. Biophys. Acta,* 813, 148, 1984.
57. **Tiffert, T., Garcia-Sancho, J., and Lew, V.,** Irreversible ATP depletion caused by low concentrations of formaldehyde and/or Ca^{2+}-chelator esters in intact human red cells, *Biochim. Biophys. Acta,* 773, 143, 1984.

Chapter 17

NEUTRAL RED ASSAY FOR TOXICOLOGY *IN VITRO*

H. Babich and E. Borenfreund

TABLE OF CONTENTS

I. INTRODUCTION

Acute toxicity tests involving the use of laboratory animals are designed to assess toxic potential, to aid in the prediction of hazards to human health or to the general biota, to generate biological data for use in risk-benefit analyses, and to provide, albeit to a limited extent, information on the mechanism of acute toxic action.[1] Within the last 15 years, however, there has been concern over the continued use of laboratory animals in biomedical research, especially in acute toxicity assays. Coupled with such socioethical concerns has been the realization of the vast numbers of chemicals, many already in commercial use, that require basic toxicological data. Acute toxicity tests with laboratory animals are costly, time-consuming, utilize much laboratory space, and require highly qualified personnel to monitor and interpret the data. Such factors have led to the development of *in vitro* assays to serve as potential alternatives to acute *in vivo* toxicity testing. One such *in vitro* approach has been the use of established cell lines in cytotoxicity assays for assessing the acute potency of chemical test agents. This chapter focuses on one such *in vitro* cytotoxicity assay, the neutral red (NR) cell viability assay.

The NR assay was developed in the Laboratory for *In Vitro* Toxicologic Assay Development, the Rockefeller University,[2,3] to serve as a potential alternative to the Draize rabbit ocular irritancy test. Prior to this, NR in cell culture cytotoxicity testing was used in viral cytopathogenicity and immunological assays.[4-9] The scope of the applicability of the NR assay to basic toxicity testing was subsequently broadened beyond that of the Draize test. Thus, the type of test agents was greatly extended from those typically evaluated as ocular irritants (e.g., surfactants,[3,10-12] cosmetic ingredients,[13] shampoos,[14,15] and detergents[16,17]), to a spectrum of test agents, including cancer chemotherapeutics,[18,19] pharmaceuticals,[20-23] biomaterials,[23] natural toxins,[24-26] food additives,[22,27] preservatives, antimicrobial agents,[28,29] industrial chemicals,[30-32] and environmental pollutants.[33-38] Similarly, a variety of cell types, including those derived from fish, rodents, and humans, have been used as the bioindicators in the NR assay.[3,25,33-36,39,40]

II. PRINCIPLE AND PROTOCOL OF THE NR ASSAY

Neutral red (3-amino-7-dimethylamino-2-methylphenazine hydrochloride) is a water-soluble, weakly basic, supravital dye that accumulates in lysosomes of viable cells. Cellular uptake of NR is accomplished either by pinocytosis or by passive transport across the plasma membrane.[41-44] Accumulation of NR within lysosomes occurs either from the trapping of the protonated form of the dye within the acid milieu of the lysosome or from the binding of NR to fixed acidic charges, such as those of acidic polysaccharides, within the lysosomal matrix.[45] In damaged cells, NR is no longer retained in cytoplasmic vacuolar membranes, and the plasma membrane does not act as a barrier to retain the dye within the cell.[46]

In the protocol for the NR cell viability assay, individual wells of a 96-well tissue culture microtiter plate are inoculated with 0.2 ml of medium containing cells (usually 1 to 2 $\times$ 10^4) to achieve 65 to 75% confluence after attachment and the addition of test agents. This seeding density allows for the target cells to complete an additional replication cycle; as such, the NR assay measures both cytotoxic and proliferative effects. After 1 or 2 days of incubation, the medium is replaced with an unamended (control) medium or with a medium amended with varied concentrations of test agents, using 4 to 8 wells per concentration. For direct-acting cytotoxicants, the cells are exposed for 24 h, whereas for metabolism-mediated cytotoxicants, longer exposures are required, so as to allow the target cells to metabolize the parent test agents to cytotoxic metabolites. An alternative approach for studying metabolism-mediated cytotoxicants, which only requires a 24 h exposure, is to include with the test agent a hepatic S9 microsomal fraction from Aroclor-induced rats or hamsters. For these studies, an S9 level of 200 to 250 μg protein per ml was sufficient. Following exposure to the test agent, the medium is replaced with a medium containing 40 μg/ml NR. This NR-containing medium was preincubated overnight at 37°C and is centrifuged (1500 × g for 10 min) prior to use, to remove fine precipitates of dye crystals. The assay plate is returned to the incubator for another 3 h to allow for uptake of the dye. The cells are then rapidly washed with a mild fixative (0.5% formaldehyde:1% $CaCl_2$). Damaged or dead cells lose the ability to retain NR, which is now removed during this wash/fixation procedure. The dye is then extracted from the intact, viable cells — i.e., those cells surviving the exposure to the test agents — with a 0.2-ml solution of 1% acetic acid:50% ethanol added to each well. The plate is left to stand at room temperature for 5 min, then agitated on a microplate shaker for 60 sec. The absorbance of the solubilized dye is then read using a scanning-well (ELISA-type) spectrophotometer equipped with a 540-nm filter. Quantitation of the extracted dye by spectrophotometry has been correlated with cell numbers, both by direct-counting with a hemacytometer and by protein determination of cell populations.[2,3,14,47-49]

Percent cell population viability, at each concentration of test agent, is calculated as:

$$\%\ \text{viability} = \frac{\text{mean absorbance of toxicant-treated wells}}{\text{mean absorbance of control wells}} \times 100$$

Individual cytotoxicity data points for each concentration of toxicant, presented as the arithmetic mean ± standard error of the mean, are used to construct concentration-response cytotoxicity curves. Figure 1 is illustrative of the types of cytotoxicity curves generated with the NR assay, with cultures exposed for 24 h to the test agents. The data for construction of such curves are used to calculate the midpoint cytotoxicity, or NR_{50}, value. The NR_{50} value is determined by linear regression analysis and is used to express the cytotoxicity data in a manner that allows for ranking the test chemicals according to their potencies. For example, with the human hepatoma HepG2 cell line as the bioindicator cell type in the NR assay, the NR_{50} values for a series of mycotoxins were 9.8 ng/ml for T-2 mycotoxin, 15.8 ng/ml for HT-2, 398.2 ng/ml for T-2 triol, and 445.3 ng/ml for T-2 tetraol.[25] NR_{50} values can also be applied to comparing the sensitivites of different cell lines to a common test agent (Table 1).

The NR assay has been compared with the MTT cytotoxicity, which is based on the reduction of a yellow tetrazolium dye to a blue formazan product by mitochondrial enzymes. Although both assays yielded comparable rankings of test agents, the optical density absorbance with the NR assay was about twice that obtained with the MTT assay and, thereby, also required fewer cells for analysis.[51,52] Furthermore, the MTT assay is greatly influenced by the availability and metabolism of glucose by the bioindicator cells, and, therefore, MTT specific activity will vary among cell lines.[53]

The NR assay, initially designed for use with a monolayer of anchorage-dependent cells, has been modified for use with a three-dimensional substrate containing several cell layers.[54] Good reproducibility of NR cytotoxicity data among different laboratories has been demonstrated.[12,55]

III. APPLICATIONS OF THE NR ASSAY

A. RANKING OF CHEMICAL POTENCIES

Chemical test agents evaluated with the NR assay can be ranked according to their respective potencies. For example, with the mycotoxins, the sequence of acute cytotoxicity was T-2 > HT-2 > T-2 triol > T-2 tetraol. The relevance of *in vitro* cytotoxicity data,

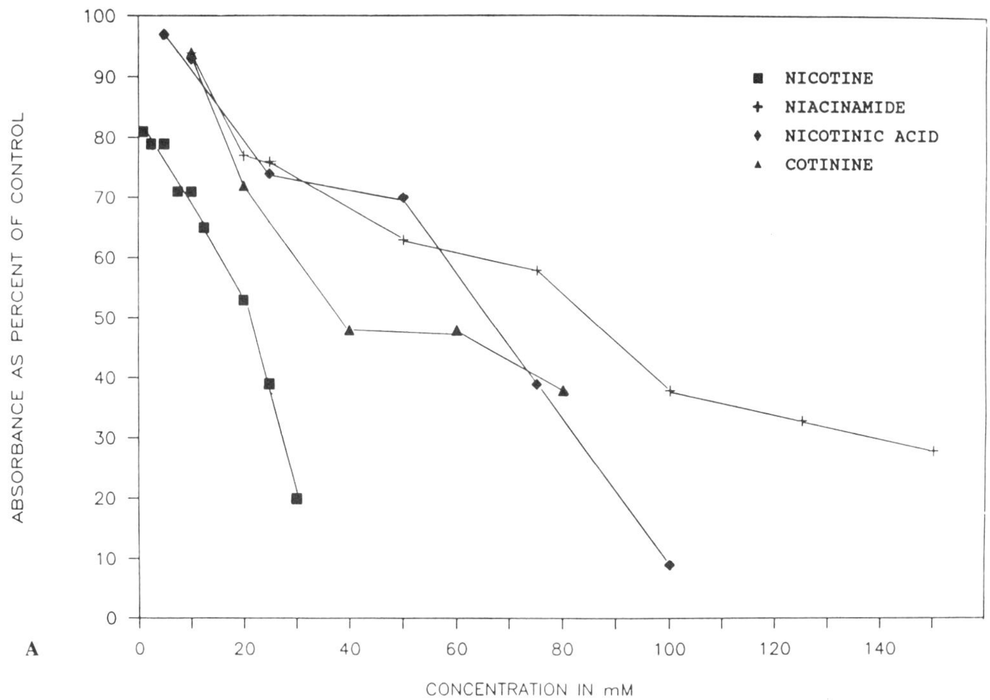

A

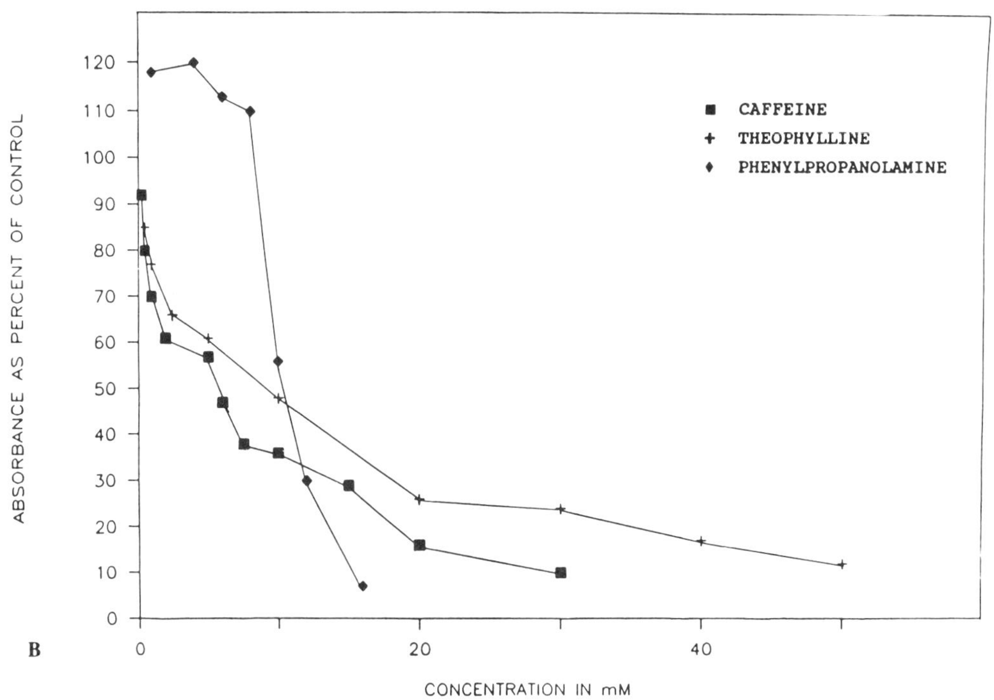

B

FIGURE 1. (a) Comparative cytotoxicities of nicotine, nicotinic acid, niacinamide (nicotinamide), and cotinine (the major metabolite of nicotine) to human keratinocytes after a 24-h exposure; (b) comparative cytotoxicities of caffeine, theophylline, and phenylpropanolamine to human endothelial cells after a 24-h exposure.

TABLE 1
Comparative Toxicities of T-2 Toxin to Human Cell Types

Designation	Description	NR_{50} (ng/ml)
SK-Mel/27	Melanoma cell line	2.8 ± 0.53
NHEK	2nd passage; keratinocytes	5.6 ± 0.66
HepG2	Hepatoma cell line	9.8 ± 1.10
CAKI	Renal carcinoma cell line	35.4 ± 2.10
HPK/1A	Keratinocyte cell line	35.7 ± 2.82
HFF	Dermal fibroblast cell line	42.3 ± 6.62
HEC	2nd passage; endothelial cells	44.8 ± 3.08
NK	2nd passage; kidney cells	72.1 ± 5.71

Note: NR_{50} = midpoint cytotoxicity value, after a 48-h exposure to T-2 mycotoxin.[25]

however, is directly related to their correlation with *in vivo* toxicity data, i.e., similar ranking of chemical potencies between *in vitro* and *in vivo* studies serves to validate the utility of the *in vitro* test as a potential surrogate for the *in vivo* test.

The ranking of the cytotoxicity of a series of surfactants, as determined with the NR assay using BALB/c mouse 3T3 fibroblasts, correlated with a similar ranking according to their Draize ocular effects.[28] Furthermore, a collaborative study involving 17 samples of surfactant-containing liquids, supplied as coded samples, was performed with a laboratory from the Procter and Gamble Company. A strong correlation was obtained between the NR cytotoxicity data using human dermal fibroblasts and low-volume rabbit eye test data.[56] Strong correlations between NR cytotoxicity data and Draize eye irritation data,[11,13,51,57–59] skin irritation data,[16,51] irritancy potential of parenteral formulations,[60] and *in vivo* renal toxicity data[29] have been reported.

Using cell lines derived from bluegill sunfish, strong correlations were noted between *in vitro* cytotoxicity data and *in vivo* acute LC_{50} data for fish and other aquatic species (e.g., *Daphnia*) for inorganic cationic metals,[61] organoleads,[62] organomercurials[63] (Table 2), diorganotins, chloroanilines, chlorobenzenes,[64,65] chlorotoluenes, and chlorophenols[31] (Table 3). A good correlation was observed with the sequence of NR cytotoxicity for a series of 15 chlorophenols towards a goldfish fibroblast cell line and *in vivo* LC_{50} toxicity data for goldfish.[66] The NR_{50} cytotoxicity data for 29 compounds (including inorganic metals, alcohols, acids, and ketones) tested with the fathead minnow FHM epithelioid cell line correlated with LC_{50} toxicity data for the fish, golden ofre.[67]

B. CANCER CHEMOTHERAPEUTICS

The comparative sensitivies of normal, transformed, and cancerous cell lines, including those representing various clinical categories of human malignancy, to cancer chemotherapeutics have been evaluated with the NR assay.[8,18,19,68–71] Based on NR_{50} values, human tumor cell lines (i.e., HepG2 hepatoma and SK-Mel/27 melanoma cells) were two to four times more sensitive than normal human cells (i.e., keratinocytes, melanocytes, and dermal fibroblasts) to doxorubicin and 5-fluorouracil.[71] For those chemotherapeutics that require metabolic activation, such as cyclophosphamide, a hepatic S9 microsomal fraction must be incorporated into the NR assay.[19,49] Without metabolic activation, cyclophosphamide exerts no cytotoxicity.[19,68]

TABLE 2
Comparative *In Vitro* and *In Vivo* Toxicities of a Series of Mercury-Containing Chemicals

Test agent	*In vitro* BG/F cells 24-h NR_{50} (μM)	Test agent	*In vivo* rainbow trout 48-h LC_{50} (μM)
Mercuric chloride	16.5	Mercuric chloride	0.77
Ethyl mercuric chloride	1.7	Ethyl mercuric phosphate	0.22
Methyl mercuric chloride	0.8	Methyl mercuric phosphate	0.15
Phenyl mercuric chloride	0.4	Phenyl mercuric acetate	0.03

Note: BG/F = epithelioid cell line derived from bluegill sunfish.

Adapted from Babich, H., Goldstein, S. H., and Borenfreund, E., *Toxicol. Lett.*, 50, 143, 1990.

TABLE 3
Comparative *In Vitro* and *In Vivo* Toxicities of a Series of Chlorinated Phenols

Test agent	*In vitro* BF-2 fibroblasts 24-h NR_{50} (μM)	*In vivo* bluegill sunfish 96-h LC_{50} (m*M*)
Phenol	6.9	143.5
2-Chlorophenol	2.4	51.1
4-Chlorophenol	1.6	29.8
2,4-Dichlorophenol	0.51	12.4
2,4,6-Trichlorophenol	0.48	1.6
2,3,5,6-Tetrachlorophenol	0.27	0.7
Pentachlorophenol	0.17	0.2

Adapted from Babich, H. and Borenfreund, E., *Environ. Res.*, 24, 229, 1987.

C. STRUCTURE-ACTIVITY RELATIONSHIPS

An important aspect of the NR assay has been its utilization in establishing structure-activity relationships (SARs) for series of related compounds. Based on NR_{50} values, the sequences of cytotoxicity for series of chlorophenols,[31,66] chlorobenzenes,[31] alkyl benzenes,[72] chlorotoluenes, chloroanilines[64] (Table 4), and phthalate diesters[72] were a direct function of their logarithmic octanol/water partition coefficients, of a series of diorganotins with their Hansch π parameters,[64,73] and of a series of divalent, inorganic metal cations with their chemical softness σ_p parameters.[47,61,74,75]

D. METABOLISM-MEDIATED CYTOTOXICITY

In regard to toxicity testing, chemical test agents can be broadly classified as (1) direct-acting toxicants and (2) indirect-acting, or metabolism-mediated, toxicants. Direct-acting toxicants are those chemicals that are toxic per se, without metabolic conversion. When evaluating direct-acting cytotoxicants in the NR assay, the choice of target cell is of minor importance. However, when evaluating metabolism-mediated cytotoxicants, the use of a target cell that lacks sufficient xenobiotic-metabolizing capacity would greatly underestimate the *in vivo* toxicity of the test compound, as noted with cyclophosphamide[19,68] and benzo[a]pyrene.[36] Two distinct approaches have been employed to incorporate a xenobiotic-metabolizing component in the NR assay. One approach focuses on the target cell, selecting a cell type with sufficient xenobiotic-metabolizing capacity. For example, the human hep-

TABLE 4
Relationship Between Cytotoxic Potencies (NR_{50}) and Log P Values for Series of Chlorinated Benzenes and Anilines

Test agent	NR_{50} (m*M*)	log P
Benzene series		
Benzene	19.46	2.13
Monochlorobenzene	5.69	2.81
1,2-Dichlorobenzene	1.53	3.53
1,3-Dichlorobenzene	1.37	3.53
1,2,3-Trichlorobenzene	0.77	4.20
1,2,4-Trichlorobenzene	0.64	4.20
1,3,5-Trichlorobenzene	0.63	4.20
1,2,3,4-Tetrachlorobenzene	0.34	4.94
Aniline series		
Aniline	16.48	0.90
4-Chloroaniline	1.90	2.02
3,5-Dichloroaniline	0.65	2.90
2,4,6-Trichloroaniline	0.51	3.41

Note: NR_{50} = midpoint cytotoxicity value, after a 24-h exposure;[64] log P = logarithmic octanol/water partition coefficient.

atoma cell line, HepG2, and low passage human keratinocytes apparently maintain sufficient endogenous levels of P450 monooxygenases to biotransform many of the polycyclic aromatic hydrocarbons, such as benzo[a]pyrene, to cytotoxic intermediate metabolites. The sensitivity of the HepG2 cells to benzo[a]pyrene was enhanced by preincubation in Aroclor-amended media, as preexposure to Aroclor elevated the intracellular levels of P450 enzymes.[33,34,76] A variation of this approach has been the use of rat and human hepatocytes in the NR assay;[77] however, this protocol requires the repeated isolation of fresh hepatocytes. Interestingly, many of the immortalized fish cell lines, both fibroblast and epithelioid cell types, maintain in culture sufficient P450 activity to detect the cytotoxic potency of benzo[a]pyrene.[78,79] In the above-noted studies, whether with mammalian or fish cells, exposure to the toxicant is usually extended from 3 to 6 days (rather than the 1 day of exposure for the direct-acting toxicants), so as to allow the target cells to biotransform sufficient quantities of the parent compound to cytotoxic metabolites.

The other approach is to incorporate into the NR assay an hepatic S9 microsomal fraction from Aroclor-induced rats or hamsters.[19,36,49] With this approach, the choice of the target cell is of secondary importance and a 1-day exposure to the test agent is sufficient to detect cytotoxicity. The hepatic S9 microsomal fraction may metabolize the parent compound to cytotoxic metabolites, as has been noted with cyclophosphamide, benzo(*a*)pyrene, acenaphthene, and *N*-nitrosodiphenylamine.[19,36,49] Conversely, the hepatic S9 microsomal fraction may detoxify some cytotoxicants, as has been shown with codeine phosphate, 6-mercaptopurine, methotrexate,[19] and the pesticide, alachlor.[36]

E. CHEMICAL INTERACTIONS

Using BALB/c mouse 3T3 fibroblasts in the NR assay, antagonistic interactions in cytotoxic potencies were noted for combinations of cadmium (Cd^{2+}) and zinc (Zn^{2+}) and Cd^{2+} and nickel (Ni^{2+}), but not copper (Cu^{2+}) and Zn^{2+} or Cu^{2+} and Ni^{2+}.[1,80] Antagonistic interactions in cytotoxic potencies were noted for selenium and arsenic compounds, when bluegill sunfish cell lines were used.[81]

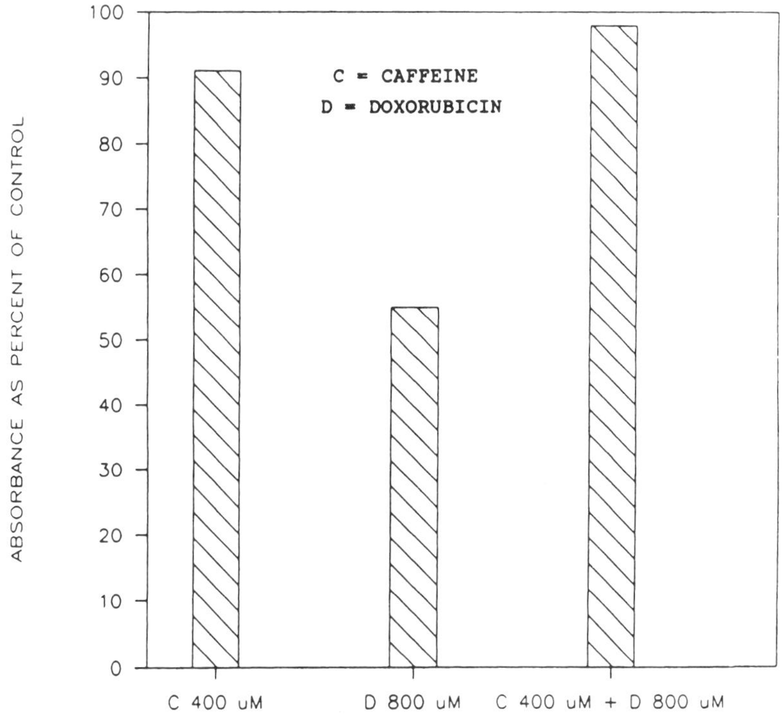

FIGURE 2. Antagonistic interactions between caffeine and the cancer chemotherapeutic agent, doxorubicin, towards human melanoma (SK-Mel/27) cells after a 24-h exposure.

The cytotoxicity of Cd^{2+} to BALB/c mouse 3T3 fibroblasts was reduced in the presence of the chelators, ethylendiaminetetraacetic acid (EDTA) and, to a lesser extent, nitrilotriacetic acid (NTA). However, EDTA was less effective in reducing the cytotoxicity of Cu^{2+} and NTA was not effective in lessening the cytotoxicity of Cu^{2+} to the 3T3 fibroblasts.[1] EDTA was also effective in reducing the cytotoxicity to 3T3 fibroblasts of a combination of cobalt (Co^{2+}) and Ni^{2+}.[17]

The reduction in the toxicity of methotrexate, a cancer chemotherapeutic, by leucovorin, a clinical "rescue agent", was also noted for 3T3 fibroblasts[52] and human hepatoma HepG2 cells[67] in the NR assay. The cytotoxicity of the cancer chemotherapeutic, doxorubicin, to SK-Mel/27 human melanoma cells was reduced by simultaneous exposure to caffeine (Figure 2).

F. TOXICITY-TEMPERATURE INTERACTIONS

Unlike mammalian cells in culture, fish cells are eurythermic and can be maintained over a wide range of temperature. The cytotoxicities of diethyltin dichloride and 4,4′-DDE to bluegill sunfish BF-2 fibroblasts and fathead minnow FHM epithelioid cells, as determined using the NR assay, were enhanced when incubation was at 34°C, as compared to 26°C.[78] The greater sensitivity of the cells to toxic agents at 34°C probably reflected their enhanced proliferation and metabolism at the higher temperature, as actively metabolizing cells are generally the most sensitive to chemical stress. Fish cells also exhibit enhanced xenobiotic-metabolizing capacity when grown at the higher temperature. This probably accounted for the greater sensitivity of BF-2 fibroblasts to the metabolism-mediated cytotoxicants, benzo[a]pyrene, 4-nitroquinoline-*N*-oxide, 2-aminoanthracene, and 2-aminofluorene, when exposures were at 34°C, as compared to 26°C[82] (Figure 3).

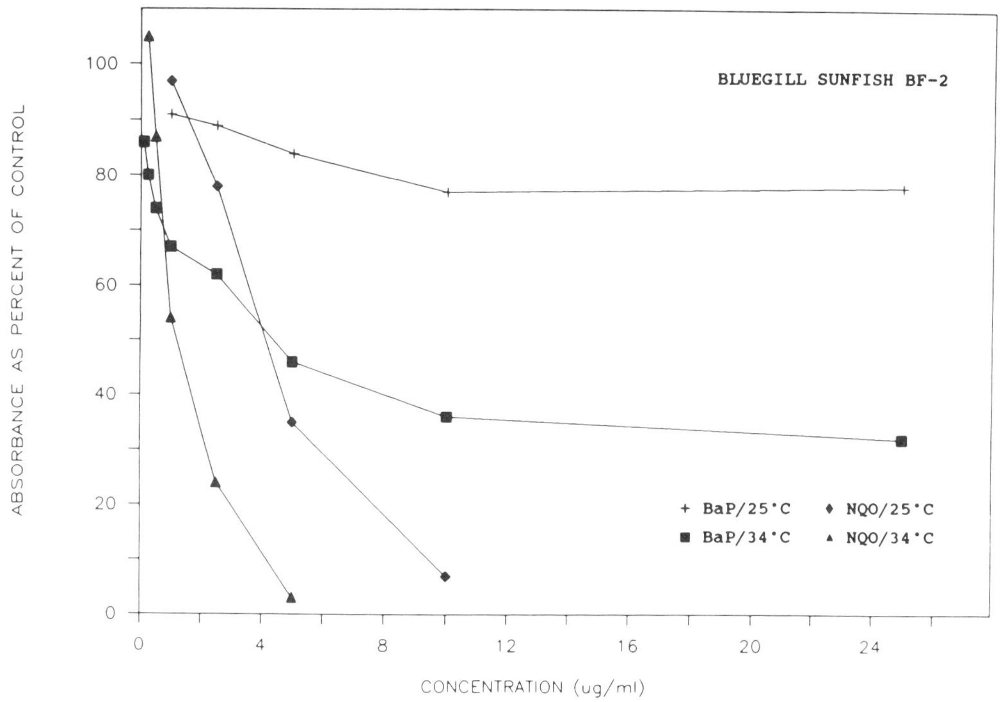

FIGURE 3. Influence of temperature on the cytotoxicity of benzo[a]pyrene (BaP) and 4-nitroquinoline-*N*-oxide (NQO) to bluegill sunfish BF-2 cells after a 24-h exposure.

G. PHOTOTOXICITY

A new application of the NR cell viability assay is in solar-simulated ultraviolet (UV) phototoxicity testing. The protocol for the NR assay to evaluate phototoxicity has been slightly modified from the procedure used for evaluating chemical toxicity. In the studies reported below, the cells were seeded into 96-well microtiter plates, but at the time of irradiation, the medium was replaced with a medium containing neither phenol red nor serum. Ultraviolet A (UVA), at 365 nm, was produced using a Blak Ray lamp fitted with 2 Sylvania, 15-watt self-filtering black light tubes. The cells were irradiated at a distance of 10 cm from the source, thereby producing energy readings for the assays of 3.3 mW/cm^2, as calibrated with an International Light IL 1700 radiometer. After irradiation, the medium was replaced with normal medium (i.e., containing phenol red and serum), the cells were then incubated for 24 h, after which the NR assay was performed. Figure 4 shows the response of different human cell types as well as of BALB/c mouse 3T3 fibroblasts to UVA for 20, 30, 40, 50, and 60 min. The percent of surviving, irradiated cells was computed by comparisons to nonirradiated controls. The SK-Mel/27 melanoma cells and the NHEM melanocytes exhibited similar sensitivites to the UVA exposure and were the most resistant of the cell types; their relative resistance was believed to be related to their pigment content. The NHEK keratinocytes exhibited intermediate sensitivity and the fibroblasts, both the mouse 3T3 and the human HFF cells, were the most sensitive to UVA (Figure 4).

Figure 5 shows the combined influence of UVA irradiation and chemical test agents on NHEK keratinocytes. The chemical test agents were tested at nontoxic concentrations and included the active components of UVA sunblockers, oxybenzone and menthyl anthranilate, and 5-methoxypsoralen; the latter is used in sunscreen preparations to induce tanning and for photoprotection against DNA damage. The keratinocytes were simultaneously exposed

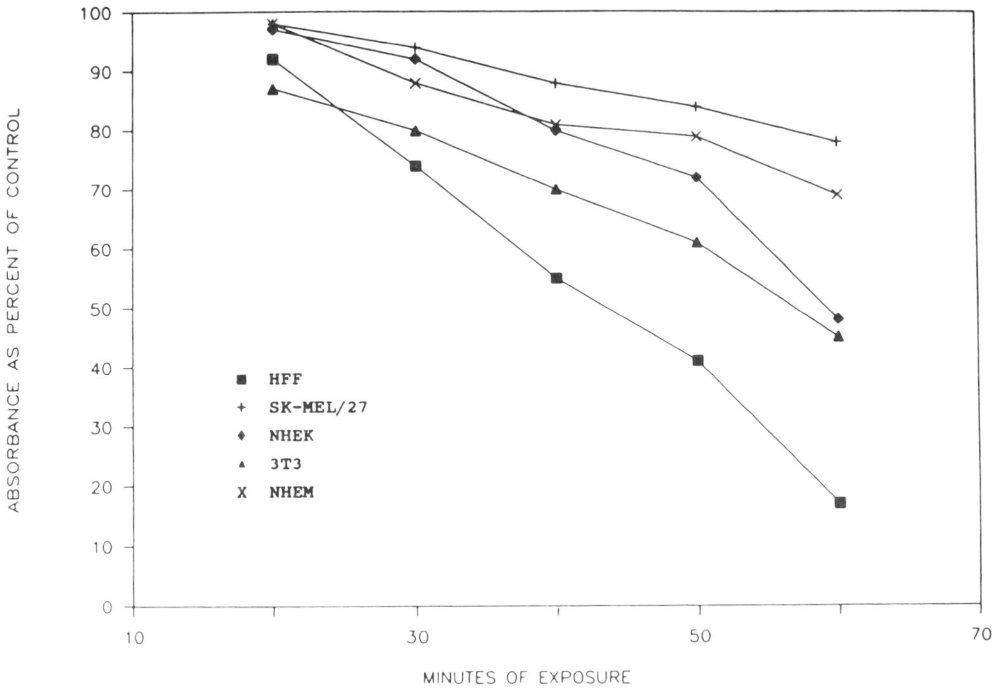

FIGURE 4. Comparative sensitivities of different cell types to radiation at 365 nm (UVA); cells were irradiated for 20, 30, 40, 50, and 60 min. HFF = human dermal fibroblasts; SK-Mel/27 = human melanoma cells; NHEK = human normal keratinocytes; NHEM = human normal melanocytes; 3T3 = BALB/c mouse embryo fibroblasts.

to radiation and to these test agents for 20 to 60 min; control NHEK cells were either exposed or nonexposed to UVA. Thereafter, the cells were maintained for another 24 h and survival was determined with the NR assay. As noted in Figure 5, the UVA sunblocker components, under the conditions of this assay, did not afford protection against UVA radiation; and exposure to 5-methoxypsoralen enhanced the sensitivity of the keratinocytes to UVA radiation. The sensitivity of the human NHEK keratinocytes, without simultaneous exposure to radiation, to various concentrations of oxybenzone, menthyl anthranilate, 5-methoxypsoralen, and the ultraviolet B (UVB) sunblockers, octyl methoxylcinnamate and octyl dimethyl *p*-aminobenzoate, over a 24-h exposure are shown in Figure 6. The relative sequence of toxicity for these test agents, which are all used in sunscreen preparations, was 5-methoxypsoralen > menthyl anthranilate > octyl dimethyl *p*-aminobenzoate > oxybenzone > octyl methoxylcinnamate.

IV. CONCLUSIONS

To best apply the NR cell viability assay to toxicology, it is most important that the investigator fully understand the scope, as well as the limitations, of an *in vitro* cytotoxicity assay. The NR assay, by its design, is an acute toxicity assay that provides information on the general, overall, toxic potential of a chemical test agent. As such, it does not reflect the sensitivity of an organ's specific physiological or secretory system. For example, the use of neural cells as the target bioindicators in the NR does not necessarily modify the assay from a cytotoxicity assay to a neurotoxicity assay. Thus, the toxicity ranking, based on NR_{50} values, for a series of di- and triorganotins was similar for BALB/c mouse 3T3 fibroblasts and mouse neuroblastoma N_2a cells.[73] Secondly, it is important to realize the limitations of

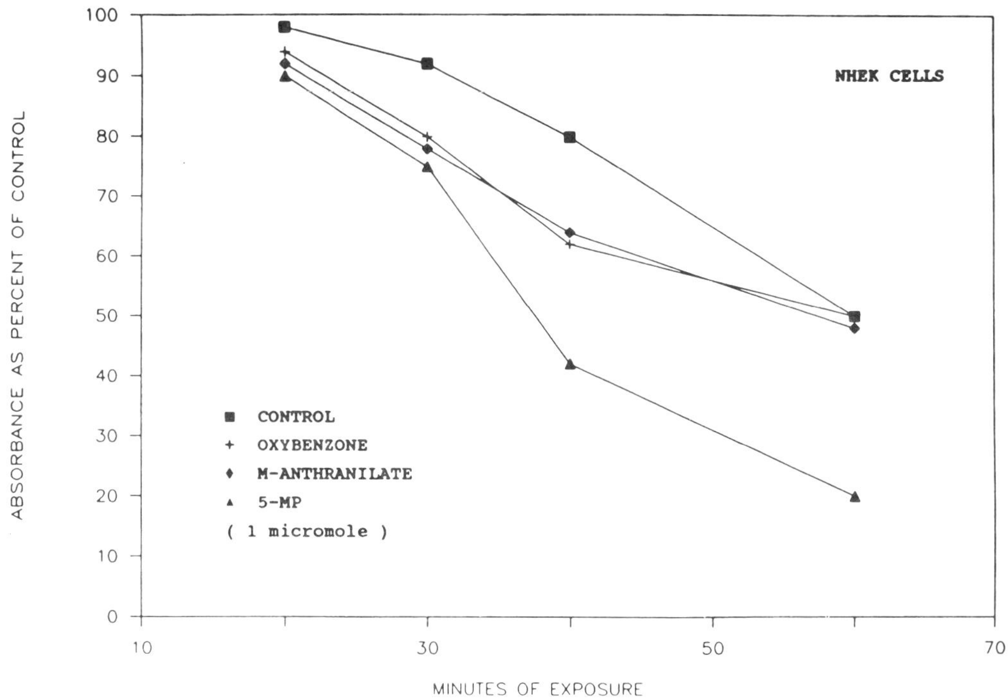

FIGURE 5. Influence of UVA radiation (365 nm), alone and in the presence of active components of sunscreen preparations and after 20, 30, 40, 50, and 60 min on human normal epithelial keratinocytes (NHEK). NR absorbance was plotted against controls, which were shielded from UVA radiation. ■, Control = radiation alone; + = oxybenzone; M-anthranilate = menthyl anthranilate; 5-MP = 5-methoxypsoralen.

the bioindicator cells. Immortalized cell lines that have been maintained in culture for many passages eventually lose some or most of their xenobiotic-metabolizing capacity. The use of such cells would underestimate the potency of metabolism-mediated cytotoxicants. For example, although the human hepatoma cell line, HepG2, maintained sufficient P450 enzymatic activity to metabolize benzo[a]pyrene, these cells were unable to metabolize cyclophosphamide, codeine phosphate, acenaphthene,[34] alachlor,[36] and eugenol. For these latter chemicals, an hepatic S9 microsomal fraction needed to be added to the test system.

The NR assay, thus, has been applied to seven aspects of acute toxicity:

1. The ranking of chemicals according to their potencies and the correlation of such *in vitro* rankings with *in vivo* rankings
2. The evaluation of the differential and selective sensitivites of normal and malignant cells to cancer chemotherapeutics
3. The formulation of SARs for series of related chemicals
4. The elucidation of antagonistic/synergistic interactions between combinations of test agents
5. The study of metabolism-mediated cytotoxicity, both for detoxification and toxification reactions
6. The determination of toxicity-temperature interactions, both for direct-acting and indirect-acting cytotoxicants and
7. The study of the phototoxic potency of various forms of radiation, alone or in combination with chemical test agents

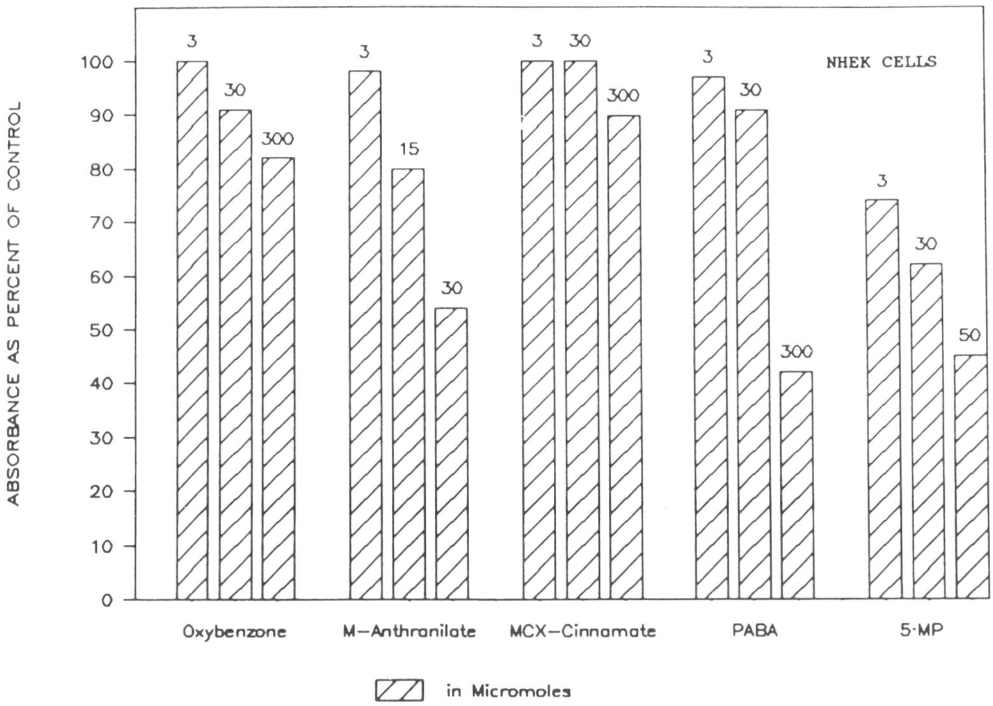

FIGURE 6. Influence of various active ingredients of sunscreen preparations on normal human epithelial keratinocytes (NHEK) after a 24-h exposure. Oxybenzone; M-anthranilate = menthyl anthranilate; MCX-cinnamate = ocytl methoxycinnamate; PABA = octyl dimethyl *p*-aminobenzoate; 5-MP = 5-methoxypsoralen.

ACKNOWLEDGMENT

Appreciation is expressed to the Clonetics Corporation for providing the normal human keratinocytes (NHEK) and serum-free keratinocyte growth medium (KGM).

REFERENCES

1. **Brown, V. K. H.,** Acute toxicity testing, in *Animals and Alternatives in Toxicity Testing,* Balls, M., Riddell, R. J., and Worden, A. N., Eds., Academic Press, New York, 1983, 1.
2. **Borenfreund, E. and Puerner, J. A.,** A simple quantitative procedure using monolayer cultures for cytotoxicity assays (HTD/NR90), *J. Tissue Cult. Meth.,* 9, 7, 1984.
3. **Borenfreund, E. and Puerner, J. A.,** Toxicity determined *in vitro* by morphological alterations and neutral red absorption, *Toxicol. Lett.,* 24, 119, 1985.
4. **Finter, N. B.,** Dye uptake methods for assessing vital cytopathogenicity and their application to interferon assays, *J. Gen. Virol.,* 5, 419, 427.
5. **Flick, D. A. and Gifford, T. E.,** Comparison of *in vitro* cell cytotoxic assays for tumor necrosis factor, *J. Immunol. Meth.,* 68, 167, 1984.
6. **Kull, F. C. and Cuatrecasas, P.,** Preliminary characterization of the tumor cell cytotoxin in tumor necrosis serum, *J. Immunol.,* 126, 1279, 1981.
7. **Parish, C. R. and Mullbacher, A.,** Automated colorimetric assay for T cell cytotoxicity, *J. Immunol. Meth.,* 58, 225, 1983.
8. **Breau, A. P., Field, L., and Mitchell, W. M.,** Thiono compounds. 4. *In vitro* mutagenic and antineoplastic activity of TEPA and thio-TEPA, *Cell Biol. Toxicol.,* 1, 21, 1984.

9. **Vastola, K. A., Ho, Y. -K., Bardos, T. J., Grossmayer, B. J., Fruck-Diviak, L., and O'Malley, J. A.,** Poly I-mercapto poly C: antiviral, anticellular, and pharmacologic effects, *Res. Commun. Chem. Pathol. Pharmacol.*, 45, 407, 1984.
10. **Borenfreund, E. and Shopsis, C.,** Toxicity monitored with a correlated set of cell culture assays, *Xenobiotica*, 15, 705, 1985.
11. **Gajjar, L. and Benford, D. J.,** Irritancy testing in cultured keratinocytes, *Mol. Toxicol.*, 1, 513, 1987/88.
12. **Triglia, D., Wegener, P. T.,Harbell, J., Wallace, K., Matheson, D. and Shopsis, C.,** Interlaboratory validation study of the keratinocyte neutral red bioassay from Clonetics Corporation, in *Alternative Methods in Toxicology*, Vol. 7, Goldberg, A. M., Ed., Mary Ann Liebert, Inc., New York, 1989, 357.
13. **Bracher, M., Faller, C., Spengler, J., and Reinhardt, C. A.,** Comparison of *in vitro* cell toxicity with *in vivo* eye irritancy, *Mol. Toxicol.*, 1, 561, 1987/88.
14. **Stark, D. M., Borenfreund, E., Walberg, J., and Shopsis, C.,** Comparisons of several alternative assays for measuring potential toxicants, in *Alternative Methods in Toxicology*, Vol. 5, Goldberg, A. M., Ed., Mary Ann Liebert, Inc., New York, 1985, 373.
15. **Cavalletti, T., Reali, E., Marangoni, C., Bader, S., and Traniello, S.,** Effects of neutral shampoos on cultures of human fibroblasts, *ATLA*, 19, 87, 1991.
16. **Sterzel, W., Bartwick, F. G., Matthies, W., Kastner, W. and Kunstler, K.,** Comparison of two *in vitro* and two *in vivo* methods for the measurement of irritancy, *Toxicol. In Vitro*, 4, 698, 1990.
17. **Babich, H. and Borenfreund, E.,** Applications of the neutral red cytotoxicity assay to *in vitro* toxicology, *ATLA*, 18, 129, 1990.
18. **Isomura, J. -I., Yoshimatsu, K., Ikeda, T., Takimoto, G. -I., and Morimoto, T.,** A dye uptake method using cultured human cancer cells and its application to a sensitivity test for anti-cancer drugs, *Yakugaku Zasshi*, 101, 227, 1981.
19. **Borenfreund, E. and Puerner, J. A.,** Short-term quantitative *in vitro* cytotoxicity assay involving an S9 activating system, *Cancer Lett.*, 34, 243, 1987.
20. **Riddell, R. J., Panacer, D. S., Wilde, S. M., Clothier, R. H., and Balls, M.,** The importance of exposure period and cell type in *in vitro* cytotoxicity tests, *ATLA*, 14, 86, 1986.
21. **Vickers, A., Guertler, J., Spaans, C., Tapparelli, C., Donatsch, P., and Fischer, V.,** Cyclosporine A nephrotoxicity studied by the combined application of kidney cell lines, hepatocytes, and endothelial-platelet cocultures, *Mol. Toxicol.*, 1, 351, 1987/88.
22. **Babich, H. and Borenfreund, E.,** Cytotoxic effects of food additives and pharmaceuticals on cells in culture as determined with the neutral red assay, *J. Pharm. Sci.*, 79, 592, 1990.
23. **Combrier, E., Metezeau, P., Ronot, X., Kiefer-Gachelin, H., and Adolphe, M.,** Comparative assessment of *in vitro* toxicity of xenobiotics using flow cytometry and spectrophotometry, *Toxicol. In Vitro*, 4, 751, 1990.
24. **Greer, C. N. and Shewen, P. E.,** Automated colorimetric assay for the detection of *Pasteurella haemolytica* leucotoxin, *Vet. Microbiol.*, 12, 33, 1986.
25. **Babich, H. and Borenfreund, E.,** Cytotoxicity of T-2 and its metabolites determined with the neutral red cell viability assay, *Appl. Environ. Microbiol.*, 57, 2101, 1991.
26. **Forsby, A., Andersson, M., and Lewan, L.,** The cytotoxicity of 22 sesquiterpenoid unsaturated dialdehydes, as determined by the neutral red absorption assay and by protein determination, *Toxicol. In Vitro*, 5, 19, 1991.
27. **Fortunati, E. and Bianchi, V.,** Spectrophotometric determination of total macromolecules for the evaluation of cellular density in cytotoxicity assays, *ATLA*, 19, 18, 1991.
28. **Shopsis, C. and Borenfreund, E.,** *In vitro* cytotoxicity assays: potential alternatives to the Draize test, in *Evaluation des Effects Cosmetiques Methods D'Aujourd'hui et de Demain*, XVemes Journees Internationales de Dermocosmetologie de Lyons, 1985, 170.
29. **Duffy, P. A. and McNae, F. R.,** *In vitro* toxicity of antibiotics to LLC-RK1 rabbit kidney cells, *Toxicol. In Vitro*, 4, 375, 1990.
30. **Babich, H. and Borenfreund, E.,** Aquatic pollutants tested *in vitro* with early passage fish cells, *ATLA*, 15, 116, 1987.
31. **Babich, H. and Borenfreund, E.,** *In vitro* cytotoxicity of organic pollutants to bluegill sunfish (BF-2) cells, *Environ. Res.*, 24, 229, 1987.
32. **Babich, H. and Borenfreund, E.,** *In vitro* cytotoxicity of polychlorinated biphenyls (PCBs) and toluenes to cultured bluegill sunfish BF-2 cells, in *Aquatic Toxicology and Hazard Assessment*, Vol. 10, Adams, W. J., Chapman, G. A., dn Landis, W. G., Eds., American Society for Testing and Materials, Philadelphia, 1988, 454.
33. **Babich, H., Martin-Alguacil, N., and Borenfreund, E.,** Mediating role of metabolic activation in *in vitro* cytotoxicity assays, *Mol. Toxicol.*, 1, 363, 1987/88.

34. **Babich, H., Sardana, M. K., and Borenfreund, E.,** Acute cytotoxicities of polynuclear aromatic hydrocarbons determined *in vitro* with the human liver tumor cell line, HepG2, *Cell Biol. Toxicol.*, 4, 295, 1988.
35. **Babich, H., Martin-Alguacil, N., and Borenfreund, E.,** Use of the rainbow trout hepatoma cell line, RTH-149, in a cytotoxicity assay, *ATLA*, 17, 67, 1989.
36. **Babich, H., Martin-Alguacil, N., Raul, C., Rosenberg, D. W., and Borenfreund, E.,** Response of human cell cultures to cytotoxicants requiring metabolic activation, in *Alternative Methods in Toxicology*, Vol. 8, Goldberg, A. M., Ed., Mary Ann Liebert, Inc., New York, 1991, 263.
37. **Jenssen, J. and Syversen, T.,** Cytotoxicity of vanadate on Chinese hamster ovary cells, *ATLA*, 14, 152, 1987.
38. **Halder, M. and Ahne, W.,** Evaluation of waste water toxicity with three cytotoxicity tests, *Z. Wasser Abwasser Forsch.*, 23, 233, 1990.
39. **Benford, D. J. and Good, S.,** Development of cytotoxicity tests for assessment of the toxicity of water samples taken from the environment, *Mol. Toxicol.*, 1, 419, 1987/88.
40. **Arranz, M. J. and Festing, M. F. W.,** Prior use of the neutral red assay and reduction of total protein determination of 96-well plate assays, *Toxicol. In Vitro*, 4, 211, 1990.
41. **Allison, A. C. and Young, M. R.,** Vital staining in fluorescence microscopy of lysosomes, in *Lysosomes in Biology and Pathology*, Vol. 2, Dingle, J. T. and Fell, H. B., Eds., Elsevier, New York, 1969, 600.
42. **Raschke, W. C., Baird, S., Ralph, P., and Nakoinz, I.,** Functional macrophage cell lines transformed by Abelson leukemia virus, *Cell*, 15, 261, 1978.
43. **Nemes, Z., Dietz, R., Lüth, J. B., Gomba, S., Hackenthal, F., and Gross, F.,** The pharmacological relevance of vital staining with neutral red, *Experientia*, 35, 1475, 1979.
44. **Hammond, M. E., Goodwin, J., and Dvorak, H. F.,** Quantitative measurements of neutral red uptake and excretion by mammalian cells, *J. Reticuloendol. Soc.*, 27, 337, 1980.
45. **Bulychev, A., Trouet, A., and Tulkens, P.,** Uptake and intracellular distribution of neutral red in cultured fibroblasts, *Exp. Cell Res.*, 115, 343, 1978.
46. **Filman, D. J., Brawn, R. J., and Dandliker, W. B.,** Intracellular supravital stain delocalization as an assay for antibody-dependent complement-mediated cell damage, *J. Immunol. Methods*, 6, 189, 1975.
47. **Borenfreund, E. and Puerner, J. A.,** Cytotoxicity of metals, metal-metal and metal-chelator combinations assayed *in vitro*, *Toxicology*, 39, 121, 1986.
48. **Babich, H. and Borenfreund, E.,** Structure-activity relationship (SAR) models established *in vitro* with the neutral red assay, *Toxicol. In Vitro*, 1,3, 1987.
49. **Babich, H. and Borenfreund, E.,** Polycyclic aromatic hydrocarbon *in vitro* cytotoxicity to bluegill BF-2 cells: mediation by S9 microsomal fraction and temperature, *Toxicol. Lett.*, 36, 107, 1987.
50. **Babich, H., Martin-Alguacil, N., and Borenfreund, E.,** Comparisons of the cytotoxicities of dermatotoxicants to human keratinocytes and fibroblasts *in vitro*, in *Alternative Methods in Toxicology*, Vol. 7, Goldberg, A. M., Ed., Mary Ann Liebert, Inc., New York, 1989, 153.
51. **Hoh, A., Maier, K., and Dreher, R. M.,** Multilayered keratinocyte culture used for *in vitro* toxicology, *Mol. Toxicol.*, 1, 537, 1987/88.
52. **Borenfreund, E., Babich, H., and Martin-Alguacil, N.,** Comparisons of two *in vitro* cytotoxicity assays: the neutral red (NR) and tetrazolium MTT tests, *Toxicol. In Vitro*, 2, 1, 1990.
53. **Vistica, D. T., Skehan, P., Scudiero, D., Monks, A., Pittman, A., and Boyd, M. R.,** Tetrazolium-based assays for cellular viability: a critical examination of selected parameters affecting formazan production, *Cancer Res.*, 51, 2515, 1991.
54. **Triglia, D., Braa, S. S., Yonan, C., and Naughton, C. K.,** *In vitro* toxicity of various classes of test agents using the neutral red assay on a human three-dimensional physiologic skin model, *In Vitro Cell Dev. Biol.*, 27A, 239, 1991.
55. **Kalweit, S., Gernet, I., and Spielmann, H.,** Validation project of alternatives for the Draize eye test, *Mol. Toxicol.*, 1, 597, 1987/88.
56. **Bruner, L. H., Kain, B. J., Roberts, D. A., and Parker, R. D.,** Evaluation of seven *in vitro* alternatives for ocular safety testing, *Fundam. Appl. Toxicol.*, 17, 136, 1991.
57. **Hockley, K. and Baxter, D.,** Use of the 3T3 cell-neutral red uptake assay for irritants as an alternative to the rabbit (Draize) test, *Food Chem. Toxicol.*, 24, 473, 1986.
58. **Gajjar, L. and Benford, D. J.,** Comparison of cultured keratinocytes and fibroblasts as models for irritancy testing, *in vitro*, *Toxicol. In Vitro*, 4, 280, 1990.
59. **Dierickx, P. J. and Gordon, V. C.,** The EYTEX™ system and the neutral red uptake inhibition assay in cultured HepG2 cells as alternative models for *in vivo* eye irritation following the EEC protocol, *ATLA*, 17, 325, 1990.
60. **Wilson, S. A., Jasiewicz, M. L., Bonner, F. W., Brown, S., and Potter, C. J.,** An *in vitro* screening test for the assessment of the irritant potential of parenteral formulations, *Toxicol. In Vitro*, 3, 335, 1989.

61. **Babich, H., Puerner, J. A., and Borenfreund, E.,** *In vitro* cytotoxicity of metals to bluegill (BF-2) cells, *Arch. Environ. Contam. Toxicol.*, 15, 31, 1987.
62. **Babich, H. and Borenfreund, E.,** *In vitro* cytotoxicities of inorganic lead and di- and trialkyl lead compounds to fish cells, *Bull. Environ. Contam. Toxicol.*, 44, 456, 1990.
63. **Babich, H., Goldstein, S. H., and Borenfreund, E.,** *In vitro* cyto- and genotoxicity of organomercurials to cells in culture, *Toxicol. Lett.*, 50, 143, 1990.
64. **Babich, H. and Borenfreund, E.,** Structure-activity relationships for diorganotins, chlorinated benzenes, and chlorinated anilines established with bluegill sunfish BF-2 cells, *Fundam. Appl. Toxicol.*, 10, 295, 1988.
65. **Babich, H. and Borenfreund, E.,** Structure-activity relationships of inorganic metals, organometals, and organic test agents determined *in vitro* with the neutral red assay, in *Alternative Methods in Toxicology*, Vol. 6, Goldberg, A. M., Ed., Mary Ann Liebert, Inc., New York, 1988, 121.
66. **Saito, H., Sudo, M., Shigeoka, T., and Yamauchi, F.,** *In vitro* cytotoxicity of chlorophenols to goldfish GF-scale (GFS) cells and quantitative structure-activity relationships, *Environ. Toxicol. Chem.*, 10, 235, 1991.
67. **Dierickx, P. J. and Van De Vyver, J. E.,** Correlation of the neutral red uptake inhibition assay of cultured fathead minnow fish cells with fish lethality tests, *Bull. Environ. Contam. Toxicol.*, 46, 649, 1991.
68. **Riddell, R. J., Clothier, R. H., and Balls, M.,** An evaluation of three *in vitro* cytotoxicity assays, *Food. Chem. Toxicol.*, 24, 469, 1986.
69. **Fiennes, A. G. T. W., Walton, J., Winterbourne, D., McGlashan, D., and Hermon-Taylor, J.,** Quantitative correlation of neutral red dye uptake with cell number in human cancer cell cultures, *Cell Biol. Int. Res.*, 11, 373, 1987.
70. **Cavanaugh, P. F., Moskwa, P. S., Donish, W. H., Pera, P. J., Richardson, D., and Andrese, A. P.,** A semiautomated neutral red based chemosensitivity assay for drug screening, *Invest. New Drugs*, 8, 347, 1990.
71. **Borenfreund, E., Babich, H., and Martin-Alguacil, N.,** Rapid chemosensitivity assay with human normal and tumor cells *in vitro*, *In Vitro Dev. Cell. Biol.*, 26, 1030, 1990.
72. **Babich, H., Rosenberg, D. W., and Borenfreund, E.,** *In vitro* cytotoxicity studies with the fish hepatoma cell line, PLHC-1 *(Poeciliopsis lucida)*, *Ecotoxicol. Environ. Saf.*, 21, 327, 1991.
73. **Borenfreund, E. and Babich, H.,** *In vitro* cytotoxicity of heavy metals, acrylamide, and organotin salts to neural cells and fibroblasts, *Cell Biol. Toxicol.*, 3, 63, 1987.
74. **Babich, H., Shopsis, C., and Borenfreund, E.,** *In vitro* cytotoxicity of aquatic pollutants (cadmium, copper, zinc, nickel) using established fish cell lines, *Ecotoxicol. Environ. Saf.*, 11, 91, 1986.
75. **Babich, H. and Borenfreund, E.,** Cultured fish cells for the ecotoxicity testing of aquatic pollutants, *Toxicol. Assess.*, 2, 119, 1987.
76. **Stark, D. M., Shopsis, C., Borenfreund, E., and Babich, H.,** Progress and problems in evaluating and validating alternative assays in toxicology, *Food. Chem. Toxicol.*, 24, 449, 1986.
77. **Zhang, S.-Z., Lipsky, M. M., Trump, B. F., and Hsu, I.-C.,** Neutral red (NR) assay for cell viability and xenobiotic-induced cytotoxicity in primary cultures of human and rat hepatocytes, *Cell Biol. Toxicol.*, 6, 219, 1990.
78. **Babich, H. and Borenfreund, E.,** Fathead minnow FHM cells for use in in vitro cytotoxicity assays of aquatic pollutants, *Ecotoxicol. Environ. Saf.*, 14, 78, 1987.
79. **Martin-Alguacil, N., Babich, H., Rosenberg, D. W., and Borenfreund, E.,** *In vitro response* of the brown bullhead catfish cell line, BB, to aquatic pollutants, *Arch. Environ. Contam. Toxicol.*, 20, 113, 1991.
80. **Babich, H., Shopsis, C., and Borenfreund, E.,** Cadmium-nickel toxicity interactions towards a bacterium, filamentous fungi, and a cultured mammalian cell line, *Bull. Environ. Contam. Toxicol.*, 37, 550, 1986.
81. **Babich, H., Martin-Alguacil, N., and Borenfreund, E.,** Arsenic-selenium interactions determined with cultured fish cell, *Toxicol. Lett.*, 45, 157, 1989.
82. **Babich, H. and Borenfreund, E.,** Applications of the neutral red cytotoxicity assay to risk assessment of aquatic contaminants, in *Environmental Toxicology and Risk Assessment*, 1st Symp., American Society for Testing and Materials, Philadelphia, in press.

Chapter 18

APPLICATIONS OF CULTURED LUNG CELLS IN TOXICOLOGY

Albert P. Li and Annette G. Teepe

TABLE OF CONTENTS

I. INTRODUCTION

From the perspectives of a toxicologist or pharmacologist, the lung is a unique organ. As an organ for gaseous exchange, the lung has direct exposure to inhaled toxicants. Examples of such toxicants include mineral dusts and fossil fuel-related combustion products. Further, regardless of the route of entrance, all xenobiotics present in the cardiac output must traverse the lungs before entering the systemic circulation. It is therefore one of the first organs exposed to pharmaceutical chemicals administered via intravenous injection. It is of no surprise that lung diseases have been linked to exposure to inhaled environmental agents and pharmaceuticals (Table 1).

The lung is a heterogenous organ known to contain more than 40 varied cell types.[58] With the recent technical advances in the isolation, culture, and characterization, *in vitro* methods for toxicity evaluation and xenobiotic metabolism have been developed for several relevant lung cell populations. In this chapter, we will describe the isolation, culture, and toxicological applications developed with purified lung cell populations: Clara cells, alveolar macrophages, alveolar epithelial cells, and pulmonary endothelial cells; and with cell systems consisting of a mixture of cell types: explants from airway epithelium, and primary lung cell cultures.

II. PURIFIED LUNG CELLS

Significant advances have been made in the past decade in the isolation and purification of differentiated cell populations from the lung. The cell types that are extensively studied include the noncilitated bronchiolar epithelial cells (Clara cells), alveolar macrophages, alveolar type II cells, and endothelial cells.

A. CLARA CELLS (NONCILIATED BRONCHIOLAR EPITHELIAL CELLS)

1. General Description

Clara cells are nonciliated cells in the epithelial lining of distal conducting pulmonary airways.[41] They are found to be located mainly in the proximal or central portion of the zone of transition between conducting airways and gas exchange areas called pulmonary acinus. While mainly present as the epithelial lining of the bronchioles, they are also found in some animal species (e.g., mouse, hamster, rabbit) in the epithelial lining of the trachea or major bronchi. Clara cells are generally described as cuboidal to columnar epithelial cells free of cilia, long apical microvilli, and dense-cored neurosecretory granules. Electron microscopy reveal the presence of extensive agranular endoplasmic reticulum, large mitochondria, and osmiophilic granules. Clara cells are believed to be one of the three major pulmonary cell types (in addition to type II alveolar cells and alveolar macrophages) responsible for xenobiotic metabolism. The high levels of cytochrome P450 monoxygenase isozymes in Clara cells have been demonstrated by immunocytochemical studies of histological sections[56] as well as isolated cells.[9] Besides xenobiotic metabolism, the Clara cells are believed to be the source of secretory material for the acellular lining of bronchioles and the progenitor for both itself and ciliated cells.[41]

2. Isolation and Culture

Clara cells can be purified from rabbit lungs using an elutriation procedure originally developed by Devereux and Fouts.[9] This procedure has also been applied successfully to rat lungs.[46] The lungs are exsanguinated by perfusion via the pulmonary artery with a Krebs-Ringer bicarbonate solution. To further remove alveolar macrophages, the lungs are lavaged several times with a cold, buffered, isotonic solution. It is important to devoid the lungs of

TABLE 1
Environmental Agents and Pharmaceuticals Believed to Be Casually Linked to Lung Disorders[a]

Agent	Lung Disorder
I. Environmental Agents	
Asbestos	Asbestosis; cancer
Coal mine dust	Coal workers' pneumoconiosis
Cigarette smoke	Chronic bronchitis; emphysema; cancer
Radiation	Emphysema; cancer
II. Pharmaceuticals	
Nitrofurantoin	Alveolitis
Aspirin	Bronchoconstriction; pulmonary edema
Thiazides	Pulmonary edema
Bleomycin	Alveolitis

[a] Contents extracted from Reference 55.

alveolar macrophages, as they are similar in size and density to Clara cells. The lavaged lungs are then instilled with a protease solution and allowed to digest at 37°C for approximately 15 min. Protease I has been found to be the most effective protease in the release of type II and Clara cells from rabbit lungs. The trachea and bronchi are then removed; the lungs are placed on ice and minced into 1- to 2-mm pieces. The minced pieces are resuspended and filtered through cheese cloth and nylon filters for the collection of the isolated cells which mainly consist of type II alveolar cells and Clara cells. The Clara cells are then separated from the type II cells by centrifugal elutriation. Being larger cells, the Clara cells are eluted later than the type II cells. To further purify the Clara cells, the enriched population is placed on a discontinuous Percoll density gradient (28% and 36% Percoll) and centrifuged. The purified Clara cells can be recovered from the 36% Percoll fraction. Using this procedure, about 1 to 2 $\times$ 10^7 Clara cells can be obtained from 4 rabbits. The purity of Clara cells at this stage is approximately 50 to 60%. With a second elutriation, the purity can be enriched to approximately 70%.[8]

Mouse Clara cells can be isolated using a procedure developed by Walker and co-workers.[4,66] With this procedure, the lungs were processed as described above, except that elastase is used to dissociate the Clara cells. The dissociated cells were then allowed to adhere for 1 h at 37°C to plastic culture dishes coated with mouse IgG. The nonadherent cells are found to be enriched for Clara cells with a purity of 75 to 80%.

Clara cells can be identified under the light microscope by staining formalin-fixed cells with nitroblue tetrazolium (NBT).[9] Air-dried smears of the purified cells are fixed in formalin and stained in a solution of 0.1% NBT and 0.1% NADPH at 37°C for approximately 10 min. The slides are then counterstained in a 1% aqueous methylene green solution. Clara cells are stained purple while non-Clara cells are blue or light pink. Trypan blue exclusion is used routinely to evaluate viability.

Relatively few studies have been performed to evaluate the culturing of Clara cells. Medium composition and attachment matrix are generally believed to be critical to maintenance. Richards et al.[45] studied the attachment efficiency of Clara cells on a variety of substrata including bovine serum albumin, fibronectin, and collagen and found that type IV collagen was the most effective, using a medium consisting of F-12 plus 2% Ultroser G. Fetal bovine serum or Ultroser G were found to be medium ingredients necessary for attachment. The percent of NBT positive cells was found to decrease with time in culture.

3. Applications in Toxicology

a. Xenobiotic Metabolism

Clara cells are believed to be the cell type in lung epithelium with the highest level of xenobiotic metabolic activities. The high level of cytochrome P450 monooxygenase activity of Clara cells is evidenced by the extensive smooth endoplasmic reticulum system in the cells, immunohistochemical staining of lung sections,[56] and immunocytochemical and biochemical studies of isolated cells.[4] Devereux et al.,[10] using a fluorescent antibody technique, showed the presence of P450-I and P450-II in the Clara cell of rabbit lung. Rietjens et al.[46] demonstrated the oxidation of P450 substrates ethoxyresorufin, pentoxyresorufin, and 7-ethoxycoumarin by microsomes prepared from rat Clara cells. Using antibodies towards specific isozymes, Domin et al.[14] showed that isolated rabbit Clara cells had higher levels of P450 isozyme 2, 5, and 6 than type II alveolar cells and alveolar macrophages. Treatment of the rabbits with 2,3,7,8-tetrachlorodibenzo-p-dioxin led to a 20-fold induction of isozyme 6. Similarly, Chichester and co-workers[4] showed that Clara cells of the mouse contain cytochrome P450 monooxygenase isozymes 2(IIB), 5(IVB), and NADPH cytochrome P450 reductase. Metabolism of a lung-specific toxicant, 4-ipomeanol, by Clara cells also has been clearly demonstrated.[11]

b. Toxicity Evaluation

While extensive studies have been performed on the xenobiotic metabolism in Clara cells, relatively few studies are available on the application of Clara cells in toxicity evaluation. Rietjens et al.[46] found that the number of Clara cells isolated from ozone-exposed rats was twice (statistically significant) that of unexposed rats, with an apparent concomitant decrease in P450 activities (measured as ethoxyresorufin-*O*-deethylase and ethoxycoumarin-*O*-deethylase activities). Richards et al.[45] found dose-dependent loss of Clara cell attachment efficiency (counting attached NBT-positive cells using an inverted microscope under different treatment conditions) upon treatment with known bronchiolar toxins including the highly toxic 4-ipomeanol, cadmium chloride, paraquat, 3-methylindole; the moderately toxic diquat, 1,4-dichlorobenzene, spermidine, naphthalene; and the minimally toxic bromobenzene, 1,2-dichlorobenzene, dichloroethylene, and trichloroethylene. The results showed a good correlation between *in vitro* TD_{50} and *in vivo* oral LD_{50} values.

B. ALVEOLAR MACROPHAGES

1. General Description*

Alveolar macrophages are found in the interstitium and epithelial surface of airways and alveoli. While their primary function is to scavenge and remove inhaled particulates, macromolecular debris, and microorganisms, they are also known to play key roles in mediating the inflammatory response and the maintenance of the integrity of the lung parenchyma. The alveolar macrophages are found to secrete a host of biologically active substances including coagulation factors, catabolic enzymes and enzyme inhibitors, bioactive lipids, chemotactic factors for neutrophils and fibroblasts, and various growth-promoting and growth-inhibitory factors.

The alveolar macrophages are relative large (diameter range from approximately 10 to 40 μm) mononuclear cells which in culture can become multinucleated cells. The cells adhere rapidly to glass or plastic after harvest. The cytoplasm of alveolar macrophages contain a large number of electron-dense secondary lysosomes. It is generally believed that alveolar macrophages have two sources of origin: migration of bone marrow-derived peripheral blood monocytes as well as local mononuclear phagocytes that replicate *in situ* in the alveolus or interstitium.

* See review, Reference 18.

Because of the diverse functions of the alveolar macrophages, damage to the cells may have significant adverse consequences in the lung. For this reason, and also because of the ease of preparation of relatively pure alveolar macrophages via pulmonary lavage, the cells are used quite extensively in toxicological studies.

2. Isolation and Culture

Alveolar macrophages can be quite easily harvested from isolated lungs in small animals such as rats, mice, and rabbits[16,24] and from larger animals such as dogs and human using an *in situ* bronchoalveolar lavage procedure.[22,44]

To isolate alveolar macrophages from small animals such as a rat, the lungs are carefully dissected out. It is important not to incur any damage to the lung lobes and the trachea for proper lavaging. In our laboratory, we place the isolated lungs on ice for approximately 30 min or longer to facilitate the dissociation of alveolar macrophages from the alveolar epithelium,[16] thus increasing the yield of macrophages. The lungs are then lavaged multiple times with ice-cold isotonic saline solution. Lavage is performed by filling the lungs via the trachea with the cold solution. The inflated lungs are massaged to facilitate release of the macrophages, and the solution is removed and collected. The cells are pelleted by centrifugation and counted using a hemocytometer. The cells removed are mainly macrophages and lymphocytes, which can be differentially counted based on size (macrophages are substantially larger) and separated by differential attachment onto tissue culture plastic (lymhocytes do not attach). From a larger animal such as man, alveolar macrophages can be obtained via bronchoalveolar lavage of anesthetized subjects with the aid of a flexible fiber-optic bronchoscope. Lavage is then performed using multiple aliquots of isotonic saline solutions delivered and recovered through the bronchoscope. The cells harvested are quantified as described above.

Alveolar macrophages can be maintained under normal tissue culture conditions for approximately 1 week in culture and still retain phagocytic activities.

3. Toxicological Applications

As the major cell type for phagocytosis, the alveolar macrophages represent a relevant cell type to evaluate cytotoxicity of inhaled gases, dusts, and particles. It is well established that macrophages play a key role in the initiation of the cascade of events leading ultimately to inflammation and lung parenchymal damage.[38] Activation of the macrophages can lead to the production of proteolytic enzymes which may lead to destruction of connective tissues. Activated macrophages can produce chemotactic factors, leading to recruitment of neutrophils and other inflammatory cells in the lung. Stimulation of fibroblast proliferation by activated macrophages may be a significant event leading towards pulmonary fibrosis.

Because of the early finding that fibrogenicity of mineral dusts, such as different forms of silica, in general parallels to their cytotoxicity *in vitro* to alveolar macrophages,[1] the cells are used extensively to evaluate biological activities of such substances. It is now generally believed that macrophages are crucial to the development of pulmonary diseases induced by inhaled toxic dusts.[2] Progressive inflammations leading to the deposition of collagen in the walls of small airways (less than 2 mm in diamter) are critical steps toward dust-induced pulmonary diseases such as chronic bronchitis and emphysema, with the alveolar macrophages playing critical roles towards disease development. Silica, for instance, is believed to induce silicotic fibrosis via toxic interactions with the plasma membrane and the secretion of fibroblast stimulating factors by alveolar macrophages.[17]

a. Toxicity Evaluation

The commonly used cytotoxicity assays involving alveolar macrophages are shown below:

1. Release of cytoplasmic enzymes — Induction of the release of cytoplasmic enzymes such as lactate dehydrogenase (LDH) is commonly used as an endpoint of cytotoxicity in cultured alveolar macrophages. In general, after isolation, alveolar macrophages are plated on tissue culture plastic and treated with the agents to be tested. After the required treatment period (usually approximately 24 h), the medium is removed to assay for LDH activity. Results are generally expressed as percent cytotoxicity, which is the LDH activity in the treated sample, expressed as a fraction of detergent-induced LDH release. Using this assay, we have studied a variety of mineral dusts including asbestos fibers, fiberglass, and a novel metaphosphate-based man-made fiber (phosphate fibers) with results which in general correlate well with known *in vivo* toxicity.[32] Our results show that phosphate fibers are less toxic than asbestos and therefore may be a safer alternative to asbestos. Other applications of this assay include the mechanistic evaluation of "hard metal disease" induced by cobalt metal powders in cobalt refineries,[33] with results demonstrating that the ground tungsten carbide-cobalt mixture has significantly higher cytotoxicity than that of cobalt metal powder. The results suggest that acceptable exposure level to cobalt metal should be different for the mixture and the pure cobalt powder.

2. Viability stain — Krueger and co-workers[28] developed an assay for viable cells based on glucose oxidation via the hexose monophosphate shunt. Alveolar macrophages are incubated with NBT chloride, and the positive (viable) cells, recognized by the presence of formazan granules, are counted. Using NBT staining coupled with a phagocytic assay (see below), Dixit et al.[12] studied alveolar macrophage functions *in vitro* after *in vivo* exposure of rats to several mineral dusts known to be generated in mining operations including corundum, mica, fly ash, and quartz, with results qualitatively similar to *in vivo* findings, showing that quartz particles were the most cytotoxic.

3. Phagocytic activity — As phagocytosis is a major function of alveolar macrophages, impairment of phagocytic activity is a relevant endpoint for cellular damage. To perform this assay, macrophages cultured in microslide chambers are incubated with polystyrene latex particles in the presence of the test agent. After the treatment period, the slides are washed, air-dried, stained, and placed in xylene to dissolve extracellular particles.[21] The number of intracellular latex particles is then counted under a microscope. Depression of phagocytic activity is expressed as a statistically significant decrease in the number of cells containing latex particles compared to negative control samples. In a similar assay,[71] phagocytosis is measured by incubation of alveolar macrophages with *E. coli* and followed by fixing, staining, and counting of cells with phagoticized bacteria. Another approach to study phagocytosis is to use [^{51}chromium]-labeled IgG-coated sheep red blood cells or [^{3}H]thymidine labeled bacteria and measure the radioactivity associated with the macrophages.[34] Using this procedure, Oosting et al.[39] studied the cytotoxicity of hydrogen peroxide *in vitro* and found that ATP depletion may be one of the major mechanisms of the induced inhibition of phagocytic functions.

4. Mutagenesis assays — Alveolar macrophages have been used as an exogenous activating system to study promutagens — mutagens that require metabolic activation to be mutagenic. The study involves the cocultivation of alveolar macrophages with an indicator cell used to measure mutations (e.g., CHO cells, V-79 cells) during the treatment period, and followed by the passaging of the indicator cells to allow for the expression of the mutated phenotype, and followed by the quantitation of mutant frequency in the indicator cells. Using this procedure, Romert and Jenssen[47] found that rabbit alveolar macrophages could metabolize benzo[a]pyrene and the 7,8-diol derivative to mutagenic products, as indicated by induction of mutations at the hypoxanthine-guanine phosphoribosyl transferase (HGPRT) gene locus. Later, using the same approach, they found that human alveolar macrophages had significantly higher promutagen activation potential than rabbit macrophages. No significant differences were found between alveolar macrophages isolated from smokers and nonsmokers.[48]

b. Xenobiotic Metabolism

An early report of Hook et al.[25] studied a variety of cytochrome P450-related enzyme activities including phase I oxidative enzymes: biphenyl 4-hydroxylase, benzpyrene hydroxylase, D-(+)-benzphetamine *N*-demethylase, total cytochrome P450; and phase II conjugative enzymes: glutathione-*S*-aryltransferase and UDP-glucuronyl transferase activities in alveolar macrophages isolated from rabbits and found extremely low activities. They concluded that alveolar macrophages might not play a significant role in xenobiotic detoxification. More recent data, however, showed that the cells possess such activities. In the laboratory of Domin et al.,[14] using specifc antibodies to various P450 isozymes, rabbit alveolar macrophages were found to contain low but detectable levels of P450 isozyme 2, 5, and 6. Treatment of the rabbits with a known P450 inducer, 2,3,7,8-tetrachlorodibenzo-*p*-dioxin, leads to a further decrease in isozyme 2, but a 90-fold induction of isozyme 6. More recently, using immunohistochemical staining, alveolar macrophages were found to contain the 4S polycyclic aromatic hydrocarbon-binding protein (PBP),[20] which is known to be present in cell types with xenobiotic metabolizing capabilities. Results of these studies are therefore consistent with the mutagenicity studies of Romert et al.[47,48] described above, showing that alveolar macrophages are capable of metabolizing xenobiotics. In general, the activities found in alveolar macrophages are significantly lower than that for alveolar type II and Clara cells.

C. TYPE II ALVEOLAR CELLS

1. General Description

The epithelium of the alveoli is composed of a thin epithelial lining consisting of type I alveolar cells where gaseous exchange occurs. The type I cells are interspersed with type II alveolar cells. Type I alveolar cells are extremely sensitive to injury and known to be injured by inhaled as well as parenterally administered toxicants including nitrogen oxides, ozone, silica, BHT, bleomycin, and cyclophosphamide. Type I alveolar cells do not undergo mitosis or repair after injury. Damage to type I alveolar cells is followed by proliferation of the type II alveolar cells which then differentiate into type I alveolar cells, restoring the integrity of the alveolar epithelium. Besides the replacement of damaged type I alveolar cells, the type II cells are also known to synthesize and secrete surfactant lipids. They are also found to have high xenobiotic metabolism capabilities.

The type II alveolar cells are therefore an extremely important cell type in pulmonary toxicology.[68] The cells have an irregular cuboidal shape and, on scanning electron micrograph, are found to be covered with numerous short microvilli. The most characteristic feature of type II alveolar cells is the lamellar bodies: highly osmiophilic multilamellar inclusions with regularly spaced lamellae. Isolated lamellar bodies are found to contain surfactant lipids, phosphatidylcholine and phosphatidylethanolamine, and are believed to be storage sites for such lipids.

2. Isolation and Culturing

Because isolated type II cells are believed to be rather unstable in culture,[15] most studies concerning these cells are performed with freshly isolated cells or cells cultured for less than

48 h. Type II alveolar cells can be isolated from the lungs of laboratory animals and humans using a procedure described earlier in this chapter for Clara cells. The isolation procedures for type II alveolar cells were mainly developed in the laboratory of Mason and co-workers.[13] To isolate the cells from laboratory animals such as rats, the lungs are isolated and lavaged several times to remove alveolar macrophages. An elastase solution is then instilled via the trachea to total lung capacity (approximately 8 to 15 ml) and incubated at 37°C. The lung is then minced and the dissociated cells collected by centrifugation through a discontinuous density gradient made with metrizamide and further purified by centrifugal elutriation. Using this procedure, an approximately 70% pure population of type II alveolar cells can be prepared, with a yield of approximately 80×10^6 cells per rat. To isolate type II alveolar cells from human, surgical specimens are used.[35] An optimal specimen is one that is bordered with pleura, preferably from the tip of a lobe. Blood is initially removed from the specimen via perfusion of a major blood vessel with a balanced salt solution. The airways are then cannulated and instilled with an elastase solution. Isotonic Percoll is used to purify the type II alveolar cells, with the cells removed from the 1.040 and 1.085 density interface. Differential attachment on tissue culture plastic in the absence of serum is used to separate the adherent alveolar macrophages from the nonadherent type II alveolar cells.

Using a similar procedure, with the exception that type I protease was used in place of elastase, and that centrifugal elutriation was performed before Percoll density gradient centrifugation, Massey et al. reported successful isolation of alveolar type II cells from mouse lungs with a yield of approximately 6×10^6 cells per mouse, with a viability of over 90%, and a purity of approximately 60%.

Type II alveolar cells can be identified by their epithelial morphology after attachment, by fluorescence after staining with phosphine 3R, by alkaline phosphatase enzyme histochemistry, and by the presence of cytokeratin.

Continuous cultures of type II alveolar cells have been found successful in several laboratories. Using trypsin digestion and clonal isolation, we have developed a putative type II alveolar cell strain from an adult Fischer 344 rat.[31] The cells are found to contain lamellar bodies at low passages, synthesize surfactant lipids, and metabolize xenobiotics.[1a] An interesting observation with the cell strain is that the cells can be cultured on collagen gel without overlying medium, therefore allowing direct exposure to gaseous agents.[30,70]

3. Toxicological Applications

Although procedures for the isolation of alveolar type II cells have been well established, the cells are not generally utilized to study chemical toxicity. Most of the studies using isolated alveolar type II cells deal with the cell biology and biochemistry of surfactants and alveolar epithelial function. The limited applications of isolated type II alveolar cells are summarized below.

a. Toxicity Evaluation

i. Cytotoxicity Evaluation

To evaluate paraquat, van der Wal et al.[65] developed a cytotoxicity assay using isolated alveolar type II cells from Wistar rats. The cells were isolated as described above and labeled overnight with [^{3}H]adenine. The cells were treated with paraquat at different concentrations, and the extent of cell injury expressed as percent ^{3}H release, with 0% representing the release from solvent control and 100% representing NaOH treated cells. using this procedure, they found that deferoxamine, an iron chelator with antioxidant capacity, could decrease both the uptake and cytotoxicity of paraquat. However, at high concentrations of paraquat, deferoxamine protection towards cytotoxicity was observed with little inhibition of paraquat uptake. Based on these data, it was concluded that one of the mechanisms of paraquat-induced cytotoxicity is via iron-catalyzed free radical generation.

Using the release of cytoplasmic lactate dehydrogenase as an indicator of cell injury, Buckley et al.[3] showed that superoxides and hydrogen peroxides generated enzymatically in culture medium were cytotoxic to isolated alveolar type II cells. They also found that enzyme release was a more reliable measurement of cytotoxicity than release of ^{51}Cr by prelabeled cells. Liposome-mediated delivery of catalase to the cultured cells led to protection against oxidant-induced cytotoxicity. Based on the results, Buckley and co-workers suggested that delivery of liposome-encapsulated antioxidants may be of therapeutic value in lung pathophysiology mediated by reactive oxygen species.

Using the putative alveolar type II epithelial cell strain, we have studied the cytotoxicity of various mineral dusts and a man-made fiber, phosphate fiber. Cytotoxicity was measured using the release of cytoplasmic lactate dehydrogenase as an endpoint, similar to that described for alveolar macrophages. Our results with the alveolar type II cell strain were in general similar to that found in alveolar macrophages.[32] Using incorporation of amino acid as a measurement of viability, a variety of vapor-phase toxicants, including nitrogen oxides and diesel automobile exhaust, has been studied in the cell strain cultured on collagen gel without overlying medium. Dose-dependent induction of cytotoxicity was observed.[30,70]

ii. Cell Proliferation In Vitro

As proliferation of alveolar type II cells is a known response of the lung upon alveolar injury, factors involved in the regulation of type II cell proliferation have been studied using the isolated cells as an experimental tool. Panos et al.[40] showed that alveolar type II cells isolated from silica-treated rats have a statistically more significant level of DNA synthesis, as measured by [^{3}H]thymidine incorporation *in vitro,* than those isolated from untreated rats. Bronchoalveolar lavage fluid from the treated animals did not increase the level of DNA synthesis in cells isolated from untreated animals. Based on this study, the authors concluded that the hypertrophic type II cells belong to a subgroup of alveolar type II cells that are committed to DNA synthesis. Using human alveolar type II cells, Mason et al.[35] showed that rat and human cells differ in the growth stimulatory effects of the bovine corneal endothelial cell-derived attachment matrix (stimulatory for rat cells but not human), concluding that there may be species-differences in growth factor requirements. This is important since it suggests that findings in laboratory animals may not necessarily be directly extrapolatable to humans.

b. Xenobiotic Metabolism

As mentioned earlier for Clara cells and alveolar macrophages, the alveolar type II cells are known to possess xenobiotic metabolism capability. An early study by Devereux et al.[11] showed that radiolabeled 4-ipomeanol, a naturally occurring furan derivative and potent pulmonary cytotoxin, could be metabolized by isolated alveolar type II cells, leading to covalent binding to cellular materials and the formation of glutathione conjugates. Using specific P450 isozyme antibodies, Devereux et al.[10] demonstrated by immunohistochemical staining that alveolar type II cells, either in whole lung sections or as isolated cells, contained the isozymes P450-I and P450-II. Jones et al.[26] showed that aryl hydrocarbon hydroxylase was barely detectable in isolated rat alveolar type II cells but the activity could be induced to detectable level after treatment of the rats *in vivo* with a known P450 inducer, β-naphthoflavone. This represents one of the initial findings of inducible cytochrome P450 monooxygenase activity in alveolar type II cells. Via the measurement of 7-ethoxycoumarin-*O*-deethylase (ECOD) and coumarin hydroxylase (CH) activities, Devereux[8] showed that rabbit alveolar type II cells had activities of approximately 30% ECOD and 3% CH that of isolated Clara cells. Domin et al.[14] demonstrated the presence of P450 isozymes 2, 5, and 6 in isolated alveolar type II cells, with 2,3,7,8-tetrachlorodibenzo-*p*-dioxin found to induce isozyme 6 by 20-fold. More recently, studies by Forkert and co-workers,[19,20] using a panel of monoclonal antibodies, showed the presence of cytochrome P_4 450, P_2 450, P450IIB1/IIB2, and the 4S polycyclic aromatic hydrocarbon-binding protein in mouse alveolar type II cells.

D. ENDOTHELIAL CELLS

1. General Description

As mentioned in the introduction, all venous blood in the human body will traverse the lung. Pulmonary endothelium is strategically situated as the first line of contact with blood-borne xenobiotics. It is surprising, however, that, comparing to alveolar macrophages, Clara cells and type II alveolar cells, pulmonary endothelial cells, have been practically ignored by toxicologists as an *in vitro* cell system to study events leading to pulmonary injury, in spite of the fact that the cells had been isolated and cultured in the 1970s.[52]

The endothelial cells in the lung are the cells lining lung blood vessels: arterial, venous, arteriolar, venular, and capillary. Even with the resolving power of the electron microscope, endothelium in transverse sections is extremely thin with very few cytoplasmic organelles. In spite of the slight frame, however, the pulmonary endothelial cells have been shown to be highly metabolically active and to be capable of processing a wide variety of circulating bioactive substances including peptides, prostaglandins, biogenic amines, nucleotides, and lipids, with a majority of the enzymes situated on the luminal surface of the cells.[50,51] The pulmonary endothelium is known to be easily damaged by partially reduced oxygen species.[6]

2. Isolation and Culture

a. Isolation

Endothelial cells can be isolated and cultured from the pulmonary artery of large animals (cow, pig, human).[52] Segments of the artery are rinsed with an antibiotic-rich isotonic saline solution such as Dulbecco's phosphate buffered saline and stripped of extraneous fatty and connective tissue. The artery is tied off at one end, filled with a collagenase solution, and followed by the clamping off of the other end with a hemostat. After incubation at 37°C, the cells dissociated by collagenase digestion are collected by centrifugation and cultured. For small laboratory animals, the lungs are perfused *in situ* via the pulmonary artery blood-free with physiological saline and followed by perfusion with a collagenase solution.[49] To avoid the use of proteolytic enzymes, cells can be harvested from large animal arteries by scraping the inner lumen gently with a scalpel.[49] For pulmonary microvascular endothelium, an ingenious technique was developed by Ryan et al.,[53] utilizing microcarriers. The micro-carriers are perfused and allowed to lodge in pulmonary capillaries in a cold saline solution containing EDTA. The endothelial cells detach from the capillaries and attach on to the microcarriers which are harvested by reversing the flow of the perfusate.

b. Culture

Endothelial cells are easily cultured. The cells divide rapidly in medium containing serum. One major contaminant of isolated endothelial cells is smooth muscle cells. By differential trypsinization, bovine endothelial cells can be selectively detached from the culture surface, thereby separated from the more trypsin-resistance smooth muscle cells.[49]

c. Identification

Pulmonary endothelial cells have a distinct cobblestone morphology upon confluence. The cells possess angiotensin-converting enzyme activity which can be assayed using bradykinin as a substrate. Angiotensin conversion enzyme is believed to be the most definitive marker for endothelial cells. Other markers include the uptake of acetyl-LDL, factor VIII, and alpha-2-macroglobulin.[49]

3. Toxicological Applications

As pulmonary endothelial cells are known to be sensitive to oxidant-induced injuries, they are used extensively *in vitro* for mechanistic studies of such events.

a. Toxicity Evaluation

Cytotoxicity of oxidants in pulmonary endothelial cells are commonly studied *in vitro* using the ^{51}Cr-release assay as described by Martin and Howard[34] for amiodarone. Amiodarone is an antiarrhythmic agent found to be associated with fatal lung toxicity. To study amiodarone, Martin and Howard prelabeled primary cultures of bovine pulmonary endothelial cells with ^{51}Cr. Cytotoxicity was measured by the induction of ^{51}Cr release into the culture medium. Cytotoxicity was expressed as a percent of the positive control, Triton X-100-induced cell lysis. Results showed that amiodarone had direct cytotoxic effects on the endothelial cells, causing cytotoxicity at a concentration as low as 10 to 20 μg/ml. Using a similar assay, Kachel et al.[27] showed that the cytotoxicity of amiodarone in human pulmonary artery endothelial cells could be protected by the addition of α-tocopherol to the culture medium.

Another assay of cytotoxicity is to measure the release of cytoplasmic enzymes. Hart et al.[23] studied the cytotoxicity of oxidants in porcine pulmonary artery endothelial cells, using lactate dehydrogenase release as an endpoint for cell injury. Using this assay, Hart and co-workers showed that supplementation of the culture medium with the fatty acid *cis*-vaccenic acid (CVA) led to an increase of CVA content in the cellular lipid and protected the cells from oxidant (hyperoxic atmosphere; hydrogen peroxide)-induced injury.

Besides the use of ^{51}Cr and enzyme release, morphological changes are also found to be a useful tool, albeit more qualitative than quantitative, in cytotoxicity studies with endothelial cells.

b. Xenobiotic Metabolism

Relative to Clara cells and alveolar type II cells, only limited studies are available concerning the xenobiotic metabolic activity of pulmonary endothelial cells. Using a panel of monoclonal antibodies, Forkert et al.[19] showed that endothelial cells in lung sections reacted with antibodies raised against 3-methylcholanthrene-induced rat hepatic cytochrome P450 (P_1450/P_3450), but found only in 3-methylcholanthrene-treated animals. P_1450 and P450b/P450e, both found in alveolar type II cells, were not detected in the pulmonary endothelium.

Although little direct measurement of xenobiotic metabolism has been studied in pulmonary endothelial cells, the presence of xenobiotic metabolism activities in these cells has been implied in earlier toxicological studies. Certain monosubstituted thiocarbamides such as α-naphthylthiourea (ANTU) have been shown to be toxic to pulmonary endothelium selectively and to disrupt endothelial cell functions.[7,37] Similar observations were also made with thiourea, the pulmonary toxicity being attributed to the generation of oxygen radicals. Since ANTU and thiourea can be metabolized by flavin-containing monooxygenases,[42,43] these studies imply that endothelial cells may have such enzymes. However, it cannot be ruled out that metabolism may occur elsewhere, for instance, in the adjacent alveolar type II cells, and that the endothelial cell damage may be a result of the metabolites generated by these adjacent cells.

It is apparent that more research needs to be performed to further understand the xenobiotic metabolism capacity of the pulmonary endothelial cells.

III. MIXED CELL POPULATIONS

Several *in vitro* experimental systems have been established not with purified cell populations as described above, but with a less defined cell population. These systems are, nevertheless, important *in vitro* systems in toxicology. These systems include epithelial cell explants from the upper airways which have been extensively applied to carcinogenesis studies and lung parenchymal explants consisting of undefined dividing cells which have been applied to mutagenesis studies.

A. AIRWAY EPITHELIAL CELLS

In an early report, Steele et al.[60] reported the first time that tracheal explants from young (10- to 12-week old) rats cultured in the presence of a potent carcinogen and mutagen, *N*-methyl-*N'*-nitro-*N*-nitrosoguanidine (MNNG), led to apparently immortal cell lines. The frequency of primary cultures and cell lines that could be established was dependent on the dose of MNNG. This observation led to extensive research towards the development of an *in vitro* cell transformation using rat tracheal epithelial explants. The *in vitro* cell transformation system is believed to be more relevant than the ones developed with fibroblasts as epithelial cells are the target cells *in vivo,* and that most human lung cancer involved the epithelium of the upper airways.

While the original study was performed with a direct-acting mutagen and carcinogen, Cohen et al.[5] subsequently showed that rat tracheal explants had the ability to metabolize benzo(*a*)pyrene, and therefore could be used to study procarcinogens. Several years after the original publication of Steele et al.,[60] Thomassen and co-workers[63] further defined the rat tracheal epithelial (RTE) cell transformation system to improve its quantitative aspects. In this defined assay, RTE cells are dissociated from the rat trachea using a method developed by Wu.[69] The cell isolation procedures involve the isolation of the trachea, ligation of one end of the isolated trachea, and instillation of pronase in the trachea, followed by the ligation of the other end of the trachea. After a digestion period of 1 to 1.5 h at room temperature, the detached RTE cells are collected, counted, and plated onto culture dishes containing a feeder layer of irradiated 3T3-J2 fibroblasts. The use of a feeder layer increases the ability of the RTE to form colonies, therefore allowing the quantitation of cytotoxicity and transformation frequencies. Exposure to carcinogens is carried out at approximately 24 h after culturing. After an exposure period of approximately 4 h, medium is changed and the cells are cultured for another 7 days. On day 7, representative dishes from each treatment group are fixed and stained for the quantitation of cytotoxicity. For the rest of the cultures, the feeder cells are removed by EDTA and vigorous pipetting. The RTE cells are then detached by trypsinization and replated into culture dishes without feeder cells. In these dishes, only the cells with enhanced growth potential, called EG variants, can form colonies. Transformation frequency can be calculated as the number of EG variants per total number of colony-forming cells surviving treatment. This procedure was further modified by Steele and Mass,[59] in which the feeder cells were entirely eliminated. With this modification, the culture medium is diluted 1:1 with 3T3-conditioned medium to support initial colony growth for the determination of cytotoxicity, after which medium is changed to that containing only 50% of the initial amount of conditioned medium for the selection of EG variants. With this procedure, Steele et al.[61] recently reported a 88% accuracy in the correlation with *in vivo* carcinogenicity data after evaluating 17 compounds with known carcinogenicity. In another recent study, Thomassen et al.[64] showed that rat trachea epithelial cells from rats exposed to cigarettes had a two- to threefold increase in the frequency of EG variants over that from air-exposed controls, demonstrating the application of the assay system in the evaluation of cells exposed *in vivo* to carcinogens.

A system similar to the RTE system is derived from human bronchial epithelium. The importance of the human bronchial epithelial system is obvious — the use of human material allows the evaluation of factors such as xenobiotic metabolic capacity, DNA repair, etc. that may be unique to the human species and not present in laboratory animals. That cells can grow out of bronchial pieces had been observed decades ago (see review, Reference 62) and is defined by Lechner and co-workers.[29] Upon obtaining human bronchial tissues as surgical samples, the bronchi are dissected into small (0.5 cm^2) pieces and incubated in explant growth medium for 3 to 5 days. The primary outgrowth is then trypsinized and replated in medium containing growth factors, on to a collagen-coated culture surface. Under this condition, human bronchial epithelial cells can grow as colonies. While the human bronchial epithelial cell system has not been used as extensively as the RTE cell system, it has been applied to study the cellular effects of various inhaled toxicants and oxidants.[54]

B. PRIMARY LUNG CULTURES

Primary lung cell cultures have been found to be useful in genotoxicity assays. An earlier study by Shimizu et al.[57] showed that primary cultures of a mixed population of dividing cells can be derived from collagenase-elastase digestion of lungs of Chinese hamsters. The lungs are perfused via the left ventricle to remove blood. The collagenase-elastase enzyme solution is then introduced through the pulmonary arterial system as well as the airways. After a brief digestion period at 37°C, the lung lobes are minced into small pieces and agitated in the enzyme solution to obtain a single cell suspension. The cells can be cultured, forming a rapidly dividing cell population with mixed cell morphology. Using this system, Shimizu et al.[57] showed the induction of sister-chromatid-exchange (SCE) frequency *in vitro* by 3-methylcholanthrene, benzo[a]pyrene, and 2-aminoanthracene. The results therefore show that the primary lung cell culture possessed the ability to metabolize xenobiotics. It is interesting to note that the hepatocarcinogen, dimethylnitrosamine, did not induce SCE in the lung cells, suggesting an organ-specific response. Primary lung cell cultures from animals exposed by nose-only inhalation to 3-methylcholanthrene had a significant increase in SCE frequency over air-exposed controls. More recently, Whong et al.[67] developed another genotoxicity endpoint, micronucleus (MN) formation with primary lung cultures similarly derived from CD rats. The mutagens mitomycin C, triethylenemelamine, and benzo[a]pyrene were found to induce MN in a dose-related manner in the primary lung cultures.

IV. CONCLUDING REMARKS

Significant progress has been made in the past years in the application of cell culture approaches in the evaluation of pulmonary toxicity. As summarized in this chapter, these include the isolation and purification of the multiple pulmonary cell populations, the functional characterization of the cell systems, and the development of relevant toxicological endpoints. These advances have definitely fueled the enthusiasm and the rapid advancement of the field of *in vitro* toxicology.

As in any other toxicological systems, it is important to bear in mind that the value of each system lies within its experimental limitations. Developers of each assay system should be vigorously researching towards these experimental limitations. Useful application of the experimental data towards the evaluation of human health risk is only possible after a thorough understanding of the assay systems.

The recent advances in molecular approaches in cell biology and toxicology, combined with the cell culture system described here, will form a yet more powerful tool to further our understanding of the induction of diseases by pulmonary toxicants.

REFERENCES

1. **Allison, A. C.,** Pathogenic effects of inhaled particles and antigens, *Ann. N.Y. Acad. Sci.*, 221, 299, 1974.

1a. **Bond, J. A., Mitchell, C. E., and Li, A. P.,** Metabolism and macromolecular covalent binding of benzo(a)pyrene in cultured Fischer-344 rat lung type II epithelial cells, *Biochem. Pharmacol.*, 32, 3771, 1983.

2. **Bowden, D. H.,** Macrophages, dust and pulmonary diseases, *Exp. Lung Res.*, 12, 89, 1987.
3. **Buckley, B. J., Tanswell, A. K., and Freeman, B. A.,** Liposome-mediated augmentation of catalase in alveolar type II cells protects against H_2O_2 injury, *J. Appl. Physiol.*, 63, 359.
4. **Chichester, C. H., Philpot, R. M., Weir, A. J., Buckpitt, A. R., and C. G. Plopper,** Characterization of the cytochrome P-450 monooxygenase system in nonciliated bronchiolar epithelial (Clara) cells isolated from mouse lung, *Am. J. Respir. Cell Mol. Biol.*, 4, 179, 1991.
5. **Cohen, G. M., Marchok, A. C., Nettesheim, P., Steele, V. E., Nelson, F., Buang, S., and Selkirk, J. K.,** Comparative metabolism of benzo(*a*)pyrene in organ and cell cultures derived from rat trachease, *Cancer Res.*, 39, 1980, 1979.
6. **Cross, C. E.,** Oxygen radicals and human disease, *Ann. Intern. Med.*, 107, 526, 1987.
7. **Cunningham, A. L. and Hurley, J. V.,** Alpha-naphthylthiourea induced pulmonary oedema in the rat: a topographical and electron microscope study, *J. Pathol.*, 106, 25, 1972.
8. **Devereux, T. R.,** Alveolar type II and Clara cells: isolation and xenobiotic metabolism, *Environ. Health Persp.*, 56, 95, 1984.
9. **Devereux, T. R. and Fouts, J. R.,** Isolation of pulmonary cells and use in studies of xenobiotic metabolism, in *Methods in Enzymology*, Vol. 77, Jakoby, W., Ed., Academic Press, New York, 1981, 147.
10. **Devereux, T. R., Serabjit-Singh, C., Slaughter, S. R., Wolf, C. R., Philpot, R. M., and Fouts, J. R.,** Identification of cytochrome P-450 isozymes in nonciliated bronchiolar epithelial (Clara) and alveolar type II cells isolated from rabbit lung, *Exp. Lung Res.*, 2, 221, 1981.
11. **Devereux, T. R., Jones, K., Bend, J., Fouts, J., Stratham, C., and Boyd, M. R.,** *In vitro* metabolic activation of the pulmonary toxin, 4-ipomeanol, in nonciliated bronchiolar epithelial (Clara) and alveolar type II cells isolated from rabbit lung, *J. Pharmacol. Exp. Ther.*, 242, 485, 1982.
12. **Dixit, R., Khanna, A. K., Waseem, M., Dogra, S. and Kaw, J. L.,** Alterations in *in vitro* functional activities of alveolar macrophages exposed *in vivo* to mineral dusts, *Vet. Hum. Toxicol.*, 32, 517, 1990.
13. **Dobbs, L. G., Geppert, E. F., Williams, M. C., Greenleaf, R. D., and Mason, R. J.,** Metabolic properties and ultrastructure of alveolar type II cells isolated with elastase, *Biochim. Biophys. Acta*, 618, 510, 1980.
14. **Domin, B. A., Devereux, T. R., and Philpot, R. M.,** The cytochrome P-450 monooxygenase system of rabbit lung: enzyme components, activities, and induction in the nonciliated bronchiolar epithelial cell, alveolar type II cell, and alveolar macrophage, *Mol. Pharmacol.*, 30, 296, 1986.
15. **Eckenhoff, R. G., Rannels, S. R., and Fisher, A. B.,** Secretory granule calcium loss after isolation of rat alveolar type II cells, *Am. J. Physiol.*, 260, L129, 1991.
16. **Engwall, K. S. and Li, A. P.,** Isolation and culturing of rat alveolar macrophages, *J. Tiss. Culture Meth.*, 8, 91, 1983.
17. **Farber, J. L.,** How do mineral dusts cause lung injury? *Lab. Invest.*, 49, 379, 1983.
18. **Fels, A. O. S. and Cohn, Z. A.,** The alveolar macrophage, *J. Appl. Physiol.*, 60, 353, 1986.
19. **Forkert, P. G., Vessey, M. L., Park, S. S., Gelboin, H. V., and Cole, S. P. C.,** Cytochrome P-450 in murine lung. An immunohistochemical study with monoclonal antibodies, *Drug Metab. Disp.*, 17, 551, 1989.
20. **Forkert, P. G., Barton, H. A., Costantini, M. G., and Marletta, M. A.,** The 4S polycyclic aromatic hydrocarbon-binding protein: immunohistochemical localization in mice, *Carcinogenesis*, 11, 1831, 1990.
21. **Gardner, D. E., Graham, J. A., Miller, F. J., Illing, J. W., and Coffin, D. L.,** Technique for differentiating particles that are cell-associated or ingested by macrophages, *Appl. Microbiol.*, 25, 471, 1973.
22. **Harris, J. O., Swenson, E. W., and Johnson, J. E.,** Human alveolar macrophages: comparison of phagocytic ability, glucose utilization, and ultrastructure in smokers and nonsmokers, *J. Clin. Invest.*, 69, 2086, 1970.
23. **Hart, C. M., Tolson, J. K., and Block, E. R.,** Fatty acid supplementation protects pulmonary artery endothelial cells from oxidant injury, *Am. J. Respir. Cell Mol. Biol.*, 3, 479, 1990.
24. **Holt, P. G.,** Alveolar macrophages. I. A simple technique for the preparation of high numbers of viable alveolar macrophages from small laboratory animals, *J. Immunol. Methods*, 27, 189, 1979.
25. **Hook, G. E. R., Bend, J. R. and Fouts, J. R.,** Mixed-function oxidases and the alveolar macrophage, *Biochem. Pharmacol.*, 21, 3267, 1972.

26. **Jones, K. G., Holland, J. F., and Fouts, J. R.,** Benzo(*a*)pyrene hydroxylase activity in enriched populations of Clara cells and alveolar type II cells from control and β-naphthoflavone-pretreated rats, *Cancer Res.*, 42, 4658, 1982.
27. **Kachel, D. L., Moyer, T. P., and Martin, W. J.,** *J. Pharmacol. Exp. Therap.*, 254, 1107, 1990.
28. **Krueger, G. G., Ogden, B. E., and Weston, W. L.,** *In vitro* quantitation of cell mediated immunity in guinea pigs by macrophage reduction of nitroblue tetrazolium, *Clin. Exp. Immunol.*, 23, 517, 1976.
29. **Lechner, J. F., Haugen, A., McClendon, I. A., and Pettis, E. W.,** Clonal growth of normal adult human bronchial epithelial cells in a serum-free medium, *In Vitro*, 18, 633, 1982.
30. **Li, A. P.,** An *in vitro* lung epithelial cell system for evaluating the toxic potential of inhaled materials, *Food. Chem. Toxic.*, 24, 527, 1986.
31. **Li, A. P., Hahn, F. F., Zamora, P. O., Shimizu, R. W., Henderson, R. F., Brooks, A. L., and Richards, R.,** Characterization of a lung epithelial cell strain with potential applications in toxicological studies, Toxicology, 27, 257, 1983.
32. **Li, A. P. and Myers, C. A.,** *In vitro* evaluation of the cytotoxic potential of a novel manmade fiber, calcium sodium metaphosphate fiber (phosphate fiber), *Fundam. Appl. Toxicol.*, 11, 21, 1988.
33. **Lison, D. and Lauwerys, R.,** *In vitro* cytotoxic effects of cobalt-containing dusts on mouse peritoneal and rat alveolar macrophages, *Environ. Res.*, 52, 187, 1990.
34. **Martin, W. J. and Howard, D. M.,** Amiodarone-induced lung toxicity. *In vitro* evidence for the direct toxicity of the drug, *Am. J. Pathol.*, 120, 344, 1985.
35. **Mason, R. J., Apostolou, S., Power, J., and Robinson, P.,** Human alveolar type II cells: stimulation of DNA synthesis by insulin and endothelial cell growth supplement, *Am. J. Respir. Cell Mol. Biol.*, 3, 571, 1990.
36. **Massey, T. E., Geddes, B. A., and Forkert, P. G.,** Isolation of nonciliated bronchiolar epithelial (Clara) cells and alveolar type II cells from mouse lungs, *Can. J. Physiol. Pharmacol.*, 65, 2368, 1987.
37. **Meyrick, B., Miller, J., and Reid, L.,** Pulmonary oedema induced by ANTU, or by high or low oxygen concentrations in the rat: an electron microscope study, *Br. J. Exp. Pathol.*, 53, 347, 1972.
38. **Nathan, C. F., Murray, H. W., and Cohn, Z. A.,** Current concepts. The macrophages as an effector cell, *New Engl. J. Med.*, 303, 622, 1980.
39. **Oosting, R. S., van Bree, L., van Iwaarden, J. F., van Golde, L. M. G., and Verhoff, J.,** Impairment of phagocytic functions of alveolar macrophages by hydrogen peroxide, *Am. J. Physiol.*, 259, L87, 1990.
40. **Panos, R. J., Suwabe, A., Leslie, C. C., and Mason, R. J.,** Hypertrophic alveolar type II cells from silica-treated rats are committed to DNA synthesis *in vitro, Am. J. Respir. Mol. Biol.*, 3, 51, 1990.
41. **Plopper, C. G.,** Comparative morphologic features of bronchiolar epithelial cells: the Clara cell, *Am. Rev. Respir. Dis.*, 128, S37, 1983.
42. **Poulsen, L. L., Hyslop, R. M., and Ziegler, D. M.,** S-oxidation of thioreylenes catalyzed by a microsomal flavoprotein mixed function oxidase, *Biochem. Pharmacol.*, 23, 3431, 1974.
43. **Poulsen, L. L., Hyslop, R. M., and Ziegler, D. M.,** S-oxidation of N-substituted thioureas catalyzed by the liver microsomal FAD-containing monooxygenase, *Arch. Biochem. Biophys.*, 198, 78, 1979.
44. **Rich, E. A., Tweardy, D. J., Fujiwara, H., and Ellner, J. J.,** Spectrum of immunoregulatory functions and properties of human alveolar macrophages, *Am. Rev. Respir. Dis.*, 136, 258, 1987.
45. **Richards, R. J., Oreffo, V. I. C., and Lewis, R. W.,** Clara cell cultures from the mouse and their reaction to bronchiolar toxins, *Environ. Health Persp.*, 85, 119, 1990.
46. **Rietjens, I. M. C. M., Dormans, J. A. M. A., Rombout, P. J. A., and van Bree, L.,** Qualitative and quantitative changes in cytochrome P-450-dependent xenobiotic metabolism in pulmonary microsomes and isolated Clara cell populations derived from ozone-derived rats, *J. Toxicol. Environ. Health*, 24, 515, 1988.
47. **Romert, L. and Jenssen, D.,** Rabbit alveolar macrophage-mediated mutagenesis of polycyclic aromatic hydrocarbons in V79 Chinese hamster cells, *Mutat. Res.*, 111, 245, 1983.
48. **Romert, L., Andersson, O., Zhang, L. -H., Ripe, E. and Jenssen, D.,** Mutagenicity studies by cocultivation of bronchoalveolar cells and blood lymphocytes with V79 Chinese hamster cells, *Mutat. Res.*, 178, 123, 1987.
49. **Ryan, U. S.,** Isolation and culture of pulmonary endothelial cells, *Environ. Health Persp.*, 56, 103, 1984.
50. **Ryan, U. S.,** Processing of angiotensin and other peptides in the lungs, *Handbook of Physiology. The Respiratory Ssytem I*, Fishman, A. P. and Fisher, A. B., Eds., American Physiological Society, Bethesda, MD, 1985, 351.
51. **Ryan, U. S.,** Metabolic activity of pulmonary endothelium: modulation of structure and function, *Annu. Rev. Physiol.*, 48, 263, 1986.
52. **Ryan, U. S., Clements, E., Habliston, D., and Ryan, J. W.,** Isolation and culture of pulmonary artery endothelial cells, *Tissue Cell*, 10, 535, 1978.
53. **Ryan, U. S., White, L. A., Lopez, M., and Ryan, J. W.,** Use of microcarriers to isolate and culture pulmonary microvascular endothelium, *Tissue Cell*, 14, 597, 1982.

54. **Saladino, A. J., Willey, J. C., Lechner, J. F., Grafstrom, R. C., La Veck, M., and Harris, C. C.,** Effects of formaldehyde, acetaldehyde, benzoyl peroxide, and hydrogen peroxide on culture normal human bronchial epithelial cells, *Cancer Res.,* 45, 2522, 1985.
55. **Seaton, A., Seaton, D., and Leitch,** *Crofton and Douglas's Respiratory Diseases,* 4th ed., Blackwell Scientific, Oxford, 1989.
56. **Serabjit-Singh, C., Wolf, C. R., Philpot, R. M., and Plopper, C. G.,** Cytochrome P-450: localization in rabbit lung, *Science,* 207, 1469, 1980.
57. **Shimizu, R. W., Sun, J. D., Li, A. P., Newton, G. J., and Brooks, A. L.,** The use of sister-chromatid exchange in Chinese hamster primary lung cell cultures to measure genotoxicity, *Mutat. Res.,* 130, 333, 1984.
58. **Sorokin, S. P.,** The cells of the lung, in *Morphology of Experiment Respiratory Carcinogenesis, Nethesheim, P., Ed., AEC Symp. Ser.,* 21, 3, 1970.
59. **Steele, V. E. and Mass, M. J.,** A rat tracheal cell culture transformation system for assessment of environmental agents as carcinogens and promoters, *Environ. Int.,* 11, 323, 1985.
60. **Steele, V. E., Marchok, A. C., and Nettesheim, P.,** Transformation of tracheal epithelium exposed *in vitro* to *N*-methyl-*N'*-nitrosoguanidine (MNNG), *Int. J. Cancer,* 20, 234, 1977.
61. **Steele, V. E., Arnold, J. T., Arnold, J. V., and Mass, M. J.,** Evaluation of a rat tracheal epithelial cell culture assay system to identify respiratory carcinogens, *Environ. Mol. Mutag.,* 14, 48, 1989.
62. **Stoner, G. D., Katoh, Y., Foidart, J. M., Myers, G. A., and Harris, C. C.,** Identification and culture of human bronchial epithelial cells, *Methods in Cell Biol.,* 21A, 15, 1980.
63. **Thomassen, D. G., Gray, T. E., Mass, M. J., and Barrett, J. C.,** High frequency of carcinogen-induced early, preneoplastic changes in rat tracheal epithelial cells in culture, *Cancer Res.,* 43, 5956, 1983.
64. **Thomassen, D. G., Chen, B. T., Mauderly, J. L., Johnson, N. F., and Griffith, W. C.,** Inhaled cigarette smoke induces preneoplastic changes in rat tracheal epithelial cells, *Carcinogenesis,* 10, 2359, 1989.
65. **Van der Wal, N. A. A., Van Oirshcot, J. F. L. M., Van Dijk, A., Verhoff, J., and Van Asbeck, B. S.,** Mechanism of protection of alveolar type II cells against paraquat induced cytotoxicity by deferoxamine, *Biochem. Pharm.,* 39, 1665, 1990.
66. **Walker, S. R., Hale, S., Malkinson, A. M., and Mason, R. J.,** Properties of isolated ciliated nonciliated bronchiolar cells from mouse lung, *Exp. Lung Res.,* 15, 533, 1989.
67. **Whong, W. Z., Stewart, J. D., and Ong, T.,** Use of rat primary lung cells for studying genotoxicity with the sister-chromatid exchange and micronucleus assays, *Mutat. Res.,* 241, 7, 1990.
68. **Witschi, H.,** Proliferation of type II alveolar cells: a review of common responses in toxic lung injury, *Toxicology,* 5, 267, 1976.
69. **Wu, R. and Smith, D.,** Continuous multiplication of rabbit tracheal epithelial cells in a defined, hormone-supplemented medium, *In Vitro,* 18, 800, 1982.
70. **Zamora, P. O., Benson, J. M., Marshall, T. C., Mokler, B. V., Li, A. P., Dahl, A. R., Brooks, A. L., and McClellan, R. O.,** Cytotoxicity and mutagenicity of vapor phase environmental pollutants in rat lung epithelial cells and Chinese hamster ovary cells, *J. Toxicol. Environ. Health,* 12, 27, 1983.
71. **Zarhower, A., Eskew, M. L., Scheuchenzuber, W. J., and Graham, J. A.,** Effects of fly ash inhalation on murine immune function: changes in macrophage-mediated activities, *Environ. Res.,* 29, 83, 1982.

Chapter 19

EVALUATING *IN VITRO* TOXICITY TO MAMMALIAN ENDOTHELIAL CELLS

Peter Borgs, Dennis L. Way, Marlys H. Witte, Todd C. Case, Geronimo Ramirez, Jr., and Charles L. Witte

TABLE OF CONTENTS

I. INTRODUCTION

A. VASCULAR TOXICITY *IN VIVO*

The endothelial lining of the blood and lymphatic vasculature comprises the extensive interface between circulating body fluids and the pericellular milieu intérieur. This vast surface area of exchange represents the initial defense against entry of toxins into the tissues and also a prime target for these injurious substances. It is not surprising, therefore, that a wide variety of vascular disorders, some lethal, are well recognized to follow administration of prescription and nonprescription drugs and exposure to an array of chemical pollutants in the environment (Figure 1).[1–7] For example, thrombosis or angioma formation targeting the hepatoportal vasculature follow use of oral contraceptives and anabolic steroids, and hepatic-venous occlusion is a complication of herbal tea (senecio alkaloid) ingestion.[1,1a] Methysergide maleate (Sansert), a prescription ergot helpful in the treatment of migraine, produces a peculiar potentially reversible vascular fibrosis[1b,2] not unlike that associated with prolonged use of the antirejection drug cyclosporin A, which has been implicated in accelerated atherosclerosis and vascular fibrosis in transplant patients.[3] Various toxic gases and halogenated hydrocarbons provoke life-threatening pulmonary vascular leak syndromes (chemical "burns"),[4,5a] and a more subtle reversible edematogenic side effect follows administration of immunomodulating cytokines interleukin-2 (IL-2) and tumor necrosis factor (TNF) in patients with advanced cancer.[5] Drugs of abuse such as heroin, methadone, and morphine also can produce fatal pulmonary edema.[5a] On the other hand, longstanding alcohol consumption is associated with chronic liver disease characterized by widespread hepatosplanchnic vascular alterations from hepatic sinusoidal capillarization to the full-blown portal hypertension syndrome manifested as ascites and esophageal varix hemorrhage and not uncommonly complicated by portal vein thrombosis.[7] Other environmental toxins and pollutants, specifically vinyl chloride, thorium dioxide, and arsenic, have been identified with vascular dysmorphogenic changes in the liver, such as peliosis and angiomas, and occasionally even malignant angiosarcomas.[8a]

Nonetheless, the cause-effect link, detailed toxicodynamics, and underlying cell-molecular mechanisms producing this vascular toxicity remain relatively unstudied and obscure. Whether or not the damage is produced directly (endothelial toxicity) by the suspect chemical or only indirectly through inflammation or parenchymal cell necrosis is unknown. *In vivo* investigations in animal models and observations in man have uncovered several distinct pathophysiologic processes damaging the vasculature, namely, thrombosis and occlusion, fibrosis and sclerosis, "capillary leak" syndromes, angiodysmorphogenesis, and neoplasia (Figures 1 and 2). These poorly understood processes may at times be interconnected and traceable to similar initiating mechanisms related to repair-regeneration-wound healing, cell necrosis, or endothelial "dysfunction".

It is the purpose of this chapter to focus on the central role of the endothelial cell, available endothelial cell culture systems, methods to delineate toxicity *in vitro,* and basic toxicological principles applicable to mammalian endothelial cell culture systems. We will then comment on the limitations and potential value of these *in vitro* models in providing insight into vascular toxicity *in vivo*.

B. ENDOTHELIUM — THE MENTOR OF THE CIRCULATION

Up until the past several decades, the endothelial lining of the vasculature was viewed as a passive membrane composed of quiescent, inert, metabolically inactive cells that formed a continuous uniform barrier or "cellophane wrapper" to contain the circulation. As a result of recent progress in uncovering the cellular and molecular biology of endothelium brought

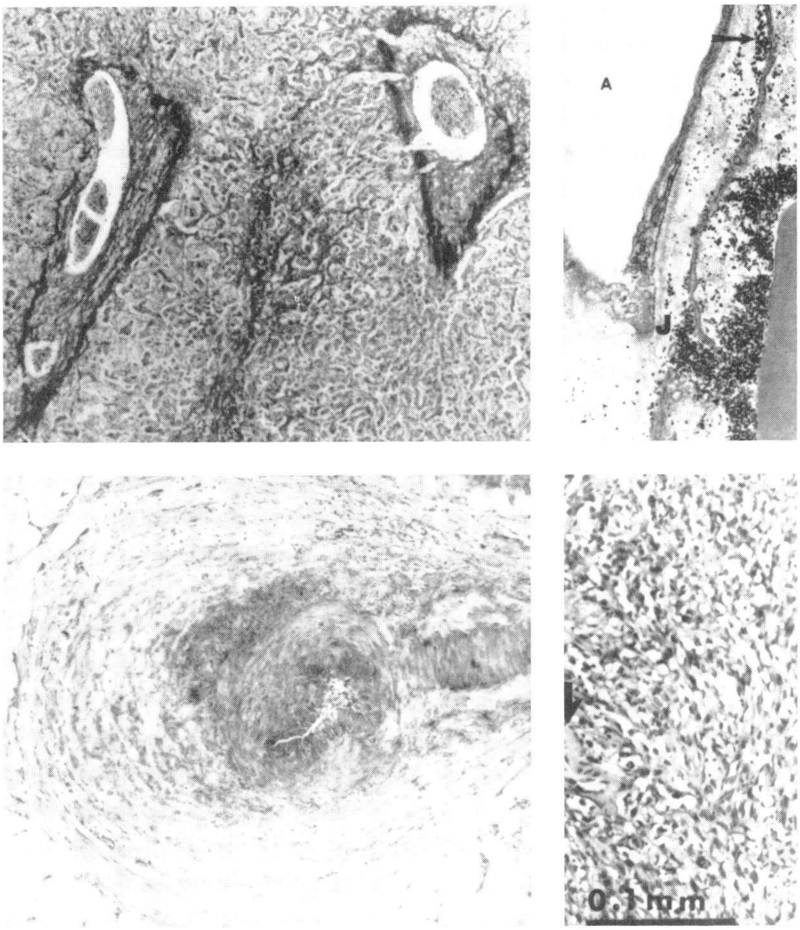

FIGURE 1. Photomicrographs of pathologic processes involved in vascular toxicity from drugs and environmental pollutants. (Upper left) occlusive hepatic venous thrombi in a horse with crotalaria poisoning (from Bras, G., Berry, D. M., and Gyorgy, P., *Lancet,* 1, 960, 1957). (Lower left) mesenteric arterial obliterative fibrosclerosis after methysergide maleate (Sansert) in patient treated for migraine headache (from Regan, J. F. and Poletti, B. J., *JAMA,* 203, 1069, 1968; copyright 1968, American Medical Association). (Upper right) transmission electron micrograph demonstrating pulmonary microvasculature with open endothelial junctions (J) and escape of particles through the basal lamina (arrow), and accumulation in the pulmonary interstitium. A, alveolus (from Wysolmerski, R., Lagunoff, D., and Dahms, T., *Am. J. Path.,* 115, 447, 1984). (Lower right) spindle cell angiosarcoma (angiotumorigenesis) with remnants of fibrotic trabeculae in hepatic nodule in worker exposed to vinyl chloride. Arrow, remnant hepatocyte (from Popper, H. et al., in *Kuppfer Cells and Other Liver Sinusoidal Cells,* Wisse, E. and Knook, D. L., Eds., Elsevier/North Holland Biomedical Press, Amsterdam, 1977, 173). Modified from originals with permission.

about primarily by the development of *in vitro* culture techniques, endothelium is now viewed as the mentor of the circulation and of tissue homeostasis. This vast endocrine organ and metabolic factory actively and dynamically maintains an intact nonthrombogenic vascular surface, modulates its own structure and function, directs the extra/intravasation of lymphocytes, monocytes and neutrophils and regulates the activities of tissue macrophages, eosinophils, mast cells, and pericytes by influencing the chemical and structural composition of the interstitial environment.[8-12] Endothelium produces and responds to an array of autocrine, paracrine, and endocrine signals, thereby mediating such diverse perturbations as inflammation, infection, wound repair, immune reactions, mechanical stress, coagulopathy,

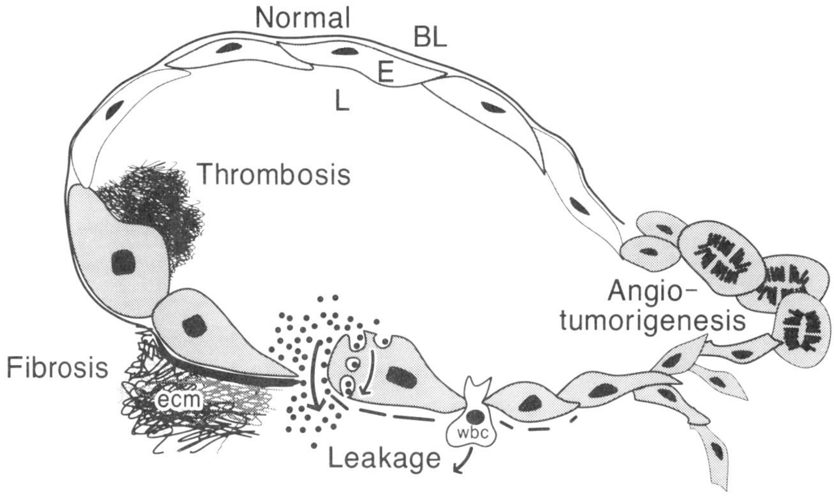

FIGURE 2. Schematic diagram illustrating putative pathophysiologic mechanisms of endothelial damage from drugs and environmental pollutants. (a) Enhanced procoagulant imbalance (thrombosis); (b) extracellular matrix (ecm) collagen deposition (fibrosis); (c) increased capillary permeability for macromolecules, cells, and particles (''leak'' syndrome); (d) enhanced angiogenesis with vascular dysmorphogenesis and neoplasia (angiotumorigenesis).

oncogenesis, and tumor dissemination. A wide variety of soluble chemicals (growth factors, procoagulants, matrix components, and proteases), mechanical forces, and genetic and environmental factors can transform the stable endothelial lining into a rapidly proliferating and organizing network of vascular structures surrounded by specialized basement membrane and extracellular matrix. Thus, endothelium can produce substances which both promote or inhibit coagulation and cell-cell adherence, vasoactive agents important in maintaining blood and lymphatic vessel tone in constricted or dilated states, and mediators which up- and downregulate the flux of fluid, macromolecules, and cells across the vessel wall by such diverse processes as convection, diffusion, pinocytosis, and phagocytosis. Other endothelial products stimulate, halt, or disorganize new vessel formation, that is, angiogenesis both *in vitro* and *in vivo*.

Furthermore, endothelium is phenotypically diverse and heterogeneous varying in morphology and distinctive markers by species, organ, vessel caliber, and segment of the circulation.[10,13,14] *In vitro*, endothelial cell phenotype expression is influenced by diverse extracellular chemical and mechanical signals as illustrated by its ''transdifferentiation'' (without mitosis) from a nonthrombogenic, nonproliferative epithelial phenotype to a migrating rapidly proliferating mesenchymal reticuloendothelial phenotype, all the while changing the surrounding extracellular matrix.[15,16] This dedifferentiation process emphasizes the pluripotential nature of the endothelial cell, recapitulating its origin from the primitive angioblast of the blood island primordium from which diverse cell types are thought to arise.

C. ASSESSING ENDOTHELIAL TOXICITY *IN VITRO* — GOALS AND PRINCIPLES

The complexity of the poorly understood events underlying vascular toxicity *in vivo* underscores the importance of applying sound toxicologic principles to develop and elucidate *in vitro* models of endothelial toxicity. Yet, little attention has been focused in this area despite the explosion of papers on endothelial cell biology and enumeration of the effects of a variety of exogenous and endogenous substances on morphology, biochemistry, and function of this cell type. Therefore, principles established in other cell culture systems need

TABLE 1
Parameters, Observations, and Techniques to Assess Endothelial Cytotoxicity and Genotoxicity *In Vitro*

Parameters	Observations	Techniques to Evaluate
1. Morphology	Monolayer conformation Angiogenesis *in vitro* Cell Shape Cytoskeletal organization Intercellular junctions Ultrastructure	Inverted light (ILM), fluorescence (FM), scanning and transmission electron microscopy
2. Biochemistry	Viability indicators of DNA and protein synthesis Enzyme leakage Permeability Dil-Ac-LDL uptake Ionic alterations Endothelial markers Endothelial synthetic products	UV, fluorescence (FS), and NMR spectroscopy, immunoassay, FM, flow cytometry (FCM), polymerase chain reaction (PCR)
3. Behavior	Migration Phagocytosis Lymphocyte adherence/trafficking	MICS chamber, videomicroscopy, ILM, FM, FCM
4. Proliferation	Doubling time, cell cycle analysis, Brd/Urd	FM, FCM, PCR

to be transferred to toxic screening of cultured endothelial cells.[17-19] Primary culture systems have distinct advantages as they best retain the longevity, differentiated functions, cell-cell contacts, and responses of intact tissues as compared to cell suspensions. Tightly controlled experimental conditions can be reproduced to isolate the effect and dose response from a specific chemical or metabolite on a purified well-identified cell type while avoiding complex interactions with other cell types, organ physiologic adjustments, and systemic messages.

Primary cultures of endothelium can be passed for many generations after the initial traumatic isolation procedures while retaining distinctive differentiated functions. The chemical and physical environment of these cultured cells can be maintained constant and simultaneous measurements repeated serially. Damage or dysfunction can then be detected by more sensitive cytotoxic indicators than cell death or dropout such as those related to deterioration in plasma membrane or metabolic integrity with associated enzyme leakage. The toxic agent must, however, be measurable and maintainable in known concentration during the evaluation. Difficulties can arise if the agent is volatile (e.g., alcohol or acetaldehyde) or rapidly metabolized. In the isolated cell system, specific molecular mechanisms of damage can be dissected in great detail and ways to reverse or prevent the effect explored in the same system.

Nonetheless, *in vitro* endothelial toxicity studies need to be based on a well-standardized set of both morphologic and functional criteria of progressive cytotoxicity and genotoxicity. Whereas such criteria have not yet been developed for endothelium, deviation from an idealized normal cell type — albeit in the face of the aforementioned heterogeneity among normal endothelial phenotypes — should include, as enumerated in Table 1, parameters of cell morphology (shape, cytoskeletal organization, and ultrastructural features); biochemical alterations including loss of endothelial-specific markers such as Factor VIII-related antigen (F8RAg), *Ulex europaeus* agglutinin (UEA) binding, acetylated low density lipoprotein (Dil-Ac-LDL), and angiotensin-converting enzyme (ACE) as well as changes in ionic composition and fluxes (potassium, calcium, pH), viability indicators of DNA and protein synthesis, permeability changes, leakage of intracellular substances such as enzymes into the culture supernatant with cell membrane disruption; and, finally, cell behavioral (functional) assays of adhesion, migration, phagocytosis, and proliferation. In this way, transdifferentiation, dedifferentiation, or transformation as well as viability of the cultured endothelial cells can be used as a measure of the presence and degree of toxic damage and its reversibility. Furthermore, it is reasonable to suppose that progressive disturbances in these structural and functional features with shifting of the cell type from the "resting" state could represent the evolving stages of endothelial toxicity that culminate in complex vascular disorders *in vivo*.

II. MATERIALS AND METHODS

A. ENDOTHELIAL CELL CULTURES

Sources include discarded human tissues such as foreskin from circumcision operations, umbilical vein at birth, excised omentum, skin and organ explants from surgical biopsy, resection and reconstruction procedures and post-mortem examination, and vascular tissues obtained similarly from other mammals (Figure 3). Primary cultures are readily available from the American Type Culture Collection (Rockville, MD) and also from large- and intermediate-size arteries, veins, and lymphatics, as well as microvascular sources through the use of collagenase-type IV enzymatic dissociation techniques as described by others. While cobblestone morphology was once considered an obligatory morphologic criterion, numerous investigators have demonstrated altered morphology of stable endothelium under various conditions.

Briefly, excised tissue is minced to $1 mm^3$ and digested at 37°C for 30 min in a solution of 100 to 400 units/ml collagenase type IV (Sigma) in isotonic phosphate-buffered magnesium and calcium-free saline (PBS-A). This solution is gently passed repeatedly through the bore of a standard pipette to increase the cell yield. Large undigested fragments are removed by a short sedimentation at unit gravity and the cell-rich supernatant collected and centrifuged at 50 × g for 10 min at room temperature. Routine culture may be carried out in supplemented or unsupplemented medium, on coated or uncoated plasticware, as desired. Except for human umbilical vein endothelium, which has an obligatory requirement for endothelial cell growth factor, other types of endothelial cells from large blood vessels, lymphatics, or of microvascular origin have been successfully cultured in supplemented medium with fetal bovine serum (FBS) and HEPES buffer.[20,22-27] A suggested milieu is 1 part HAMS' F12 to 1 part DMEM (high glucose) with 10 to 20% FBS and 25 m*M* HEPES. Additional stimulation to endothelial cell proliferation is attained by increasing CO_2 content of the humid atmosphere water-jacketed incubator from the routine 5% to a hypoxic-like environment of almost 10%. Trypsin passage or feeding is routinely performed once per week since endothelial cells tolerate maximum confluence for as long as 2 weeks until passage becomes necessary. Endothelial culture is also particularly amenable to techniques of nonenzymatic passage where collagen-coated microcarrier beads are added to a confluent culture, incubated for several days under routine conditions allowing the cells to coat the beads, then transferred to new flasks followed by routine culture allowing the cells to migrate onto the second plastic surface.[26] By repeating the process, it is possible to establish cultures on microcarrier beads for such purposes as permeability assay and propagation of cultures that have not been exposed to the trauma of enzymatic dissociation, a constant source of potential error for *in vitro* assays. The endothelial cell phenotype is confirmed by positivity for endothelial markers, F8RAg, UEA, ACE, and Dil-Ac-LDL.[25,27,28]

Experiments are performed in a containment system such as 24- or 96-well plates where concentrations of the suspected toxic agent are varied and observations made on multiple samples over defined periods of time. In the case of volatile substances such as alcohol, measures must be undertaken to prevent changing concentrations over time.

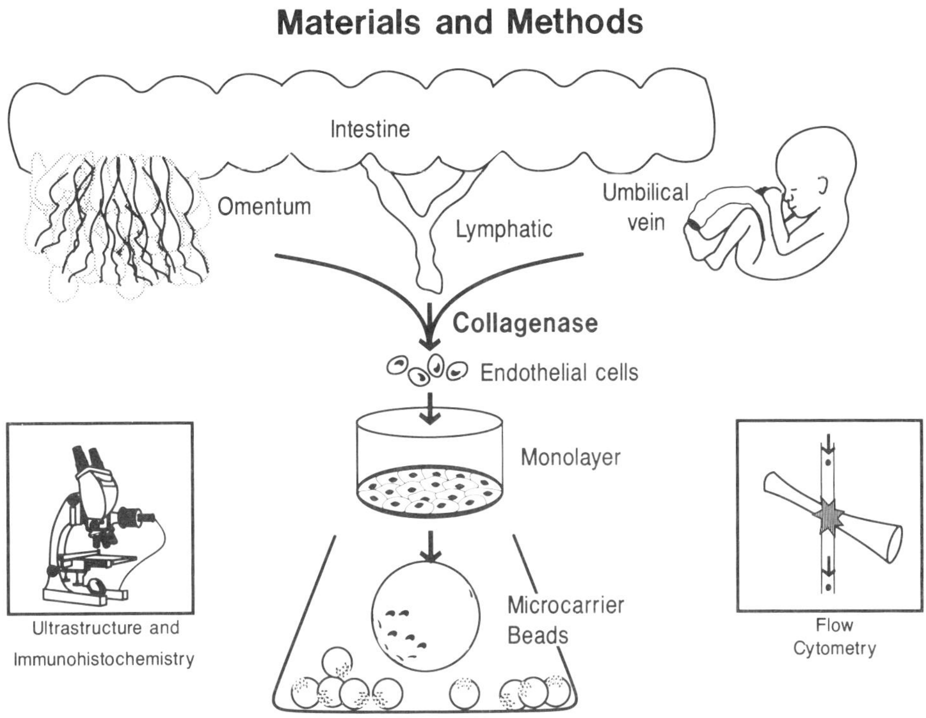

FIGURE 3. Techniques for isolation and study of endothelial cell toxicity. After enzyme digestion techniques, cultured blood vascular and lymphatic endothelial cells are examined both as monolayers and after uptake onto microcarrier beads for the effect of toxic agents on cell structure, biochemistry, and behavior (see text for details).

Before considering parameters of toxicity, a word of introduction to flow cytometry will be provided as this technique is used extensively in Section II, particularly in evaluating biochemical, behavioral, and proliferative responses. The availability of flow cytometry (FCM) for both qualitative and quantitative evaluation of photometric-based parameters allows sophisticated objective collection of multiparameter data. Coherent monochromatic light for excitation is centered on a hydrodynamically focused stream consisting of an outer water sheath and an inner injection core presenting a flow of suspended single cells in isotonic solution. Through the use of specific fluorochromes, lectins, mono- and polyclonal antibodies, and scattered light, specific identifiable parameters unique to the cell are measured. An array of photomultipliers and diodes attached to amplifiers and analog-to-digital converters, interfaced with a computer and its operating software, comprise the electronic detection, storage, and analysis system. A necessary requirement for the use of this instrument is hardy, reasonably ''clean'', single cell suspensions of the endothelial cell population of interest. Furthermore, the choice of fluorochrome is restricted to the output modes (available wave lengths for excitation) of the laser configuration and the emission detection capability of the photomultipliers and their associated filter arrangement.

B. PARAMETERS OF CYTOTOXICITY AND GENOTOXICITY

1. Altered Morphology

Morphologic changes evaluated by inverted light, fluorescence, and scanning-transmission electron microscopy include piling up with loss of contact inhibition or disruption of the monolayer, cyst, or tube formation (angiogenesis or dysmorphogenesis *in vitro*), alterations in cell shape, cytoskeletal orientation and content, intercellular junctional complex

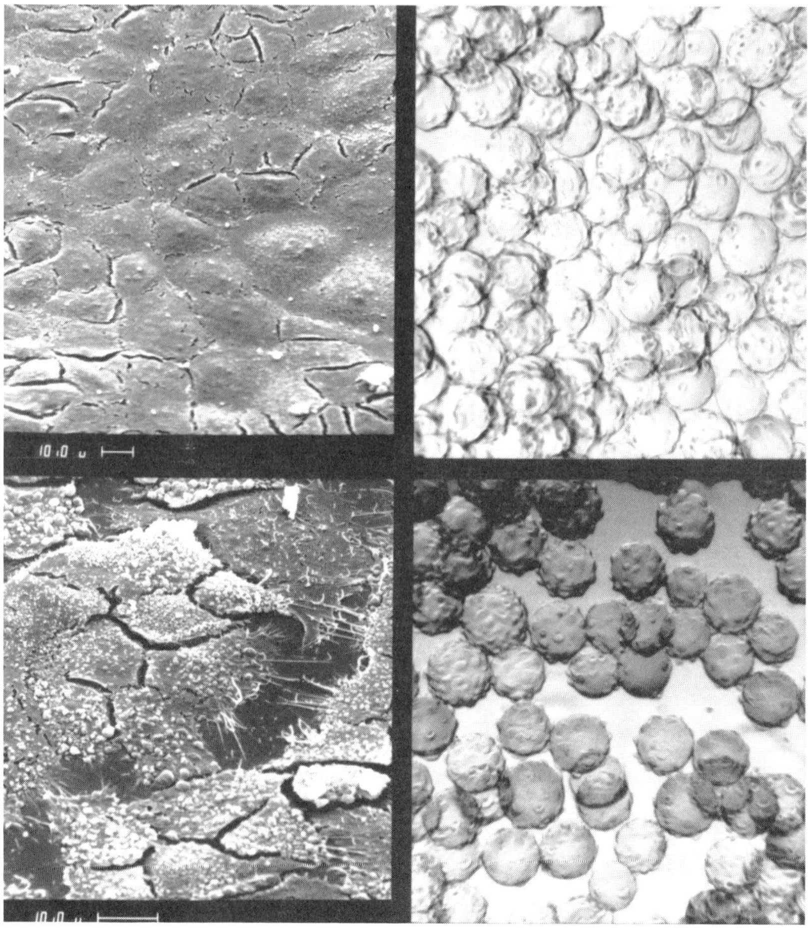

FIGURE 4. Toxic effects of alcohol on endothelial cells cultured to monolayer confluence and grown on microcarrier beads. After application of 2% ethanol, there is disruption of endothelial monolayer integrity (lower left) and increased accumulation of Evans blue-labeled albumin (lower right) in the microcarrier beads (compare with upper panels without alcohol).

type and number, vesicle formation or loss, and specific loss of Weibel-Palade bodies, which may occur early in the transdifferentiation process.[15,20,24,29-31] As an example of altered morphology, endothelial cells exposed to 2% EtOH *in vitro* display reversible toxic changes such as pleomorphic surface protrusions and retraction of cell margins (Figure 4). However, not all cells are similarly affected.

Fluorescent 7-nitrobenz-2-oxa-1,3-diazole (NBD)-phallacidin selectively stains F-actin and is useful in revealing alterations in cytoskeletal architecture, contractility, and, with the use of FCM, quantity of whole cell F-actin content. For static determinations of cellular F-actin distribution, single point monolayer cultures are prepared on coverslips and exposed to medium with or without the toxic agent for various times. The coverslips are washed in isotonic PBS-A and fixed in formalin for 10 min at 37°C followed by permeabilization with acetone at -20°C for 5 min, stained with 0.15 μg/ml (NBD)-phallacidin in PBS-A, and visualized using routine fluorescence microscopy for red fluorescence. For FCM evaluation of total cellular F-actin content, trypsin-harvested experimental and control cells are fixed, permeabilized, and stained as above and analyzed for total fluorescence in the 515 nm range after 488 nm excitation. For assessment of dynamic F-actin structural alterations, unfixed viable monolayers are labeled with (NBD)-phallacidin and exposed to the experimental or control medium with constant observation and video documentation on the heated stage of an epifluorescent microscope.

2. Biochemical Abnormalities

a. Membrane Integrity

Traditionally, viability has been measured using any of several dye exclusion methods [e.g., trypan blue, fluorescent erythrosin B, propidium iodide (PI), eosin].[22,32,33] It is commonly accepted that positive staining is synonymous with a loss of membrane integrity and equatable with eventual cell death. However, transitory changes in membrane integrity occur in normal uncompromised intact cells.[34] To account for this, simultaneous multiparameter determinations using FCM, scanning cytometry (SCM), or fluorescent microscopy (FM) with both fluorescein diacetate (FDA) and PI staining may be carried out to determine the number of nonviable cells and those with transitory leaky membranes.[35] Briefly, after exposure to a toxic agent, cells or monolayers are incubated at 37°C with 1-2 μg/ml PI and 50 μg/ml FDA. Red fluorescent cells with no green fluorescence are considered nonviable; red fluorescent cells with green fluorescence are viable but transiently permeable, while green fluorescent cells are viable without transient permeability. The advantages of this technique over trypan blue dye exclusion or radioactive chromium release are in the assessment of viability by transitory permeability changes (membrane integrity) and avoidance of biohazardous radioisotopes.

b. Enzyme Leakage

The release of lactate dehydrogenase (LDH) activity from endothelial cells as a result of toxic exposure is assayed to evaluate loss of membrane integrity, associated with cell death. A 50-μl sample of culture supernatant is added to a 1 ml volume of 0.2 *M* Tris-HCl, pH 8.2, buffer containing 1.5 m*M* β-nicotinamide adenine dinucleotide (NAD) co-factor and 1.4 m*M* lactic acid substrate in an optical cuvette and agitated manually to ensure thorough mixing. The cuvette is immediately placed in a fluorescence spectrophotometer which is adjusted to detect the reduced form of NAD (excitation at 365 nm and emission at 430 nm) as it is formed in the LDH-mediated reaction. Measurements taken every 30 sec for 120 to 180 sec are recorded and used to assess the rate of the reaction. Results are expressed as a percentage of the total LDH activity in a similar but severely damaged population of cells where LDH is released after cell lysis, e.g., repeated freeze-thawing.[35a]

c. Transendothelial Permeability

The ability of endothelial cell monolayers to selectively exclude or pass macromolecules *in vitro* is an attempt to directly correlate with cellular and tissue permeability or molecular sieving *in vivo*. Qualitative and quantitative evaluation of this process requires endothelial cell culture on semipermeable membranes or collagen-coated dextran microcarrier beads.[22,23,28,36]

When permeability to specific compounds of defined molecular weights (e.g., sucrose, albumin, IgG, or IgM) is used to assess the selectivity of small solute or macromolecular passage, semipermeable membrane-supported monolayers are the method of choice. The test is carried out in well cups designed with an upper and lower chamber separated by a confluent endothelial cell monolayer grown on gelatin-coated acetate or polycarbonate membranes. Reference membranes without monolayers are handled similarly for normalization. The experimental milieu consisting of fresh medium containing the indicator macromolecules with or without the toxic agent is added to the upper chamber. A small amount of medium, typically 100 to 500 μl, is removed from the lower chamber at several time points for detection and quantitation of the indicator macromolecules and the toxic agent. Typical indicator compounds include fluorescein isothiocyanate-hydroxyethyl starch (FITC-HES) analyzed by high-performance size-exclusion chromatography (HPSEC), radio-labeled sucrose, and albumin or immunoglobulin classes analyzed by radioactive decay counters and polyacrylamide gel electrophoresis under reducing conditions (SDS/PAGE). In this way, the kinetic pattern of macromolecular permeability and the effect of the toxic agent on this pattern is assayed.

By increasing the pore size to 40 μm or greater, it is possible to document transendothelial leukocyte trafficking (a model of *in vivo* extravasation) using radioisotope (^{51}Cr, ^{111}In), Hoechst 33342, BrdUrd, FDA, or even unlabeled cells. Leukocytes are added to the upper chambers with the toxic compound or with control diluent and sequential samples removed from the lower chambers for cell traffic analysis. Radioisotope-containing samples are quantitated using a gamma counter while fluorochrome-labeled samples are detected using FCM or FM, but in the case of unlabeled cells simple phase microscopy is sufficient. By comparing controls to experimental wells, a simple percent transit is determined. It is important to perform several trials of the test to obtain significantly comparable groups and to include control trials on reference membranes without monolayers in order to evaluate the efficiency of the cellular transmigration and to correctly interpret the data.

Another permeability assay designed to quantitate albumin transport uses endothelial cells cultured on collagen-coated dextran microcarrier beads. Beads (60 mg per T75 flask) added to a confluent endothelial cell monolayer are covered in most cases in 3 to 5 days due to normal endothelial migration. Agitation (vigorous shaking) is sufficient to dislodge the beads, and a further wash and culture for 3 days in a spinner flask apparatus is sufficient to complete the bead coverage process.[23] Experiments are generally conducted in 1 ml of medium using 1 mg of cell-covered beads in multiple wells of a 24-well culture plate. The beads are incubated in culture medium with or without the toxic agent for between 10 min at 72 h as necessary. After incubation, the permeability of the monolayer is assessed by adding Evans blue-albumin (EB) to a final concentration of 50 μg/ml for a further incubation of 10 min at 37°C. The solution is then carefully evacuated and the beads are washed in PBS-A three times until all traces of blue are absent. The EB is extracted from the beads with 10% BSA in PBS-A by mixing on an orbital shaker at 200 rpm for 24 h at room temperature. Extracted EB is quantitated spectrophotometrically (A_{610}) and expressed as mg EB/mg microcarrier beads.

d. Acetylated Low Density Lipoprotein Uptake

Dil-Ac-LDL uptake is a well-differentiated function of endothelial cells potentially lost after cell damage. To evaluate this process, endothelial cell monolayers are incubated in 10 μg Dil-Ac-LDL per mililiter medium for various time points, e.g., 4 h. For FCM, washed cells are trypsin harvested and fixed with 10% formalin while coverslips for FM are washed, fixed, and mounted with glycerol and viewed. Washed and fixed cells for FCM are analyzed using the 514-nm mode of an argon laser for excitation and evaluating emissions at 590 nm or greater. By subtracting control (background) fluorescence from the positive population, a percent activity value is determined.

e. Other Indicators of Cell Damage

i. Ionic Alterations

Assessments can be made of potassium leakage, alterations in intracellular calcium, and pH (fluorescent spectroscopy and FCM).[37,38]

ii. Loss of Endothelial Markers

Specific markers of endothelium, namely, surface and cytoplasmic F8RAg, UEA, DiI-Ac-LDL, and ACE are determined by FM or more quantitatively by FCM techniques.

iii. Abnormalities in Endothelial Synthetic Activity

Synthesis of prostacyclin, endothelin, endothelium-derived relaxing factor (EDRF), procoagulants and anticoagulants, and extracellular matrix-integrin components can be assessed, thereby evaluating, through this profile, metabolic integrity of the cell and leakage of cell components as well as maintenance of the characteristic differentiated endothelial phenotype.

3. Behavioral Dysfunction

Endothelial cell migration is studied using time-lapsed video images of cells by heated stage-inverted videomicroscopy and analyzing in detail on a cell track S-motion analyzer equipped with a VP-110 video processor for migratory patterns and rates. Alternatively, the membrane invasion culture system (MICS) chamber can be used as described by Hendrix.[39]

Phagocytosis of particulates is assessed after the addition of 1 to 10 μm diameter fluorescent latex beads, usually as ~1200 beads per cell, *in vitro* in complete medium for between 1 and 48 h. Evaluation by FM is expressed as the number of phagocytes per culture and as the number of beads per phagocyte. Flow cytometric evaluation, where monolayer cultures are harvested using trypsin digestion, frozen in complete medium and 10% DMSO at −20°C, thawed, and analyzed after DNA staining with 50 μg PI/ml, is expressed as the number of cells containing beads and the number of beads per cell in a population of 10,000 cell events.[40,41]

Leukocyte adhesion and transendothelial lymphoid cell trafficking is assessed in a dual-chambered transmembrane system. The upper and lower chambers are delineated by a semipermeable membrane, such as Gortex, which supports a viable endothelial cell monolayer. After incubating labeled or unlabeled leukocytes in the upper chamber for 1 to 48 h, evaluation of leukocyte extravasation into the lower chamber is done by cell count or, as in the above immunoanalysis, by FCM or FM of FDA or Hoescht 33342-labeled sucrose gradient-separated leukocytes. Briefly, 1×10^5 labeled autologous leukocytes per ml are added to the endothelial cell coated transmembrane chambers incubated at 37°C in a CO_2 humid atmosphere incubator, nonattached leukocytes are removed by washing with PBS-A, and the remaining labeled leukocytes are harvested using trypsin-EDTA, frozen in complete medium and 10% DMSO at −20°C. Following thawing and labeling of all nuclei, samples are analyzed by FCM. Cytometric analysis involves triggering on cells containing nuclei to determine the percentage of attached leukocytes identified by their dual positivity for nuclear and leukocyte staining labels.

4. Proliferative Disturbances

Proliferation of endothelium can be targeted by toxic agents through promotion, suppression, or disorganization, including direct killing. The evaluation is carried out by FCM methods to assess DNA cell cycle transit. Recently it has been shown that DNA compartmental analysis is accurately determined by FCM eliminating the need for biohazardous tritiated radio-tracers.[34] The stoichiometric binding of PI to DNA and monoclonal antibodies directed against BrdUrd and to cell cycle-related proteins makes it possible to determine the precise quantity of cellular DNA and the rate kinetics of cell cycle transit, respectively.[42-47]

Briefly, endothelial cell monolayers, exposed and not exposed to a toxic agent, are trypsin harvested, washed in PBS-A, and frozen at −20°C in medium containing 10% FBS and 10% DMSO. Immediately prior to DNA compartmental analysis, these samples are quick thawed, washed in PBS-A, and resuspended in a solution of 0.1% NP40, 0.1% NaCi and 50 μg/ml PI with 0.1 mg/ml RNase for 30 min at room temperature and analyzed as described previously.[34]

For rate kinetics analysis, endothelial cell monolayers, during or after toxic agent or control exposure, are cultured with BrdUrd for several time intervals, the first for approximately 30 min, followed by increasingly longer incubations for up to 16 or more hours. Samples are trypsin harvested, washed, and frozen as before, thawed, fixed in 3% paraformaldehyde, and incubated in 0.1 *N* HCL and detergent (NP40) to lyse the plasma membrane and destabilize the DNA so as to expose the complexed BrdUrd. Attachment of anti-BrdUrd antibody is at room temperature and the preparation is counterstained with 20 μg/ml PI. Comparison of the percentage of the population moving from G_1 through S to the G_2 phase is carried out to determine a rate as described previously.[48]

Cell cycle-related proteins and their temporal appearance within the cycle are qualitatively evaluated by FCM and immunoprecipitation using monoclonal antibodies to specific cell cycle-related proteins. Nuclear cell cycle-related protein immunofluorescence is carried out on detergent or enzyme-released cell isolates from endothelial cell culture monolayers which have been treated with or without toxic agents. The cells are paraformaldehyde (0.5% in PBS-A) or ethanol (70%) fixed for 30 min on ice, washed in PBS-A, and permeabilized in 0.1% Triton X-100 PBS-A for 3 min on ice and labeled with a primary or irrelevant monoclonal antibody for 60 min in PBS-A 0.1% BSA at 4°C. The labeled nuclei are then washed in PBS-A 0.1% BSA and incubated with a biotinylated second antibody. Staining is completed by the addition of FCM grade FITC-labeled avidin followed by a final wash and resuspension in PBS-A and 0.1% BSA.

In situations where FCM is not available or inappropriate, immunoblotting techniques may be used. Briefly, detergent lysate protein extracts of primary or synchronized toxic agent-incubated, endothelial cell monolayers are electrophoresed under reducing conditions in an SDS/PAGE gel. Separated proteins are electrophoretically transferred to a nitrocellulose membrane, washed, and stained with antibody probes to p53, $p34^{cdc2}$, PCNA, c-*sis*, c-*fos*, c-*myb*, c-*ras*, and c-*myc*. Stained band optical density is determined by densitometry and quantitated protein concentrations compared against normal control cultures and tissues.

Message transmission by competitive mRNA PCR may be used to examine endothelial cell nuclear and cytoplasmic cell cycle protein mRNA. Briefly, reaction tubes are salted with increasing known concentrations of control RNA template and undergo reverse transcription into cDNA upon addition of the RNA sample of interest. Using one ^{32}P-labeled primer, 25 PCR cycles are completed, and the resulting bands are separated by SDS/PAGE electrophoresis and stained with ethidium bromide. Identified bands are excised and ^{32}P activity determined using standard scintillation techniques. Activities of known control bands are compared to experimental sample bands and the concentration of unknown mRNA is quantitated in the unknown sample.[49,50]

III. COMMENT — EXAMPLES AND PROSPECTS

Although well-focused studies on *in vitro* endothelial toxicity have been limited, primary cultures of mammalian endothelial cells are readily available and parameters potentially useful in defining and quantitating cytotoxicity and genotoxicity are being vigorously pursued. What remains is to standardize these techniques and determine the range of normal response values among the heterogenous endothelial cell types under defined basal growth conditions.

Several examples of applications of this approach have yielded preliminary information, albeit incomplete and at times conflicting, but nonetheless illustrating the potential value and utility of more rigorous toxicologic screening *in vitro*. Postulated as an expression of ''endothelial toxicity'', the edematogenic side effect of cytokine IL-2 (in the presence or absence of lymphokine-activated killer lymphocytes [LAK cells]) for immunotherapy of advanced cancer manifests as life-threatening pulmonary edema and anasarca. Indeed, some *in vitro* studies suggest that while IL-2 alone fails to produce endothelial damage (defined using the extreme endpoint of cell lysis), addition of LAK cells causes disruption of the endothelial monolayer and cell death.[51] Yet, *in vivo* studies, which have shown prompt recovery from the edema syndrome in patients after cessation of IL-2 therapy,[6] suggest that endothelial desquamation is not a likely mechanism. Furthermore, *in vivo* studies in experimental animals have shown that during IL-2 therapy, the normal restriction to macromolecular transendothelial passage is maintained consistent with no disruption in the endothelial sieving property but rather an overall increase in transport of normally sieved proteins.[52] Clearly, more comprehensive standardized toxicity studies of IL-2 and TNF *in vitro,* including biochemical and functional parameters short of cell death, need to be carried out with and without LAK cell coculture. As another example, *in vitro* studies of alcohol toxicity to endothelial cells have pointed out the shortcomings of the standard multiple-well culture plate for use with volatile substances and led us to design a mechanical plate-sealing system to maintain constant alcohol concentrations during the test period.[53] Alterations in macromolecular permeability of the endothelial monolayers derived from different sources (omentum, microvasculature, lymphatic, hepatic sinusoid) (Figure 4) have been detected at high alcohol concentrations seldom attainable in systemic blood of alcoholic subjects but documented in first-pass portal blood entering the liver, perhaps rendering this regional vasculature particularly susceptible to damage from ethanol.[54] Another example, ethchlorvynol, which produces pulmonary edema in animal models (Figure 1), directly applied to endothelial cells *in vitro* causes reversible widening of the intercellular junctional gaps, a morphologic counterpart of enhanced capillary permeability.[55] Several agents appear to exert their toxic effect by inhibiting proliferation of endothelium and thereby impeding regenerative and reparative processes. These antiproliferative effects can be measured after BrdUrd incorporation and cell cycle analysis by flow cytometry to assess suppression of cell cycle events. In this light, endothelial cells contain less antioxidant activity and are more sensitive than fibroblasts to the killing effect of high concentrations of oxygen, presumably underlying the destruction of pulmonary capillaries associated with long-term fibrosis and diffusion defect from hy peroxia.[56] X-ray contrast media also suppress endothelial proliferation.[21] Cyclosporin A, a mainstay of immunosuppressive therapy in control of transplant rejection, produces myocardial fibrosis and accelerated allograft atherosclerosis in heart transplant recipients as well as glomerular thrombosis and renal vascular sclerosis in kidney transplant recipients. This drug has been found *in vitro* to inhibit the growth of both endothelial and vascular smooth muscle cells in a dose-dependent fashion.[3] On the other hand, a variety of drugs are known to stimulate endothelial proliferation ranging from angiogenesis to neoplasia, including, in the case of several environmental pollutants, promotion of malignant vascular tumors (angiosarcomas).[1] To our knowledge, no *in vitro* studies have been done from a comprehensive standardized toxicologic viewpoint to document and delineate the progression of structural, biochemical, and functional alterations in endothelial cells from increased mitogenesis to vascular neoplasia.

Thus, the tools are ready and the time is ripe to develop *in vitro* models of endothelial toxicity in mammalian tissues. Direct toxic effects on the vascular lining cells can be evaluated under basal conditions with standardized and sensitive measurements of cytotoxicity and genotoxicity. In addition,the *in vivo* environment of the vasculature can be simulated using coculture techniques and varying ambient chemical and mechanical signals. A plethora of prescription and nonprescription drugs and environmental pollutants can be screened rapidly, economically, and efficiently *in vitro* for endothelial toxicity prior to *in vivo* testing in animal models for vascular toxicity before clinical testing. Agents known to be associated with vascular disorders such as oral contraceptives, anabolic steroids, estrogens, IL-2, Sansert, cyclosporin A, chemotherapeutic agents, X-ray contrast media, oxygen, vinyl chloride, and thorium dioxide should be investigated *in vitro* for the mechanism of vascular injury and potential therapeutic approaches. How do these agents affect endothelial (and accessory vascular cell) structure, biochemistry, behavior, and proliferation so as to produce thrombosis and occlusion, fibrosis and sclerosis, heightened permeability, dysmorphogenesis, and neoplasia? The developing approach of *in vitro* vascular simulation by coculture with other cell types and variation of ambient chemical and mechanical signals should shed light on how endothelium interacts with other cell types to produce or protect against organ dysfunction and how these processes relate to wound healing, repair, embryogenesis, and neoplasia. *In vitro* studies of endothelial toxicity should thereby offer fresh insights into these fundamental biologic processes intimately involving the vasculature and indirectly the accessory and parenchymal cells that the fluid circulation nourishes, drains, and modulates. Based upon this information, rational therapeutic approaches can be developed to prevent or reverse the vascular disorders that result when these processes go awry.

ACKNOWLEDGMENTS

This investigation was supported by grants from NIH (ADAMHA) Program Projects #P50 AA08037 (MHW) and -S1 (GR); Arizona Disease Control Research Commission Contracts 82-2707 — #1-053 (MHW), 8277-000000-1-0-WF-9314 (MHW), and -WE-9313 (CLW); and UNDP/World Bank/WHO Special Program for Research and Training in Tropical Diseases (ID No. 870051) (MHW).

REFERENCES

1. **Zafrani, E., Pinandeau, Y., and Dhumeaux, D.,** Drug induced vascular lesions of the liver, *Arch. Int. Med.*, 143, 495, 1983.
1a. **Bras, G., Berry, D. M., and Gyorgy, P.,** Plants as etiologic factor in veno-occlusive disease of the liver, *Lancet*, 1, 960, 1957.
1b. **Regan, J. F. and Poletti, B. J.,** Vascular adventitial fibrosis in a patient taking methysergide maleate, *JAMA*, 203, 1069, 1968.
2. **Kunkel, R. S.,** Fibrotic syndromes with chronic use of methysergide, *Headache*, 11, 1, 1971.
3. **Ferns, G., Reidy, M., and Ross, R.,** Vascular effects of cyclosporine A *in vivo* and *in vitro, Am. J. Pathol.*, 137, 403, 1990.
4. **Staub, N. C.,** Pathophysiology of pulmonary edema, in *Edema*, Staub, N. C. and Taylor, A. E., Eds., Raven Press, New York, 1984, 719.
5. **Rosenberg, S. A., Lotze, M. T., Yang, Y. C., Aebersold, P. M., Marston, W., Seipp, C. A., and White, R. E.,** Experience with the use of high dose interleukin-2 in the treatment of 652 cancer patients, *Ann. Surg.*, 210, 474, 1989.
5a. **Wysolmerski, R., Lagunoff, D., and Dahms, T.,** Ethchlorvynol-induced pulmonary edema in rats, *Am. J. Path.*, 115, 447, 1984.
6. **Ingram, R. H., Jr. and Braunwald, E.,** Dyspnea and pulmonary edema, in *Harrison's Principles of Internal Medicine*, 11th ed., Braunwald, E., Isselbacker, Petersdorf, R., Wilson, J., Martin, J., and Fauci, A., Eds., McGraw-Hill, New York, 1987, 144.
7. **Witte, C. L., Witte, M. H., and Krone, C. L.,** Contrasting hemodynamic patterns of portal hypertension, *Ann. Surg.*, 176, 68, 1972.
8. **Shepro, D. and D'Amore, P. A.,** Physiology and biochemistry of the vascular wall endothelium, in *Handbook of Physiology — The Cardiovascular System IV*, American Physiological Society, Washington, D.C., 1984, 103.

8a. **Popper, H., Thomas, L. B., Schaffner, F., Maltoni, C., and Selikoff, I. J.,** Interaction between sinusoidal cells and hepatocytes in human and experimental angiosarcoma induced by environmental factors, in *Kuppfer Cells and Other Liver Sinusoidal Cells,* Wisse, E., and Knook, D. L., Eds., Elsevier, Amsterdam, 1977, 173.
9. **Ryan, U. S., Ed.,** *Endothelial Cells,* Vol 1–3, CRC Press, Boca Raton, FL, 1988.
10. **Witte, M. H. and Witte, C. L., Eds.,** Are lymphatics different from blood vessels? *Lymphology,* 20, 167, 1987.
11. **Vane, J. R., Änggård, E. E., and Botting, R. M.,** Regulatory functions of the vascular endothelium, *N. Engl. J. Med.,* 323, 27, 1990.
12. **D'Amore, P. A. and Braunhut, S. J.,** Stimulatory and inhibitory factors in vascular growth control, in *Endothelial Cells,* Vol. 2, Ryan, U. S., Ed., CRC Press, Boca Raton, FL, 1987, 13.
13. **Turner, R. R., Beckstead, J. H., Warnke, R. A., and Wood, G. S.,** Endothelial cell diversity: *in situ* demonstration of immunologic and enzymatic heterogeneity that correlates with specific morphologic subtypes, *Am. J. Clin. Pathol.,* 87, 569, 1987.
14. **Zetter, B. R.,** Endothelial heterogeneity: influence of vessel size, organ localization, and species specificity on the properties of cultured endothelial cells, in *Endothelial Cells,* Vol. 2, Ryan, U. S., Ed., CRC Press, Boca Raton, FL, 1987, 63.
15. **Lipton, B. H., Bensch, K. G., and Karasek, M. A.,** Microvessel endothelial cell transdifferentiation: phenotypic characterization, *Differentiation,* 46, 117, 1991.
16. **Ryan, T. J.,** Biochemical consequences of mechanical forces generated by distention and distortion, *J. Am. Acad. Derm.,* 21, 115, 1989.
17. **Goldberg, A. M. and Frazier, J. M.,** Alternatives to animals and toxicity testing, *Sci. Am.,* 261, 24, 1989.
18. **Acosta, D., Sorenson, E., Anufora, D., Mitchell, D., Ramos, K., Santone, K., and Smith, M.,** An *in vitro* approach to the study of target organ toxicity of drugs and chemicals, *In Vitro,* 21, 495, 1985.
19. **Bull, H. A.,** The use of cultured endothelial cells in the study of platelet-vessel wall interactions, in *Platelet-Vessel Wall Interactions,* Pittilo, R. M. and Machin, S. J., Eds., Springer-Verlag, London, 1988, chap. 3.
20. **Montesano, R., Orci, L., and Vassalli, P.,** Human endothelial cell cultures: phenotypic modulation by leukocyte interleukins, *J. Cell. Physiol.,* 122, 424, 1985.
21. **Morgan, D. M. L. and Bettmann, M. A.,** Effects of X-ray contrast media and radiation on human vascular endothelial cells *in vitro, Cardiovasc. Intervent. Radiol.,* 12, 154, 1989.
22. **Siflinger-Birnhoim, A., Copper, J. A., Del Vecchio, P. J., Lum, H., and Malik, A. B.,** Selectivity of the endothelial monolayer: effects of increased permeability, *Microvasc. Res.,* 36, 216, 1988.
23. **Killackey, J. J., Johnston, M. G., and Movat, H. Z.,** Increased permeability of microcarrier-cultured endothelial monolayers in response to histamine and thrombin, *Am. J. Pathol.,* 122, 50, 1986.
24. **Phillips, P. G., Higgins, P. J., Malik, A. B., and Tsan, M. -F.,** Effect of hyperoxia on the cytoarchitecture of cultured endothelial cells, *Am. J. Pathol.,* 132, 59, 1988.
25. **Voyta, J. C., Via, D. P., Butterfield, C. E., and Zetter, B. R.,** Identification and isolation of endothelial cells based on their increased uptake on acetylated-low density lipoprotein, *J. Cell Biol.,* 99, 2034, 1984.
26. **Ryan, U. S., Mortara, M., and Whitaker, C.,** Methods for microcarrier culture of bovine pulmonary artery endothelial cells avoiding the use of enzymes, *Tissue Cell,* 12, 619, 1980.
27. **Launder, T. M., Gregen, N. W., Knedler, A., and Harbeck, R. J.,** The isolation and characterization of enriched microvascular endothelial cells from mouse adipose tissue, *J. Immunol. Methods,* 102, 435, 1987.
28. **Holthöfer, H., Virtanen, I., Kariniemi, A. -L., Hormia, M., Linder, E., and Miettinen, A.,** *Ulex europeaus* I lectin as a marker for vascular endothelium in human tissues, *Lab. Invest.,* 47, 60, 1982.
29. **Wallace, P. J., Wersto, R. P., Packman, C. H., and Lichtman, M. A.,** Chemotactic peptide-induced changes in neutrophil actin conformation, *J. Cell Biol.,* 99, 1060, 1984.
30. **Wong, A. J., Pollard, T. D., and Herman, I. M.,** Actin filament stress fibers in vascular endothelial cells *in vivo, Science,* 219, 867, 1983.
31. **Toth, B. and Malick, L.,** Scanning electron-microscopic study of the surface characteristics of neoplastic endothelial cells of blood vessels, *J. Pathol.,* 118, 59, 1976.
32. **Krause, A. W., Carley, W. W., and Webb, W. W.,** Fluorescent erythrosin B is preferable to trypan blue as a vital exclusion dye for mammalian cells in monolayer culture, *J. Histochem. Cytochem.,* 32, 1081, 1984.
33. **Jacobs, D. B. and Pipho, C.,** Use of propidium iodide staining and flow cytometry to measure antibody-mediated cytotoxicity: resolution of complement-sensitive and resistant target cells, *J. Immunol. Methods,* 62, 101, 1983.
34. **Shapiro, H. M.,** *Practical Flow Cytometry,* 2nd Ed., Alan R. Liss, New York, 1988.

35. **Jones, K. H. and Senft, J. A.,** An improved method to determine cell viability by simultaneous staining with fluorescein diacetate — propidium iodide, *J. Histochem. Cytochem.*, 33, 77, 1985.
35a. **Pirozhkov, S. V.,** personal communication.
36. **Schaeffer, R. C., Jr., Renkiewicz, R. R., Chilton, S. -M., Marsh, D., and Carlson, R. W.,** Preparation and high-performance size-exclusion chromatographic (HPSEC) analysis of fluorescein isothiocyanate-hydroxyethyl isothiocyanate-hydroxyethyl starch-macromolecular probes of the blood-lymph barrier, *Microvasc. Res.*, 32, 230, 1986.
37. **Martínez-Zaguilán, R., Martinez, G. M., Latanzio, R., and Gillies, R. J.,** Simultaneous measurement of intracellular pH and Ca^{2+} using the fluorescence of Snarf-1 and Fura-2, *Am. J. Physiol.*, 2, 297, 1991.
38. **Martínez-Zaguilán, R.,** Measurement of intracellular Ca^{2+} and pH_{in} in cultured cells by fluorescence spectroscopy, in *In Vitro Methods of Toxicology,* Watson, R. R., Ed., CRC Press, Boca Raton, FL, 1992, 16.
39. **Hendrix, M. J. C.,** *In vitro* models for the study of cancer, in *In Vitro Methods of Toxicology,* Watson, R. R., Ed., CRC Press, Boca Raton, FL, 1992, chap. 1.
40. **Ramirez, G., Case, T., Borgs, P., Way, D., Witte, M. H., and Witte, C. L.,** *In vitro* phagocytosis by endothelial cell lines of different origins, *Clin. Res.*, 39, 274A, 1991.
41. **Chen, G.-J., Watzl, B., Huang, D. S., Tachibana, K., Way, D., and Watson, R.,** *In vitro* measures of mononuclear phagocyte functions, in *In Vitro Methods of Toxicology,* Watson, R. R., Ed., CRC Press, Boca Raton, FL, 1992, chap. 6.
42. **Dolbeare, F., Kuo, W., Beisker, W., Vanderlaan, M., and Gray, J.,** Using monoclonal antibodies in bromodeoxyuridine-DNA analysis, in *Methods in Cell Biology,* Vol. 33, Darzynkiewicz, Z. and Crissman, H. A., Eds., Academic Press, San Diego, 1990, 207.
43. **Kung, A. L., Sherwood, S. W., and Schimke, R. T.,** Cell line-specific differences in the control of cell cycle progression in the absence of mitosis, *Proc. Natl. Acad. Sci. U.S.A.*, 87, 9553, 1990.
44. **Laemmli, U.,** Cleavage of structural proteins during the assembly of the head of Bacteriophage T4, *Nature,* 227, 680, 1970.
45. **Sambrook, J., Fritsch, E., Maniatis, T.,** *Molecular Cloning: A Laboratory Manual,* 2nd ed., Cold Spring Harbor Laboratory Press, Cold Spring Harbor, NY, 1989, 18.30.
46. **Towbin, H., Staehelin, T., and Gordon, J.,** Electrophoretic transfer of proteins from polyacrylamide gels to nitrocellulose sheets: procedure and some applications, *Proc. Natl. Acad. Sci. U.S.A.*, 76, 4350, 1979.
47. **Crissman, H. and Steinkamp, J.,** *Cytochemical Techniques for Multivariate Analysis of DNA and Other Cellular Constituents: Flow Cytometry and Sorting,* 2nd ed., Melamed, M. R., Lindmo, T., and Mendelsohn, N. L., Eds., Wiley-Liss, New York, 1990, chap. 13.
48. **Traganos, F. and Kimmel, M.,** The stathmokinetic experiment: a single-parameter and multi-parameter flow cytometric analysis, in *Methods in Cell Biology,* Vol. 33, Darzynkiewicz, Z. and Crissman, H. A., Eds., Academic Press, San Diego, 1990, 249.
49. **Wang, A., Doyle, M., and Mark, D.,** Quantitation of mRNA by the polymerase chain reaction, *Proc. Natl. Acad. Sci. U.S.A.*, 86, 9717, 1989.
50. **Gilliland, G., Perrin, S., Blanchard, K., and Bunn, H.,** Analysis of cytokine mRNA and DNA: detection and quantitation by competitive polymerase chain reaction, *Proc. Natl. Acad. Sci. U.S.A.*, 87, 2725, 1990.
51. **Damle, N. K., Doyle, L. V., Bender, J. R., and Bradley, E. C.,** Interleukin-2 activated human lymphocytes exhibit enhanced adhesion to normal vascular endothelial cells and cause their lysis, *J. Immunol.*, 138, 1779, 1987.
52. **Stuntz, M. E., Witte, M. H., Witte, C. L., Way, D. L., Champsi, J. H., and Finley, P. R.,** Effect of interleukin-2 on microvascular liquid and protein transport in the rat small intestine, *Lymphology,* 23, 149, 1990.
53. **Borgs, P., Witte, M., Way, D., and Watzl, B.,** Inter-well diffusion of ethanol in multiple well tissue culture plates: an important source of experimental error, *Clin. Res.*, 39, 426A, 1991.
54. **Way, D., Stuntz, M., Witte, M., Johnston, M., Witte, C., and Finley, P.,** Effect of ethanol on the permeability of cultured microvascular and lymphatic endothelium, *Clin. Res.*, 38, 319A, 1990.
55. **Wysolmerski, R. and Lagunoff, D.,** The effect of ethchlorvynol on cultured endothelial cells: a model for the study of the mechanism of increased vascular permeability, *Am. J. Path.* 119, 505, 1985.
56. **Michiels, C., Toussaint, O., and Remacle, J.,** Comparative study of oxygen toxicity in human fibroblasts and endothelial cells, *J. Cell. Physiol.*, 144, 295, 1990.

INDEX

A

D

E

F

I

J

K

L

M

N

O

P

Q

R

S

T

U

V

W

X

Y

Z